Bilirubin

Volume I

Chemistry

Editors

Karel P. M. Heirwegh, Ph.D.
Professor of Analytical Chemistry
Laboratory of Hepatology
Catholic University of Leuven
Leuven, Belgium

Stanley B. Brown, Ph.D.
Reader in Biochemistry
University of Leeds
Leeds, England

CRC Press, Inc.
Boca Raton, Florida

Library of Congress Cataloging in Publication Data
Main entry under title:

Bilirubin.

Bibliography: p.
Includes index.
Contents: v. 1. Chemistry -- v. 2. Metabolism.
I. Heirwegh, Karel P. M. II. Brown, S. B.
(Stanley B.)
QP671.B55B54 612'.01528 82-1324
ISBN 0-8493-6155-9 (v.1) AACR2
ISBN 0-8493-6156-7 (v.2)

Direct all inquiries to CRC Press, Inc., 2000 Corporate Blvd., N.W., Boca Raton, Florida, 33431.

International Standard Book Number 0-8493-6155-9 (vol. 1)
International Standard Book Number 0-8493-6156-7 (vol. 2)

Library of Congress Card Number 82-1324
Printed in the United States

PREFACE

Bilirubin* is formed in large amounts by many animals containing hemoglobin. It appears to have no specific function other than participation in a pathway for the elimination of unwanted heme from the organism. Nevertheless, the structure and metabolism of bilirubin have been extensively studied for many years. Clinical and biochemical studies have been inspired largely because of their diagnostic value in a wide range of normal and disease states. More recently, the application of techniques such as X-ray crystallography and nuclear magnetic resonance spectroscopy has revealed novel chemical features in the structure of bilirubin which appear to be implicated in its physiological behavior. In parallel with recent developments on clinical, biochemical and physicochemical work much progress has been made in methodological studies, especially relating to analytical chemistry and the isolation and identification of pure bile pigments and their various derivatives. For example, it is now possible to synthesize (or isolate from natural sources) pure samples of various bilirubin conjugates. Indeed, the development of these methods has shed new light on much previous experimentation and laid a foundation for more rigorous future developments.

The book appears in two volumes, the first dealing primarily with chemical and structural aspects, and the second with metabolic aspects. The purpose is not only to review recent work on chemical and physiological aspects of bilirubin structure and metabolism, but also to emphasize the importance of methodological advances and their potential in future studies. An attempt has been made to present the advances in techniques and physicochemical studies in a manner which will be useful to clinicians, physiologists, and biochemists as well as those directly concerned with these more fundamental aspects. In this way, it is hoped that the book will assist in the integration of what is becoming an increasingly diverse field. Moreover, it has become apparent that certain aspects of the metabolism and transport of biliverdin and its binding to proteins, may be useful in setting up more general models for the binding and transport of metabolites.

Each chapter is devoted to a specific aspect of the structure or metabolism of bilirubin and its derivatives. The contributors are all actively concerned with research in one or more areas within the field. In a multiauthor text, differences in style and some overlap in coverage is inevitable. However, by the use of extensive cross-referencing, it is hoped that such overlap will enhance rather than detract from the text.

* In agreement with the proposal of the joint commission of IUPAC and IUB, bilirubin-IXα will be denoted throughout the book as bilirubin, unless it is desirable to stress the isomeric structure.

THE EDITORS

Karel P. M. Heirwegh, Ph.D., received his undergraduate degree in 1950 from the University of Leuven, Leuven, Belgium, and his Ph.D. degree in 1952 from that same university. Dr. Heirwegh is currently Professor of Analytical Chemistry and Research Director of the Laboratory of Hepatology at the Catholic University of Leuven.

Prior to his current position, Dr. Heirwegh was a Research Fellow of the Institute for Industrial and Agricultural Research of Belgium (1954-1956) and a Research Fellow of the National Foundation for Scientific Research of Belgium (1957-1959).

Stanley B. Brown, Ph.D., received his B.Sc. degree from the University of Durham in 1963 and his Ph.D. degree in 1966 from the University of Newcastle. Dr. Brown is currently a Reader in Biochemistry at the University of Leeds, England.

Dr. Brown is a member of the Biochemical Society, the British Biophysical Society, and the Tetrapyrrole Group.

CONTRIBUTORS

Paul D. Berk, M.D.
Professor of Medicine and Director
Polly Annenberg Levee Hematology Center
Department of Medicine
Mount Sinai School of Medicine
New York, New York

Pierre Berthelot, M.D.
Unite d'Hepatologie
Hopital Laennec
Paris, France

B. H. Billing, M.D.
Professor of Biochemistry Applied to Medicine
Academic Department of Medicine
Royal Free Hospital
London, England

N. Blanckaert, M.D., A.H.O.
Research Associate
National Fund for Scientific Research (Belgium)
Lecturer, Catholic University of Leuven
Leuven, Belgium

Rolf Brodersen, D.Phil.
Professor of Medical Biochemistry
University of Aarhus
Aarhus, Denmark

S. B. Brown, Ph.D.
Department of Biochemistry
University of Leeds
Leeds, England

Ewart R. Carson, Ph.D.
Reader in Systems Sciences
Department of Systems Science
The City University
London, England

Frans Compernole, Ph.D.
Laboratory of Hepatology
Lecturer, Catholic University of Leuven
Leuven, Belgium

Ph. Duvaldestin, M.D.
Unite de Recherches INSERM
Hopital Henri Mondor
Creteil, France

J. Fevery, M.D., A.H.O.
Professor of Medicine
Laboratory of Hepatology
Catholic University of Leuven
Leuven, Belgium

Karel P. M. Heirwegh, Ph.D.
Professor of Analytical Chemistry
Laboratory of Hepatology
Catholic University of Leuven
Leuven, Belgium

E. Anthony Jones, M.D., F.R.C.P.
Chief, Liver Diseases Section
Digestive Diseases Branch
National Institute of Arthritis, Diabetes and Digestive and Kidney Diseases
National Institutes of Health
Bethesda, Maryland

David A. Lightner, Ph.D.
Professor of Chemistry
University of Nevada
Reno, Nevada

Jules A. T. P. Meuwissen, M.D., M.Med.Sc.
Research Associate
National Fund for Scientific Research (Belgium)
Lecturer, Catholic University of Leuven
Leuven, Belgium

Mark S. Stoll, Ph.D.
Division of Clinical Chemistry
Clinical Research Centre
Middlesex, United Kingdom

R. F. Troxler, Ph.D.
School of Medicine
Boston University Medical School
Boston, Massachusetts

ACKNOWLEDGMENTS

The editors and contributors are grateful for the support and guidance given by their families and colleagues during the preparation of these volumes. The editors also wish to express their appreciation to the authors for their cooperation and understanding during the planning and editing processes.

Bilirubin

Karel P. M. Heirwegh and Stanley B. Brown

VOLUME I: CHEMISTRY

Structure, Photochemistry, and Organic Chemistry of Bilirubin
Bilirubin Conjugates: Isolation, Structure Analysis, and Snythesis
Physical Chemistry of Bilirubin: Binding to Macomolecules and Membranes
Analytical Chemistry of Rubins

VOLUME II: METABOLISM

Heme Degradation and Bilirubin Formation
Aspects of Bilirubin Transport
The Role of Conjugating Enzymes in the Biliary Excretion of Bilirubin
Formation, Metabolism, and Properties of Pyrrolic Compounds Appearing in the Gut
The Role of Kinetic Analysis and Mathematical Modeling in the Study of Bilirubin Metabolism In Vivo
Physiology and Disorders of Human Bilirubin Metabolism

TABLE OF CONTENTS

Volume I

Chapter 1

STRUCTURE, PHOTOCHEMISTRY, AND ORGANIC CHEMISTRY OF BILIRUBIN*

David A. Lightner

TABLE OF CONTENTS

* Although aspects of bilirubin chemistry, photochemistry and biochemistry have been reviewed from time to time, the most complete, comprehensive, and highly useful recent review has been provided by McDonagh.[1] The present work, completed in summer 1980, is less comprehensive and is oriented specifically toward the structure of bilirubin and its photochemistry.

I. NOMENCLATURE

A. Bilirubin and Its Conjugates

Attempts have been made to produce a useful, systematic naming system for tetrapyrroles. The IUPAC-IUB Joint Commission on Biochemical Nomenclature has proposed[2] that linear tetrapyrrole names should be based on a fundamental carbon/nitrogen skeletal structure called "bilin" as illustrated in Figure 1. Chemical Abstracts currently uses a variation of this nomenclature with a root name 21*H*-biline as opposed to bilin in the 22*H*-form. In either case, it should be noted that position 20 does not appear; it corresponds to the extra main atom, e.g., carbon, that would be required to transform the linear tetrapyrrole into a macrocyclic porphyrin structure. Fortunately, bilirubin-IXα is allowed to retain the common name "bilirubin" (here meaning specifically the IXα structure),[2] although Chemical Abstracts currently indexes it under the cumbersome systematic name: 2,17-diethenyl-1,10,19,22,23,24-hexahydro-3,7,13,18-tetramethyl-1,19-dioxo-21*H*-biline-8,12-dipropanoic acid. (Note that in the latter name, vinyl is given priority over methyl, thus bilirubin is 2,17-diethenyl and not 3,18-diethenyl.) The IUPAC-IUB proposal[2] leaves the less natural bilirubins, e.g., bilirubin-IIIα or bilirubin-IXβ, to be named systematically. In view of their simplicity, common names will no doubt continue to be preferred in many instances.

Further designations are required in order to specify stereochemical features of the molecules. In particular, one should note that geometric configurational isomers exist at the carbon-carbon double bonds located between atoms 4 and 5, 10 and 11, and 15 and 16. To distinguish between the two possible geometric isomers at each carbon-carbon double bond, the standard notations Z (zusammen) and E (entgegen)[3] are used. In this nomenclature, priorities are assigned to each atom (or group) attached to each carbon atom of the carbon-carbon double bond: at position 4, N(21) is higher priority than C(3) because N has a larger atomic number than C; at position 5, C(6) is higher priority than H because C has a larger atomic number than H. When the higher priority atoms (groups) are on the *same* side of the carbon-carbon double bond, the configuration is Z; when they are on opposite sides, the configuration is E. The stereochemical designations are illustrated in Figure 2 with the four possible different geometric isomers of bilirubin.

Additional recognizable stereochemical features may be found through rotations about the carbon-carbon single bonds between 5 and 6, 9 and 10, and 14 and 15. When imposed on the configurational isomers recognized and designated as above, two more forms obtain for each Z and E isomer. This is true because focal points, viz., the N atoms, may appear near *(syn)* or away *(anti)* from each other in the planar projections.[4] This is illustrated in Figure 3.

Another nomenclature which is specifically directed toward bilirubin and biliverdin structures has been submitted to the IUPAC-IUB Joint Commission on Biochemical Nomenclature and is acceptable to Chemical Abstracts.[5] The retention of the core names bilirubin (for bilirubin-IXα) and biliverdin (for biliverdin-IXα) is proposed. For other isomers of bilirubin or biliverdin, the core names are used in conjunction with designations for the locations of vinyl and propionic acid groups, as illustrated in Figure 4. This nomenclature allows for easy designation of conjugates, e.g., bilirubin glucuronides, according to the tetrapyrrole structure and the sugar derivatives that are shown in Figure 5. In most instances the sugar is in the pyranose form and is attached through the β-linkage at the anomeric carbon (C-1′). It is proposed that the mode of linkage not be specified unless it is different from β, and that the pyranose symbol (p) be deleted in the abbreviation because the sugars have not been observed to occur naturally in a different form. Thus ordinary bilirubin-IXα diglucuronide would become named bilirubin-8,12(GlcU; GlcU). The nomenclature differentiates between the

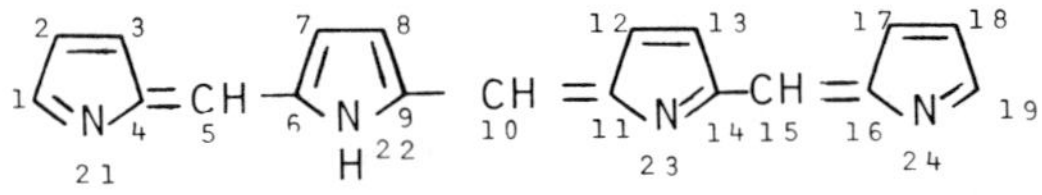

BILIN (22H FORM)

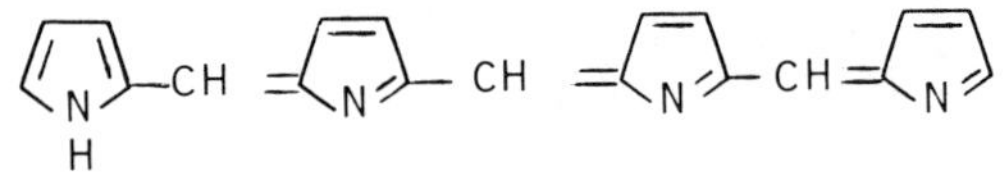

21H-BILINE

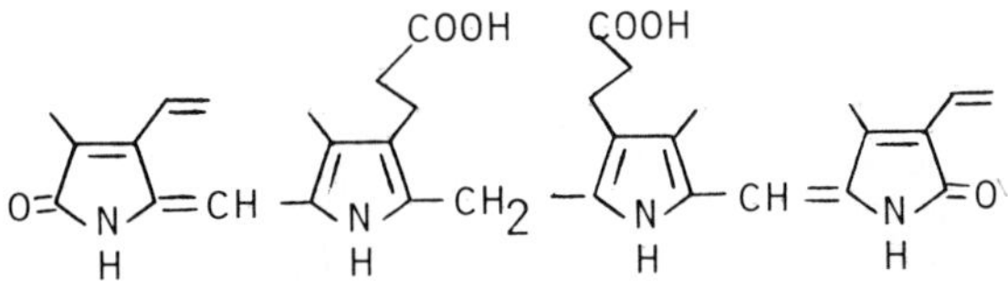

BILIRUBIN (BILIRUBIN-IXα)

FIGURE 1. (Upper) Proposed systematic nomenclature for linear tetrapyrroles.[2] (Middle) Chemical Abstracts nomenclature. (Lower) Bilirubin-IXα has the systematic names: 1,10,19,21,23,24-hexahydro-2,7,13,17-tetramethyl-1,19-dioxo-3,18-divinylbilin-8,12-dipropanoic acid[2], or 8,12-bis(2-carboxyethyl)-10,21,23,24-tetrahydro-2,7,13,17-tetramethyl-3,18-divinyl-bilin-1,19-dione (Ref. 2 proposed) or 8,12-*bis* (carboxyethyl)-2,7,13,17-tetramethyl-3,18-divinyl (10 H, 21 H, 24 H) bilin-1,19-dione (Ref. 2, proposed), or 2,17-diethenyl-1,10,19,22,23,24-hexahydro-3,7,13,18-tetramethyl-1,19-dioxo-21H-biline-8,12-dipropanoic acid (Chemical Abstracts).

two possible position isomers of bilirubin monoglucuronide by italicizing or underlining the *number* of the propionic acid side chain to which the sugar is attached. When the isomeric position is unknown, the number is not italicized or underlined. If two different sugars are attached, that, too, may be indicated in the bracketed part of the name. Synthetic esters can also be named in this system: bilirubin dimethyl ester becomes bilirubin-8,12(Me; Me). Examples of applications of the nomenclature may be found in Figure 6 and Table 1, and more varied examples are shown in Reference 5.

B. Dipyrrole Azo Derivatives from Bilirubin

Bilirubins react with aromatic diazonium salts to give dipyrrole azo derivatives (azopyrromethenes) which are useful in characterization, especially the ordering of the pyrrole β-substituents. For example, diazotized ethyl anthranilate reacts with bilirubin at

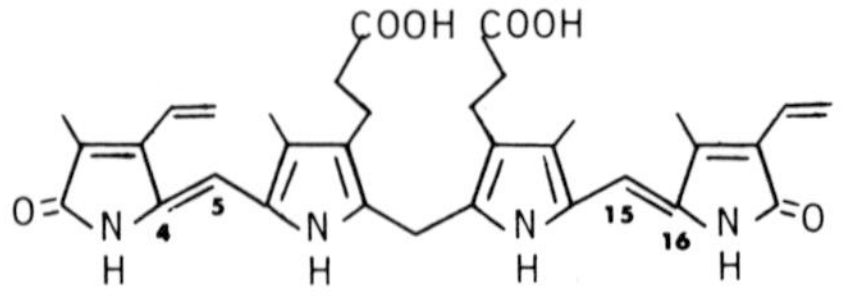

4Z,15Z

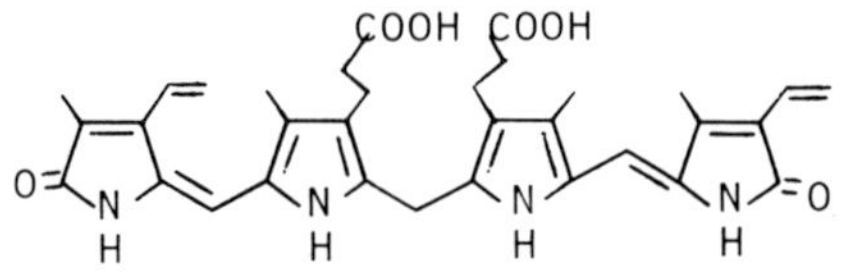

4E,15Z

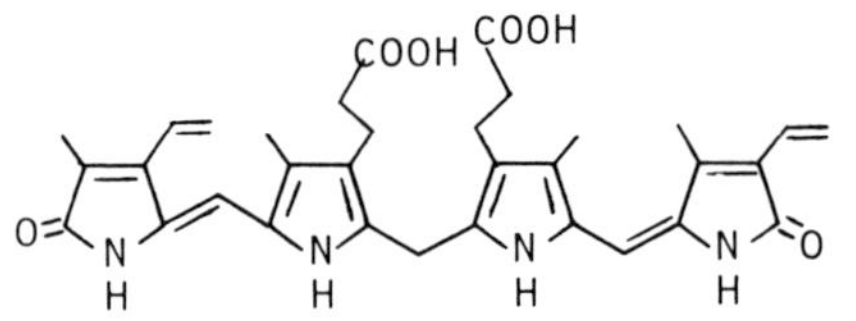

4Z,15E

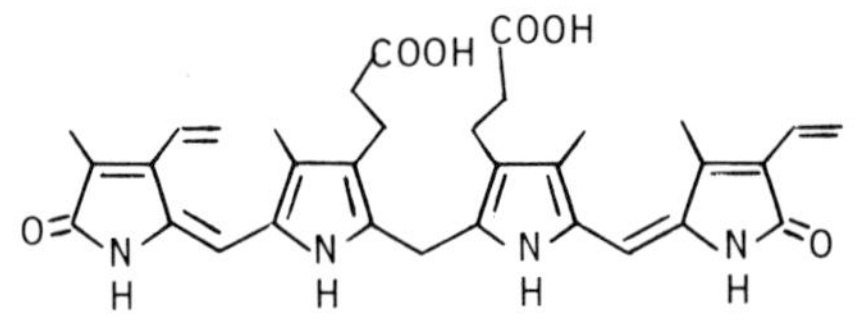

4E,15E

FIGURE 2. Double bond geometric configurational isomers of bilirubin-IXα.

positions 9 and 11 to give the two isomeric azopyrromethenes as shown in Figure 7. In the suggested nomenclature[5] for these substances, azopyrromethene is abbreviated "azpm". The type of diazonium salt used is indicated in parentheses, e.g., (*o*-CO_2Et)azpm is the azo derivative from reaction of diazotized ethyl *o*-anthranilate, if needed to distinguish one type of diazonium reagent from another. If it can be assumed that one is dealing only with azo pigment derivatives of the IXα, IXβ, IXγ and IXδ isomers of blirubin, the nomenclature is handled simply by designating the location(s) of the propionic acid group(s), or if none are present, by denoting the locations of the vinyl groups. Examples are provided in Table 2, and it should be noted that some difficulty may be encountered (each β-substituent might have to be indicated) with "unnatural" bilirubins. Conjugates, esters, and amides of azopyrromethenes may be named by adding the appropriate suffix to the name. Thus, if the two azopyrromethenes shown in Figure 7 had been derived from bilirubin diglucuronide [bilirubin-8,12(GlcU; GlcU)], they would be named Azpm-8(GlcU) and Azpm-12(GlcU). Examples of the nomenclature discussed herein and proposed by Bergstrom and Blumenthal[5] are shown in Table 3.

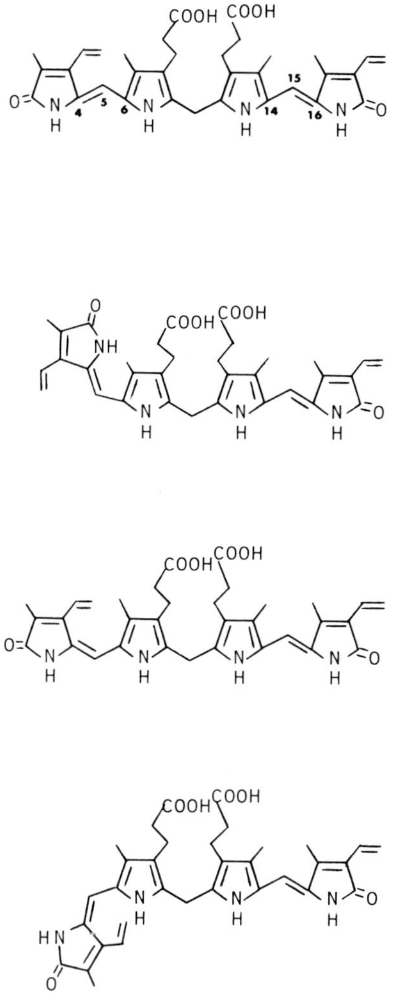

SYN-4Z, SYN-15Z

ANTI-4Z, SYN-15Z

SYN-4E, SYN-15Z

ANTI-4E, SYN-15Z

FIGURE 3. Double bond geometric configurational (C_4-C_5) and rotational isomers (C_5-C_6) of bilirubin-IXα. Similar representations (not shown) are possible about C_{14}-C_{15} and C_{15}-C_{16} because the structures are not flat.

II. STRUCTURE

A. Primary Structure

1. Degradation

a. Resorcinol Melt

Bilirubin-IXα, derived from heme catabolism, was determined to have the molecular formula: $C_{33}H_{36}O_6N_4$.[6] It therefore has one less carbon atom and two more oxygen atoms than the protoporphyrin-IX ($C_{34}H_{34}O_4N_4$) precursor. Its structure was deduced as having a "tetrapyrrane" skeleton on the basis of work done with mesobilirubin-IXα (Figure 8). Mesobilirubin is a tetrahydro derivative of bilirubin with ethyl groups in place of vinyl groups. It is prepared by controlled catalytic hydrogenation of bilirubin.[7] Treatment of mesobilirubin-IXα for brief periods in molten resorcinol leads to the formation of oxodipyrromethene derivatives. At first, two types of oxodipyrromethenes were isolated: one with an unsubstituted pyrrole α-position and one with a methyl-substituted pyrrole α-position. The former belongs to the class neoxanthobili-

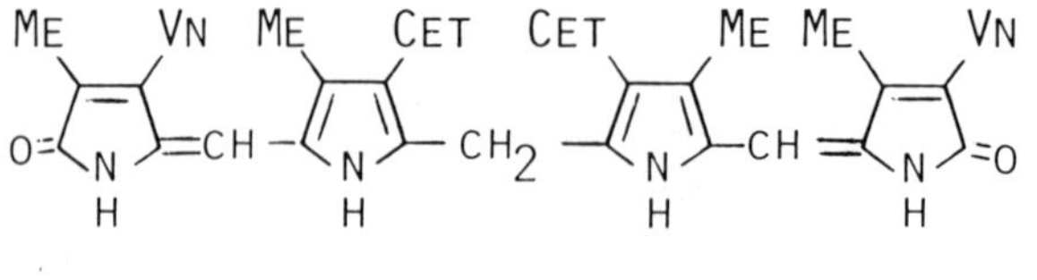

BILIRUBIN (BILIRUBIN-IXα)

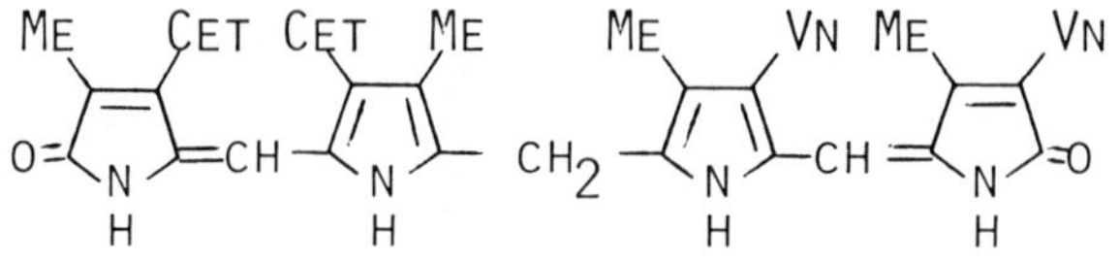

13,18-$\underline{VN}_2$-BILIRUBIN-3,7 (BILIRUBIN-IXβ)

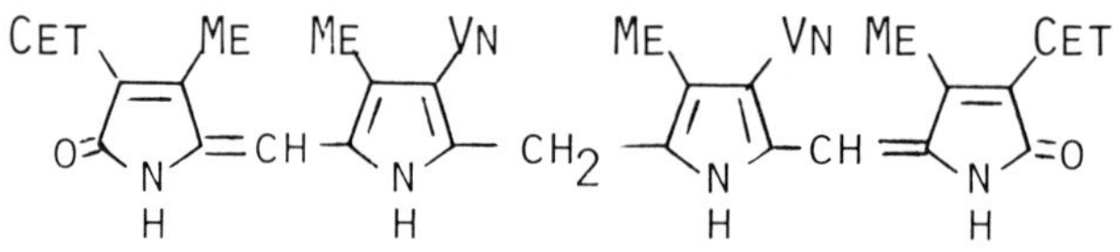

8,13-$\underline{VN}_2$-BILIRUBIN-2,18 (BILIRUBIN-IXγ)

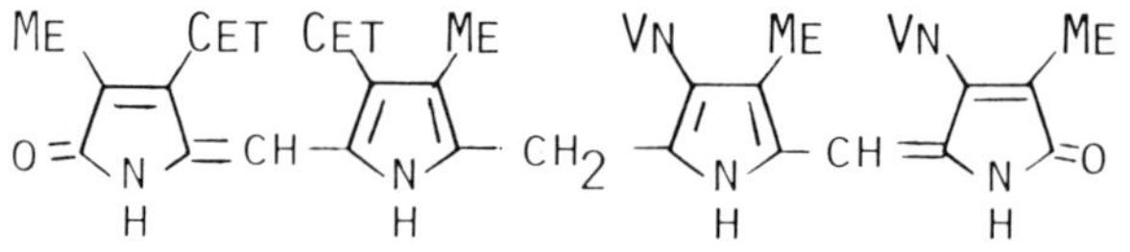

12,17-VN_2-BILIRUBIN-3,7 (BILIRUBIN-IXδ)

FIGURE 4. Proposed nomenclature of Bergstrom and Blumenthal[5] for bilirubins and biliverdins as illustrated for various bilirubin isomers. (ME, methyl; VN, vinyl; CET, carboxyethyl).

rubinic acid, the latter to xanthobilirubinic acid (Figure 8). The methyl group was thought to have originated from the central methylene group of mesobilirubin; thus, two parts fit together nicely as a tetrapyrrole of the now well-recognized skeleton. However, Fischer and Hess[8] concluded that mesobilirubin-IX*α* and its precursor bilirubin-IX*α* must have the symmetrical ordering of *β*-substituents, as dictated by reassembling xanthobilirubinic and neoxanthobilirubinic acid to give what is now known as the XIII*α* structure. Subsequently, Fischer and Siedel[9] determined that each oxodipyrromethene type consisted, in fact, of two substances: that with an unsubstituted pyrrole *α*-position was a mixture of neoxanthobilirubinic acid and isoneoxanthobilirubinic acid; that with a methyl-substituted pyrrole *α*-position consisted of a mixture of xanthobilirubinic acid and isoxanthobilirubinic acid (Figure 8). Thus, they concluded (correctly) that an unsymmetric ordering of the end ring substituents must ob-

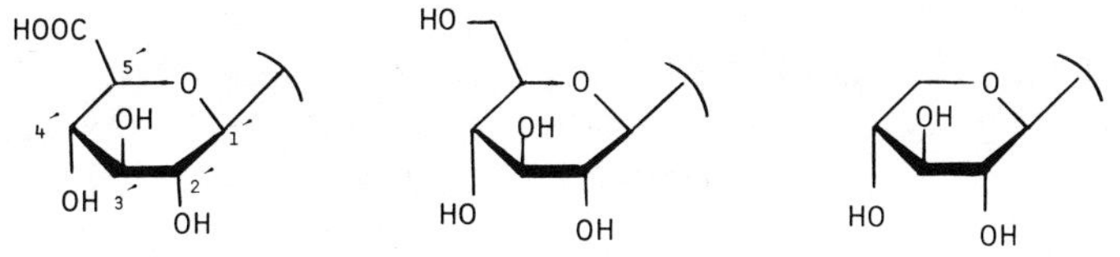

β-D-GLUCOPYRANURONOSYL β-D-GLUCOPYRANOSYL β-D-XYLOPYRANOSYL

GLCUP GLCP XYLP

FIGURE 5. Conjugating sugars (for bilirubin) and their abbreviations according to Bergstrom and Blumenthal.[5]

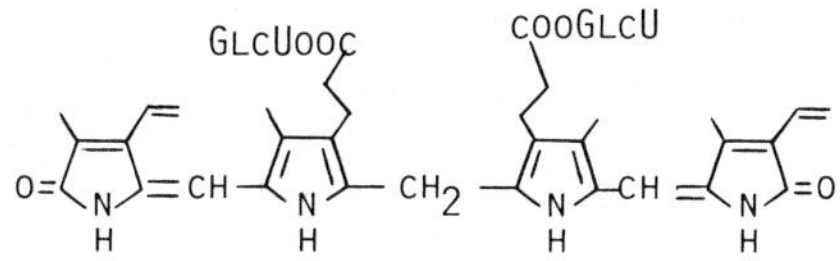

BILIRUBIN-8,12(GLCU;GLCU)

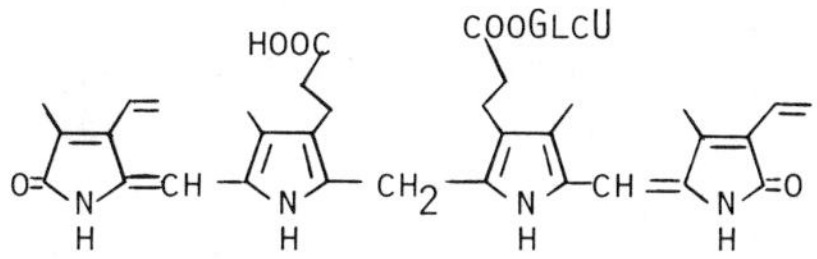

BILIRUBIN-8,12(GLCU)

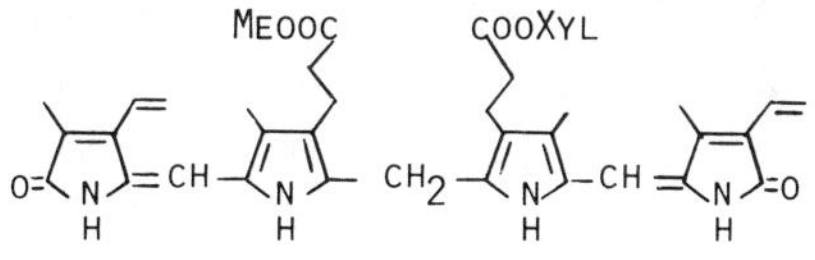

BILIRUBIN-8,12(ME;XYL)

FIGURE 6. Esters of bilirubin-IXα illustrating the proposed nomenclature of Bergstrom and Blumenthal.[5]

tain for mesobilirubin-IXα and therefore for bilirubin-IXα. The various xanthobilirubinic acid structures (Figure 8) were proved unequivocally by total synthesis,[10] and it became established that the arrangement of the pyrrole β-substituents (side chains) is the same in bilirubin-IXα (nonsymmetrical) as in protoporphyrin-IX and hematin.

b. Oxidation

Oxidative degradation of bile pigments can lead to monopyrrole derivatives. Identification of the derivatives is useful in elucidation of the nature of the pyrrole β-substituents. A particularly useful method is that developed by Rüdiger using dichromate-chromic acid to yield cyclic imides and formyl pyrroles.[11,12] Bilirubin-IXα with chromic acid would yield the cyclic imide products shown in Figure 9, but so would any of the

Table 1
EXAMPLES USING ABBREVIATIONS FOR DESIGNATING THE ANOMERIC CONFIGURATION AND SUGAR FORM ILLUSTRATED FOR BILIRUBIN-8,12 MONOXYLOSIDE

Abbreviation	
Bilirubin-*8*,12(Xyl)	Xylose in pyranose form; β configuration at anomeric carbon; attached to carboxyethyl in position 8(8-Cet).
Bilirubin-*8*,12(αXyl)	Pyranose form; α configuration; attached at 8-Cet.
Bilirubin-*8*,*12*(αXylf)	Furanose form; α configuration; attached at 12-Cet.
Bilirubin-*8*,12(α,βXyl)	Pyranose form; mixture of α and β configuration; attached at 8-Cet.

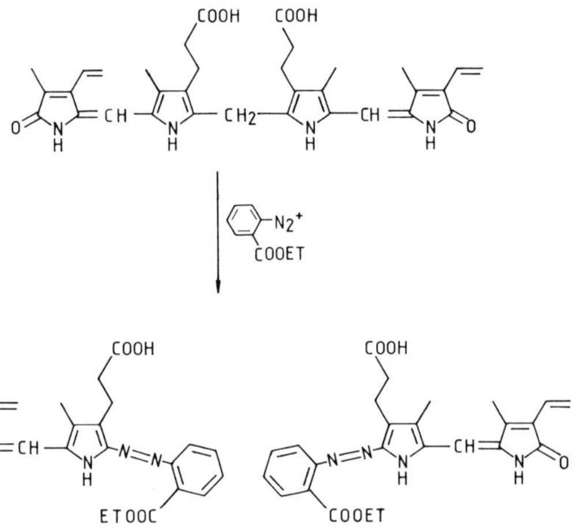

FIGURE 7. Reaction of bilirubin-IXα with diazotized ethyl anthranilate to yield two isomeric azopyrromethenes.

Table 2
AZOPYRROMETHENES DERIVED FROM REACTION OF FOUR BILIRUBIN ISOMERS WITH DIAZOTIZED ETHYL ANTHRANILATE

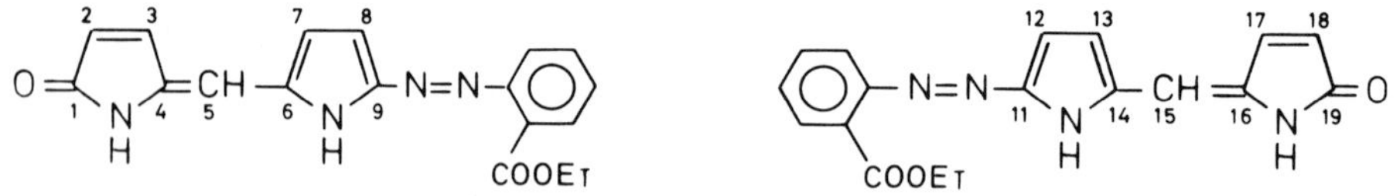

Originating bilirubin	Azopyrromethene abbreviation	2	3	7	8	12	13	17	18
		Substituents and locations							
IXα	Azpm-8	Me	Vn	Me	Cet				
	Azpm-12					Cet	Me	Me	Vn
IXβ	Azpm-3,7[a]	Me	Cet	Cet	Me				
	13,18-*Vn*$_2$-Azpm					Me	Vn	Me	Vn
IXγ	Azpm-2	Cet	Me	Me	Vn				
	Azpm-18					Me	Vn	Me	Cet
	Azpm-3,7	Me	Cet	Cet	Me				
IXδ	12,17-*Vn*$_2$-Azpm					Vn	Me	Vn	Me

[a] Can be obtained from either the IXβ or IXδ isomer.

Table 3
EXAMPLES ILLUSTRATING THE PROPOSED NOMENCLATURE OF BERGSTROM AND BLUMENTHAL[5]

Trivial name	Systematic name	Position of designated substituents
Bilirubin-IXα	Bilirubin	
Bilirubin-IXβ	13,18- Vn_2-Bilirubin-3,7	
Bilirubin-IXγ	8,13- Vn_2-Bilirubin-2,18	
Bilirubin-IXδ	12,17- Vn_2-Bilirubin-3,7	
Azopigment α_F	13,18- Vn_2-Azpm	
Azopigment α_F	12,17- Vn_2-Azpm	
Azopigment α_O	Azpm-12	
Azopigment α_O	Azpm-8	
Azopigment α_{OM}	Azpm-12(Me)	12 - $CH_2CH_2CO_2Me$
Azopigment α_{OM}	Azpm-8(Me)	2 - $CH_2CH_2CO_2Me$
Azopigment α_{ON}	Azpm-12(amide)	12 - $CH_2CH_2CONH_2$
Azopigment α_{ON}	Azpm-8(amide)	2 - $CH_2CH_2CONH_2$
Azopigment α_2	Azpm-12(Xyl)	12 - $CH_2CH_2CO_2$-β-D-Xyl
Azopigment α_2	Azpm-8(Xyl)	2 - $CH_2CH_2CO_2$-β-D-Xyl
Azopigment α_3	Azpm-12(Glc)	12 - $CH_2CH_2CO_2$-β-D-Glc
Azopigment α_3	Azpm-8(Glc)	2 - $CH_2CH_2CO_2$-β-D-Glc
Azipigment β_x	Azpm-3,7	
Azopigment δ	Azpm-12(GlcU)	12 - $CH_2CH_2CO_2$-β-D-GlcU
Azopigment δ	Azpm-8(GlcU)	2 - $CH_2CH_2CO_2$-β-D-GlcU

other isomers of bilirubin, e.g., XIIIα, IXγ, etc. Dichromate oxidation can be more informative. With dichromate, methylvinylmaleimide and the pyrrole dialdehyde (Figure 9) are formed, an observation which would indicate clearly that the bile pigment has at least one central ring with methyl and propionic acid groups, and at least one end ring with methyl and vinyl substituents. Assuming that other cyclic imides and pyrrole dialdehydes were incapable of being formed, a tetrapyrrole would have end rings possessing only one methyl and one vinyl group (per end ring) and central rings possessing only one methyl and one propionic acid group per ring. Only the IIIα, IXα, and XIIIα isomers of bilirubin satisfy those criteria. Other oxidative degradation methods have been employed. Alkaline permanganate gives pyrrole-2,5-dicarboxylic acid (from the central rings),[13,14] and paraperiodic acid can yield cyclic imides and pyrrole dialdehydes.[15]

c. Diazo Cleavage

Bilirubin and other 4,15-biladienes react with diazotized aromatic amines to give red to violet colored oxodipyrromethene azo compounds which can be useful in structure determination. Thus, as illustrated in Figure 10, bilirubin-IXα is capable of giving one mole equivalent of each of two isomeric azodipyrroles (isomerism due to differently located vinyl substituents;[16-19] the theoretical number of isomers is eight when the geometric *cis-trans* and *syn-anti-* isomers are included). On the other hand, the symmetrical bilirubin-IIIα and XIIIα isomers each can give only one of the azo pigments (two mole equivalents), as shown, and other isomers of bilirubin, e.g., IXβ, IXγ, IXδ have been shown to give the expected different isomeric azo pigments (Table 2).[20]

A reasonable reaction mechanism has been postulated to involve electrophilic attack by diazonium ion on a central pyrrole ring at either position 9 or 11 (Step 1, Figure 11) in a manner similar to that of aromatic azo dye formation.[21] The initially formed tetrapyrrolic azo intermediate can decay with C-C bond cleavage to yield (Step 2) the "vinyl" azo pigment[19] when the initial point of electrophilic attack is position 9 (or the "isovinyl" azo pigment[19] from initial attack at position 11). The remaining oxodi-

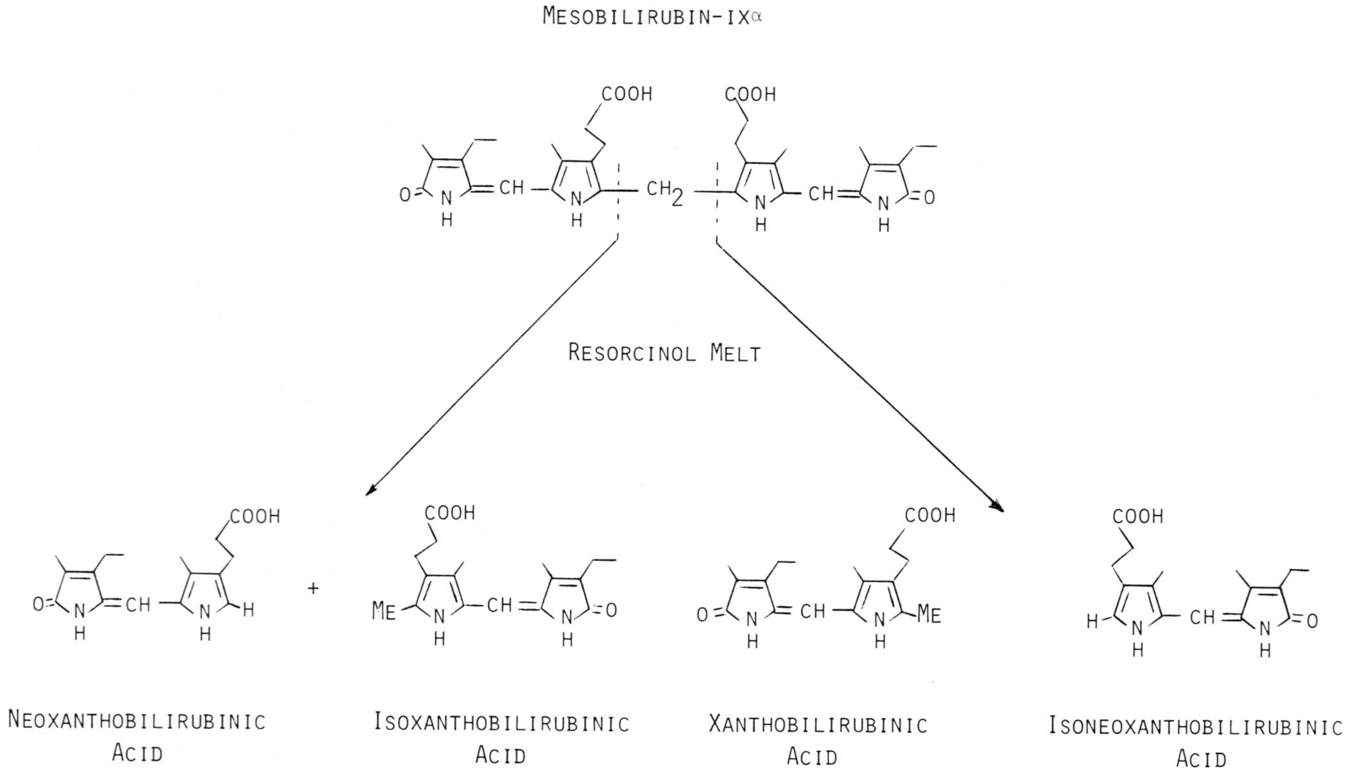

FIGURE 8. Products of the reaction of mesobilirubin-IXα in melted resorcinol.[6,9]

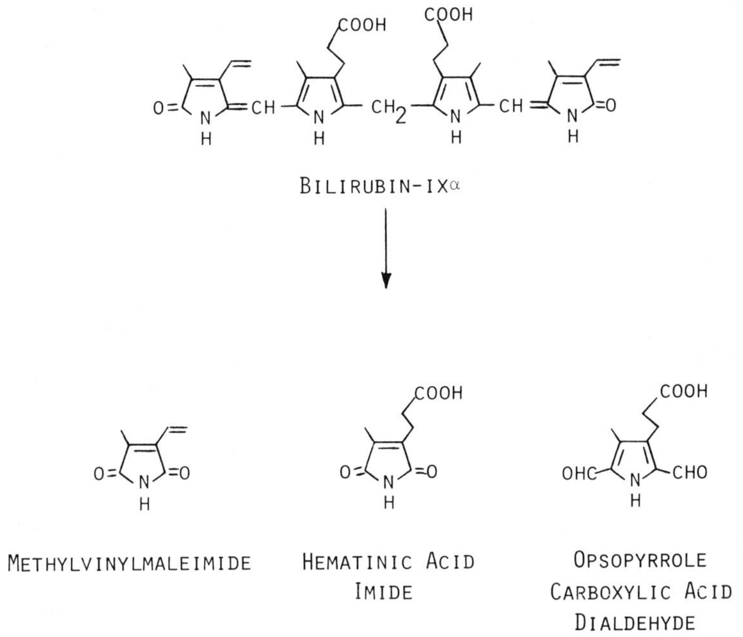

FIGURE 9. Monopyrrolic oxidation products from reaction of bilirubin-IX*α* with chromic acid and dichromate.

pyrromethene half of bilirubin is potentially reactive with an additional mole equivalent of diazonium ion in the way shown in Step 3 leading to formation of (in this scheme) the "isovinyl" azo pigment and one equivalent of formaldehyde. In support of this overall mechanism, formaldehyde has been proven to be a reaction product (isolated as its dimedone derivative)[21] along with the two isomeric azodipyrroles. The azo pigment products thus convey the same sort of structural information, viz., ordering of the pyrrole *β*-substituents, that the previously described resorcinol melt degradation does. It must be stressed, however, that although either method involves the degradation of a tetrapyrrole to a structurally simpler dipyrrole, the structure of the azodipyrrole must still be ascertained, either by synthesis or by spectroscopic analysis.

In addition to the often extremely useful structural information imparted by analysis of the azo pigment from the diazo reaction, it has been used for many years in the clinical quantitation of serum bilirubin (van den Bergh reaction)[1,22] with particular notice paid to the differing reactivities of bilirubin and its conjugates. Thus, the diazo reaction was placed on a reasonably quantitative basis using visible spectroscopy, and distinction could be made between the faster reacting ("direct-reacting") conjugated serum bilirubin and the slower ("indirect-reacting") unconjugated serum bilirubin. Addition of "accelerators", e.g., ethyl alcohol, to the serum samples causes the slower reacting bilirubin to react considerably faster, probably because its state of aggregation is reduced (see below and Chapter 3).

2. *Total Synthesis*

The structure of bilirubin-IX*α* was proved conclusively by total synthesis and reported in 1942 by Fischer and Plieninger.[23] The presence of vinyl groups and the nonsymmetrical ordering of the side chains (pyrrole *β*-substituents) made the synthesis difficult and tedious. In its time, it represented one of the monumental accomplishments of natural products total synthesis and is outlined in Figures 12 to 15. Bilirubin was obtained by bisulfite reduction of biliverdin, a reduction which is commonly car-

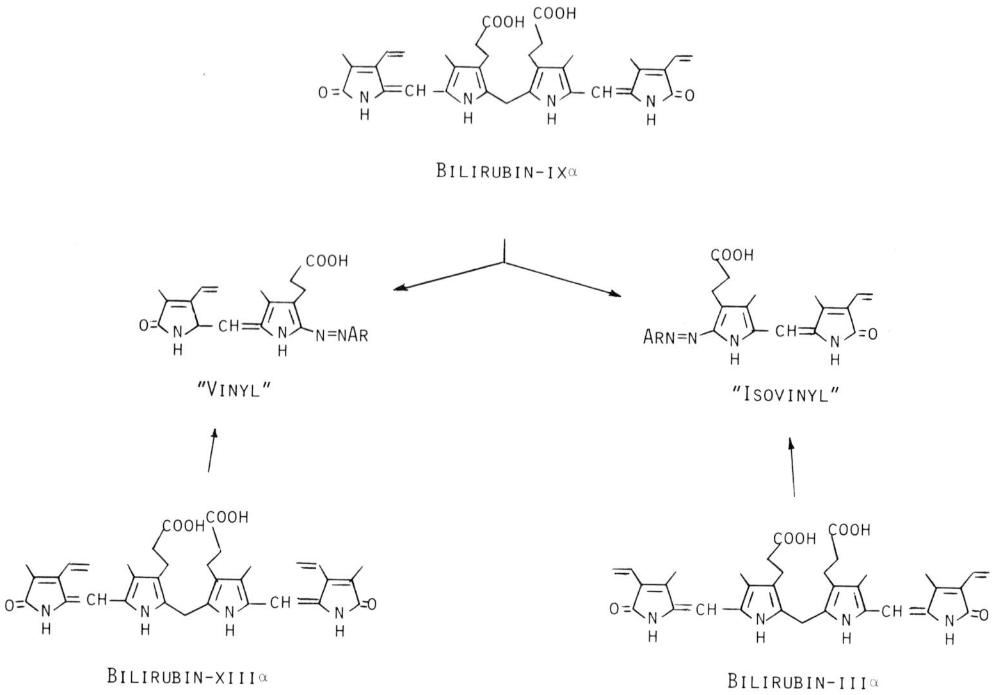

FIGURE 10. Azo pigments derived from bilirubin-IXα and the symmetrical constitutional isomers bilirubin-IIIα and bilirubin-XIIIα.

ried out today by use of sodium borohydride.[1,24] One of the key synthetic steps involved coupling two different oxodipyrromethene "halves" to afford a biliverdinoid tetrapyrrole. This solved the problem of making an unsymmetrical tetrapyrrole because in the acid-catalyzed coupling shown in Figure 12, the oxodipyrromethene aldehyde must react with an "unsubstituted" oxodipyrromethene half and, under the reaction conditions employed, neither oxodipyrromethene can react with itself (and lead to a symmetrically substituted tetrapyrrole). In this procedure, the two oxodipyrromethene "halves" can (with the proper ordering of their pyrrole β-substituents) provide the desired unsymmetrical ordering of β-substituents in the final tetrapyrrole. The other key step overcame difficulties associated with the preparation of material with (reactive) vinyl substituents by masking the incipient vinyl group as a urethane derivative. The urethane group was hydrolyzed in due course to an amine which was permethylated and eliminated under Hoffmann conditions as described in Figure 12.

The key synthetic intermediates were the oxodipyromethenes shown in Figure 12. Their syntheses are outlined in Figure 13 and involve coupling of monopyrrole units. Thus, base-catalyzed condensation of a pyrrole aldehyde (α-formyl pyrrole) with a 3-pyrrolin-2-one gave the desired oxodipyrromethene in high yield. Preparation of the appropriately substituted 3-pyrrolin-2-one was accomplished by alkaline hydrogen peroxide oxidation of opsopyrrole carboxylic acid (3-carboxyethyl-4-methylpyrrole) and separation of the two isomers by fractional crystallization, with the less alcohol-soluble (and more easily obtained) isomer being 3-methyl-4-carboxyethyl-3-pyrrolin-2-one (the upper compound of Figure 14). The propionic acid group was converted to urethane by means of a Curtius rearrangement.

Preparation of opsopyrrole carboxylic acid and its corresponding aldehyde are shown in Figure 15 and are accomplished in a straightforward way from the structurally simple, inexpensive ethyl acetoacetate.

More recent syntheses of bilirubin have been described.[25]

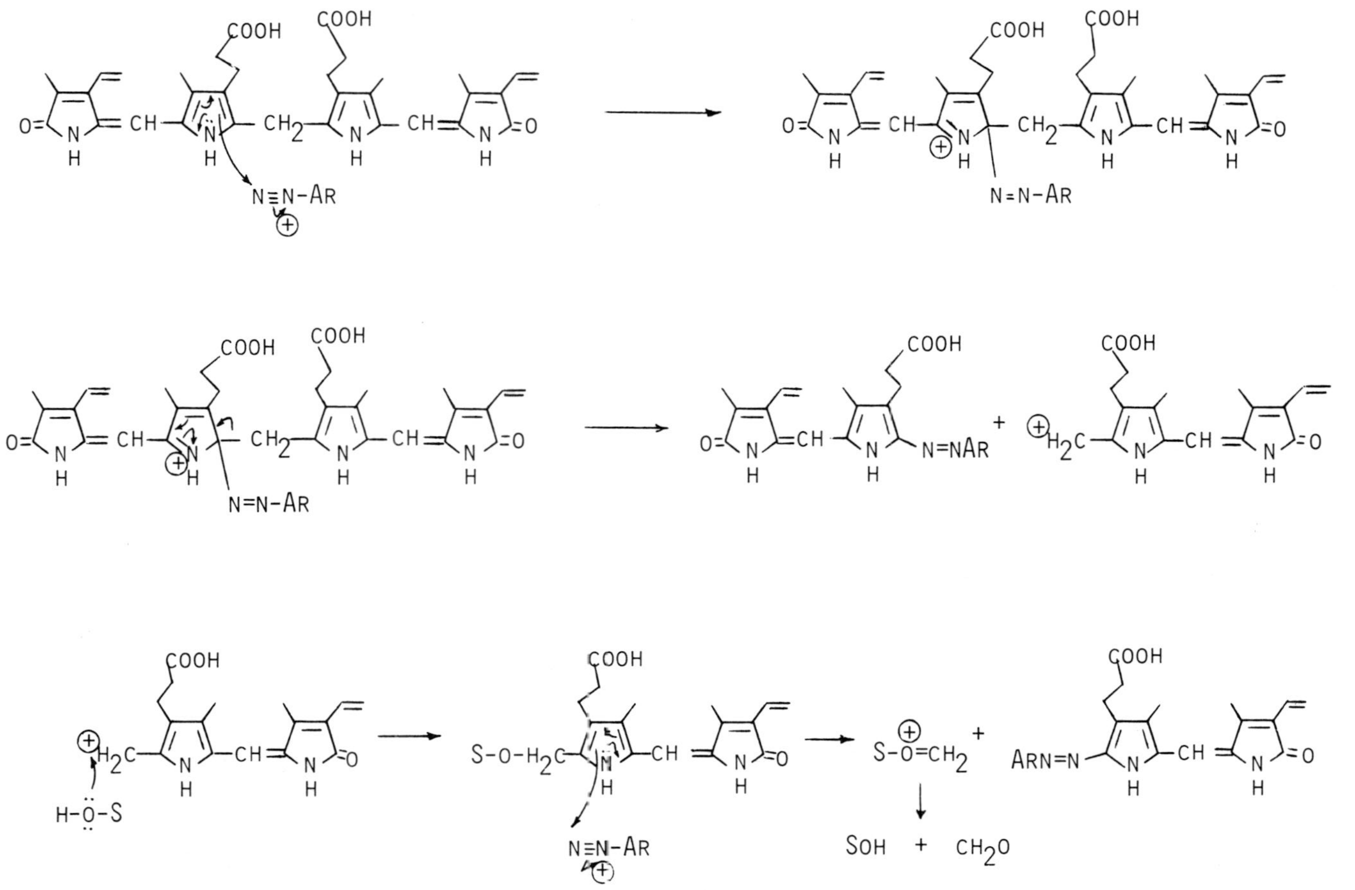

FIGURE 11. Mechanism of reaction of bilirubin-IXα with an aromatic diazonium ion to give azodipyrroles: upper line-step 1, middle line-step 2, bottom line-step 3. SOH is hydroxylic solvent.

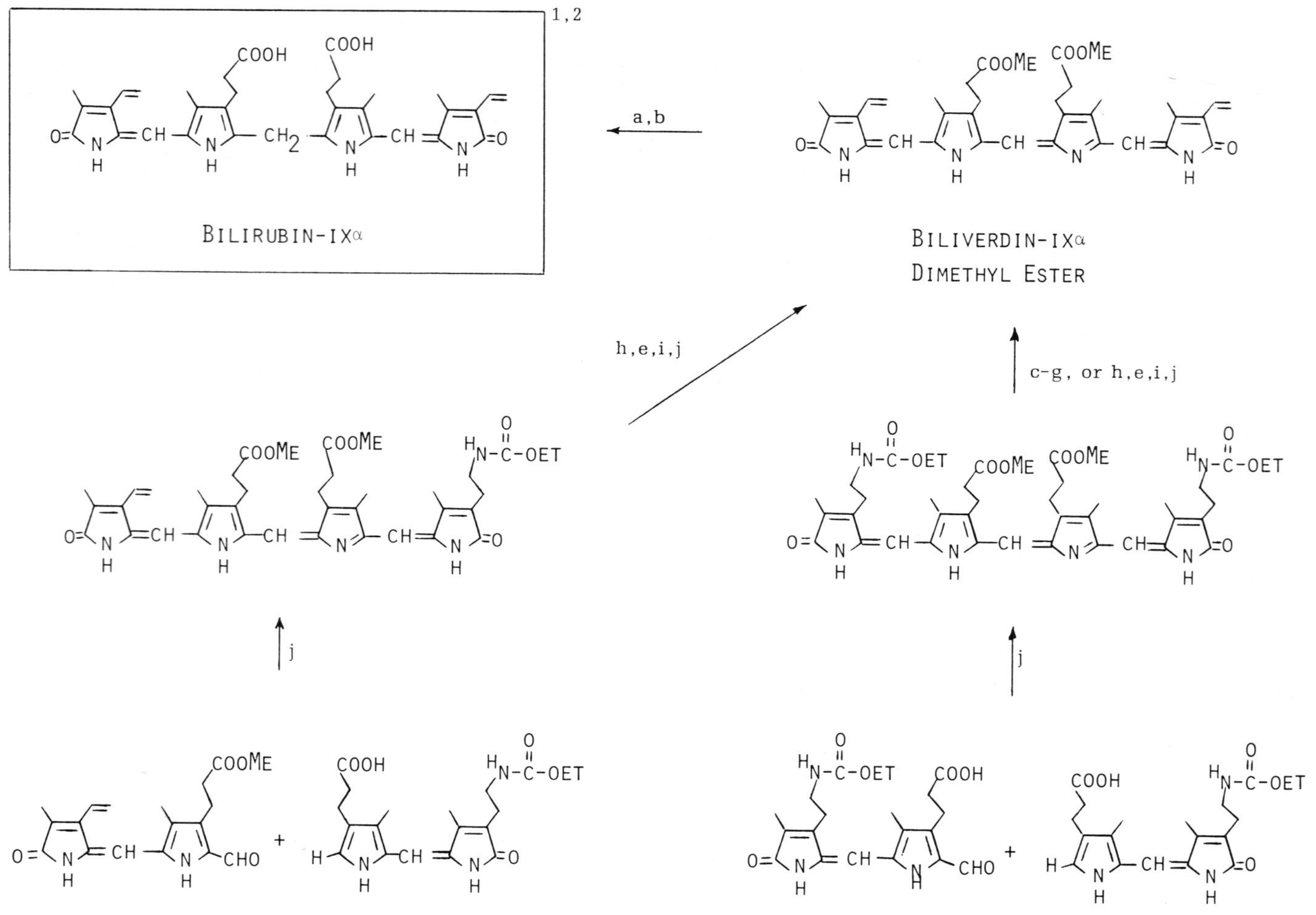

FIGURE 12. Synthetic scheme for the preparation of bilirubin-IXα and biliverdin-IXα from oxopyrromethenes[23] The reagents are: a, KOH/aq CH_3OH; b, cold aq. $NaHSO_3$; c, conc. HCl/100°C; d, KOH/CH_3OH; e, $Zn(OAc)_2$; f, CH_3I; g, conc $KOH-CH_3OH$, boil; h, $NaOH/H_2O$; i, $(CH_3O)_2SO_2$; j, 48% aq $HBr-CH_3OH$/reflux 1: Ref. 23a, 2: Ref. 236.

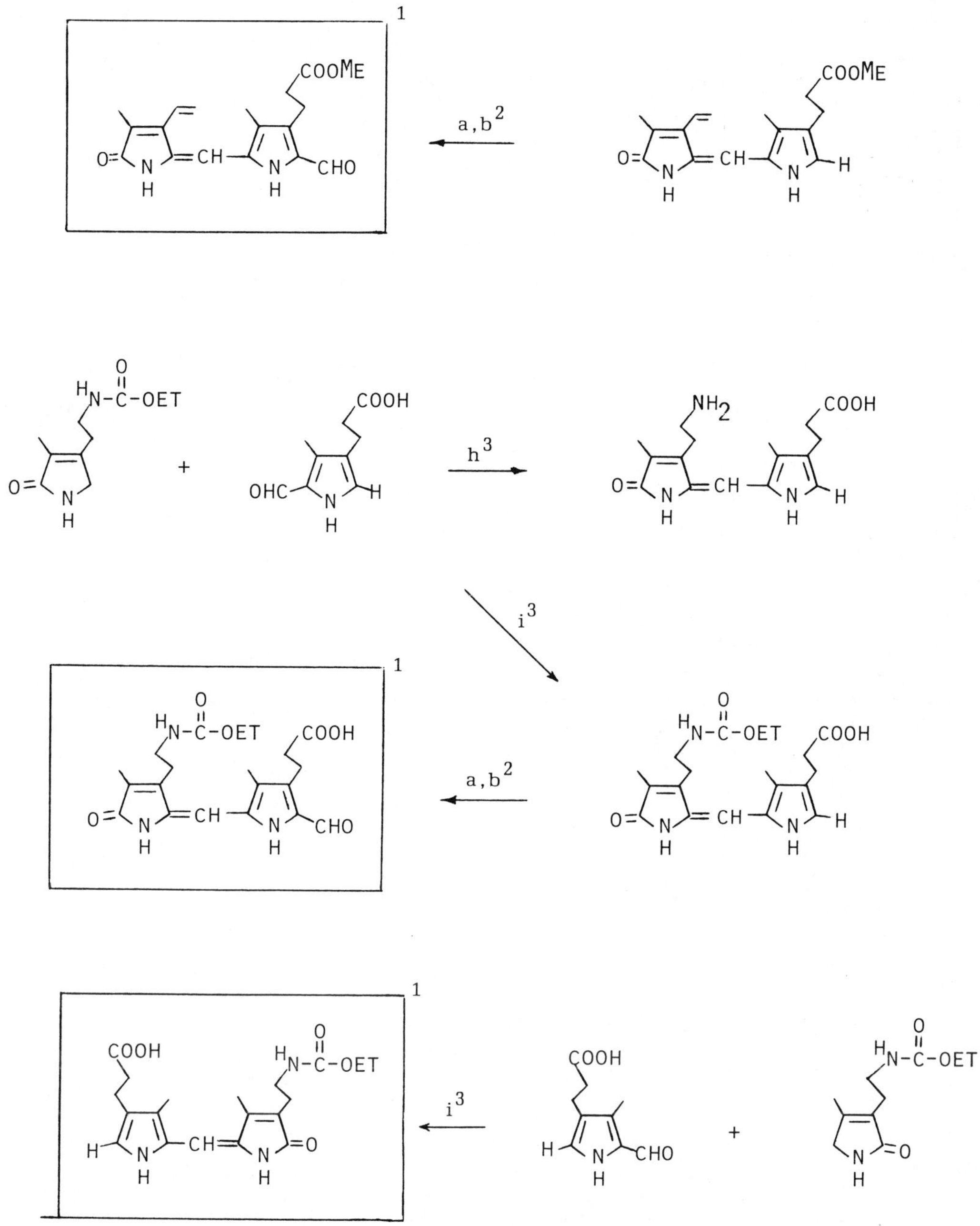

FIGURE 13. Reaction schemes for the preparation of oxopyrromethene synthetic precursors to bilirubin-IXα. The reagents are: a, $CHCl_3$-HCN; b, dry HCl; C, NaOH-H_2O; d, $Zn(OAc)_2$; e, $(CH_3O)_2SO_2$; f, NaOH/CH_3OH/boil; g, HCl-CH_3OH; h, NaOH-aq. CH_3OH, reflux; i, NaOH-aq CH_3OH. 1: Ref. 23b, 2: Ref. 23a, 3; Ref. 148.

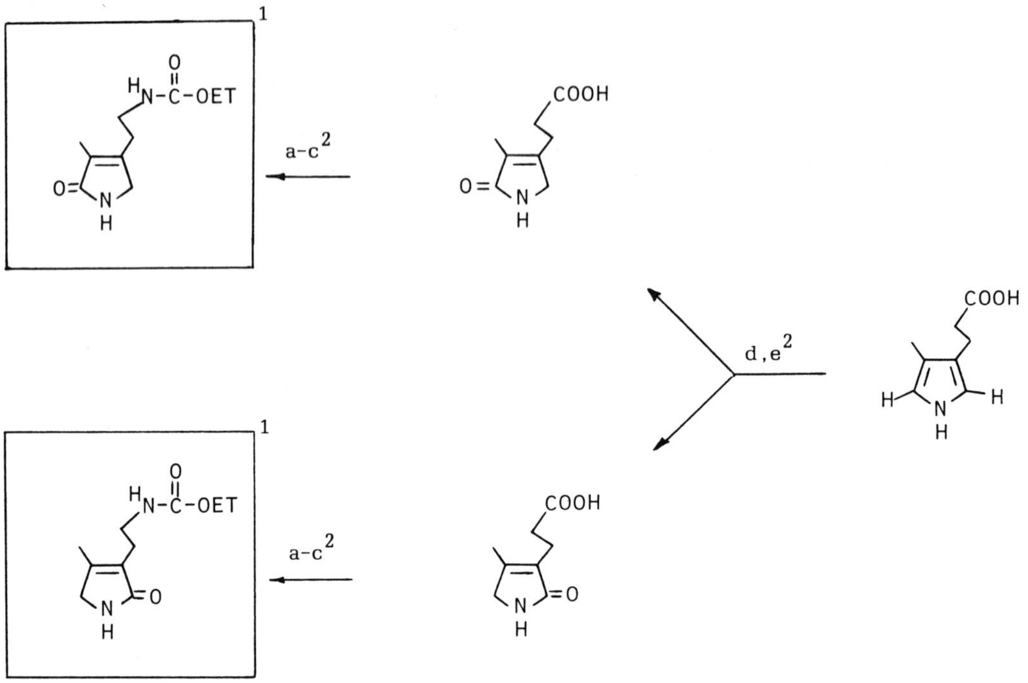

FIGURE 14. Reaction schemes for the preparation of monopyrrole synthetic precursors to bilirubin-IXα.[23] The reagents are: a, CH_3OH-HCl; b, H_2NNH_2/CH_3OH; c, HNO_3-$NaNO_2$; d, H_2O_2-pyridine/55°C; e, fractional crystallization from ethanol. 1: Ref. 23b, 2: Ref. 23a.

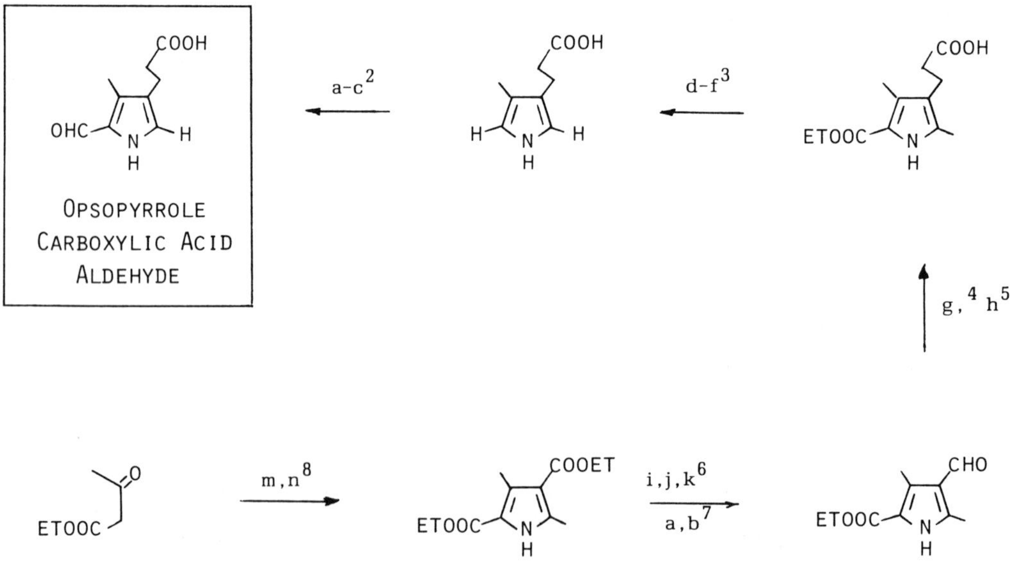

FIGURE 15. Reaction scheme for the synthesis of opsopyrrole carboxylic acid aldhyde used in the synthesis of bilirubin-IXα. The reagents are: a, HCl-HCN(g)/$CHCl_3$-ether/0°C; b, aq. HCl; c, aq. NaOH; d, SO_2Cl_2; e, H_2O/Δ; f, aq. NaOH/175-180° (autoclave); g, $CH_2(CO_2H)_2$/aniline/Δ; h, Na(Hg)/NaOH; i, conc. H_2SO_4; j, ice/NaOH; k, Δ; m, aq. $NaNO_2/CH_3CO_2H$/50°C; n, Zn dust/reflux in AcOH. The steps in the synthesis are described in Fischer, H. and Orth, H., *Die Chemie des Pyrrols,* Vol. I, Akademische Verlagsgesellschaft, MBH, Leipzig, 1934 and Johnson Reprint Corp., New York, 1968, as follows: a-c, p. 171; d-f, p. 282; g, p. 267; h, p. 276; i-k, p. 239; a, b, p. 164; m, n, p. 255.

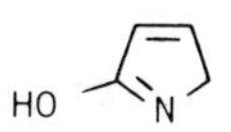

LACTIM

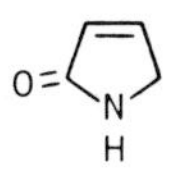

LACTAM

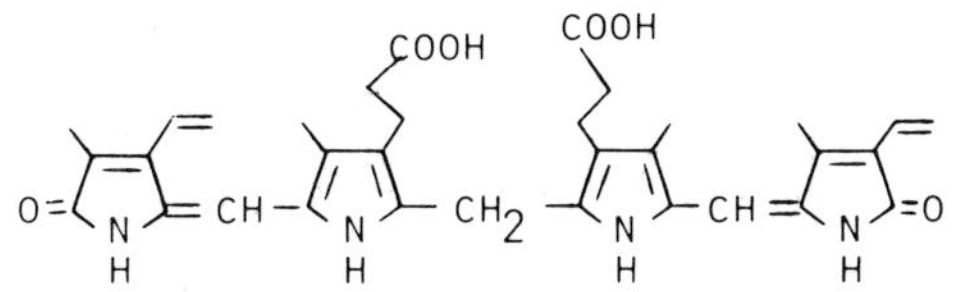

BISLACTAM STRUCTURE OF BILIRUBIN-IXα

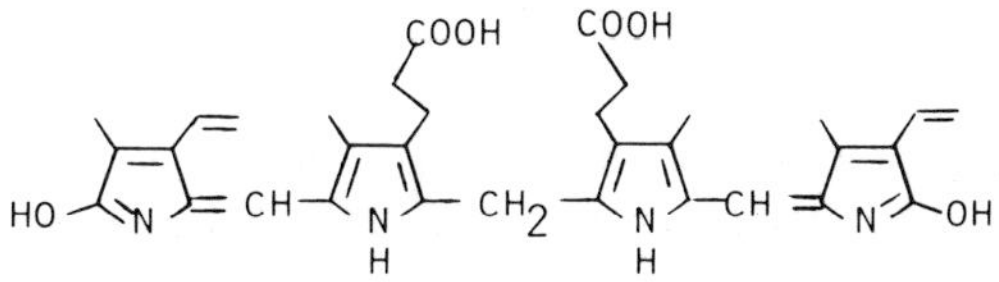

BISLACTIM STRUCTURE OF BILIRUBIN-IXα

FIGURE 16. Structures showing lactim (enol) and lactam (keto) forms of cyclic amides and their incorporation into the bilirubin-IXα structure. The two different, possible lactim-lactam structures, e.g., 1-hydroxy, 19-oxo and 1-oxo, 19-hydroxy are not shown.

B. Secondary Structure

1. Lactam-Lactim Tautomerism

Keto-enol tautomerism between lactam and lactim forms of the 3-pyrrolin-2-one end rings of bilirubin and other bile pigments (Figure 16) was mentioned by Kuster over 60 years ago,[26] but the issue was not resolved until nearly 40 years later. The Fischer School favored the lactim tautomer; consequently, most bile pigment structures drawn in books and in research publications conveyed that preference. Even today one occasionally finds bile pigment structures drawn in the lactim form. However, considerable evidence has been marshaled to show that the lactam tautomer is in fact the predominant, if not exclusive tautomeric form in both neutral solution and in the solid. Falk[27] showed that the lactam form is more stable by a large factor (10^4 for bilirubin) in some carefully done equilibrium studies using optical-pK methods. Birch[28] first recognized that infrared spectroscopy might distinguish between a lactim and lactam form. The former would have =C−O stretching and O−H stretching; whereas, the latter would have C=O stretching bands. He successfully concluded that stercobilin was in the more stable lactam form using infrared spectroscopy.

Considerable spectroscopic evidence, including X-ray crystallography,[29] infrared spectroscopy,[30-33] and nuclear magnetic resonance spectroscopy,[16,30-40] has been brought to bear on the question of lactim-lactam tautomeric structures for bilirubin.

Table 4
SELECTED BOND DISTANCES (Å) FROM CRYSTALLOGRAPHIC STRUCTURES

Compound	C(1) - O(1)	C(4) - C(5)	C(5) - C(6)	Ref.
Bilirubin-IXα	1.25-1.28	1.30	1.45	29
Bilirubin-IXα Bis-isopropyl Ammonium Salt	1.24	1.35	1.43	41
Mesobilirubin-IXα	1.253	1.318	1.486	42a
Biliverdin-IXα Dimethyl Ester	1.219	1.351	1.477	43
3,8-12-Triethyl-14-formyl-2,7,13-trimethyl-1(15 H)-tripyrrinone	1.227	1.356	1.433	44
3,4,4′-Triethyl-3′,5′-dimethyl-2Z,2′-pyrromethen-5(1 H)-one	1.216	1.354	1.431	4
3,4-Dimethyl-2,2′-pyrromethen-5(1 H)-one	1.248	1.354	1.431	45
5′-Ethoxycarbonyl-3,4-dihydro-3′,4′-dimethyl-5(1 H)-2Z,2′-pyrromethenone	1.223	1.321	1.466	46
5′-Ethoxycarbonyl-3,4-dihydro-3′,4′-dimethyl-5(1 H)-2E,2′-pyrromethenone	1.241	1.324	1.444	46
5-Ethoxy-5′-Ethoxycarbonyl-3,4-dihydro-3′,4′-dimethyl-27,2′-pyrromethenone	1.326	1.356	1.454	46
Dimethoxybilirubin dimethyl ester	1.357 1.347(C_{19}-O_{19})	1.361 1.348(C_{15}-C_{16})	1.387 1.425(C_{14}-C_{15})	42b

The conclusion reached is that bilirubin exists essentially completely in the bislactam form (Figure 16). The methods are considered in the following.

a. X-ray Crystallography

In the recently available crystallographic data for bilirubin[29] the observed end ring (3-pyrrolin-2-one) carbon-oxygen bond distances were 1.25-1.28 Å—in good agreement with lactam structures found in related cyclic amides (Table 4) structures[4,41-46] — but considerably shorter than the carbon-oxygen single bond distance in lactims (1.33 Å).[45] The lactam carbonyl bond distance appears to be relatively insensitive to (C−C) saturation-(C=C) unsaturation in the five-membered ring as well as to substitution on the ring(s) (Table 4).

b. Infrared Spectroscopy

Complete or partial infrared spectra of bilirubin have been published over the years.[1,32,47-50] However, most spectra were determined on solid bilirubin dispersed in the solid (KBr) phase or nujol (mineral oil) mulls. A partial chloroform solution spectrum of bilirubin was reported,[49] but it lacks resolution, and it is unclear whether the chloroform contained the usual ethanol stabilizer. Infrared spectra of bilirubin in solution and as a solid dispersion are shown in Figure 17.[51] It is especially instructive to examine the N-H/O-H and C=O bond stretching regions of the spectra of Figure 17. Commercial bilirubin (Sigma) crystallized from dimethylsulfoxide (DMSO)-acetone shows what is believed to be N−H stretching[1] near 3410 cm^{-1} (lactam) and 3265 cm^{-1} (pyrrole) when dispersed in pressed KBr or Teflon® discs, or in nujol mulls. However, the intensities of those bands are variable. They are more easily seen in the dispersed solid spectra (Figures 17A, 17B, 17C, and 17D) and more difficult to recognize in the solution spectra (Figures 17E and 17F). The location of the expected O−H (COOH) stretching band is obscure; it has been suggested[1] to be quite broad in the region 2500 to 3000 cm^{-1}.

It is unclear what role aggregation or interstitial water plays in the dispersed solid spectra. In the KBr spectra (Figure 17A) it is exceedingly difficult to remove the last traces of water from the KBr itself. Consequently, the compressed powdered Teflon®

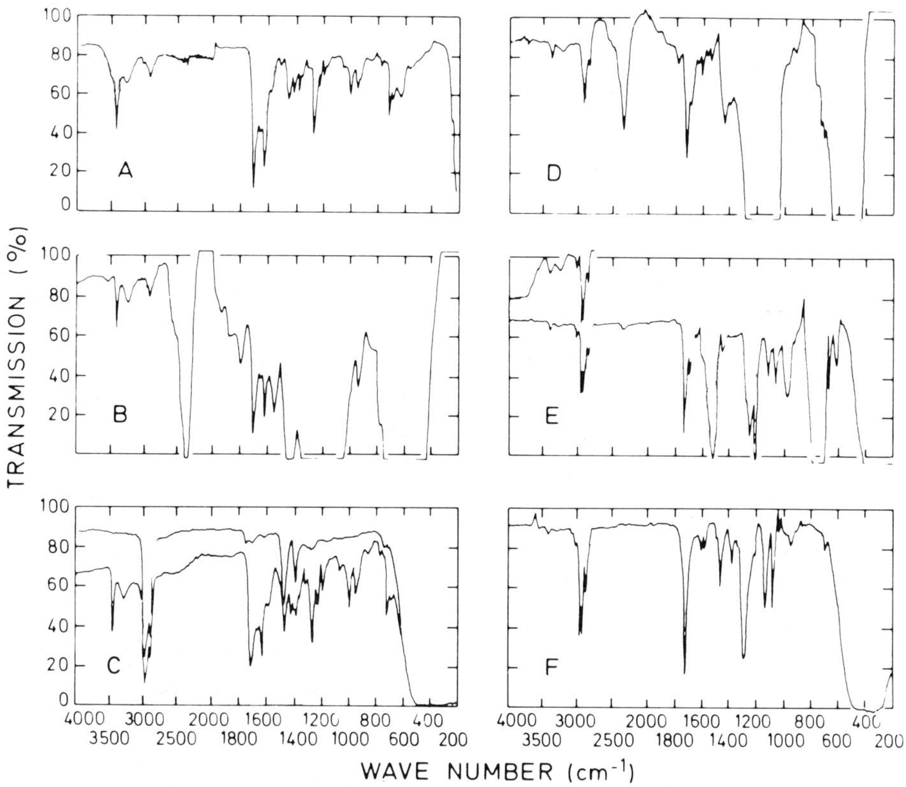

FIGURE 17. Infrared spectra of bilirubin-IXα: A, in KBr disc; B, in compressed Fluoropak® 80 (powdered Teflon®); C, in Nujol (the upper curve is a Nujol reference); D, in compressed Fluoropak® 80 (powdered Teflon®); E, in dry carbon tetrachloride (the upper partial spectrum is run at increased sensitivity); and F, in dry, ethanol-free chloroform. The spectra were run by W. P. Linnane, this laboratory.

discs (Figures 17B and 17D) are more reliable when considering the 3000 to 4000 cm^{-1} region. Their disadvantages are associated with their strongly absorbing regions near 2400 cm^{-1} and <1500 cm^{-1}. Nujol mulls (Figure 17C) perhaps offer a good compromise. Solution spectra (Figures 17E and 17F) bring forth the sp^3 C—H stretching bands which are not as easily seen in the solid phase, except in the less concentrated Teflon® disc spectrum (Figure 17D), whereas the alleged N—H stretching is not as readily seen. Thus, it would seem that, whereas the relatively high concentrations of bilirubin to KBr facilitate observation of the (inherently weak) O—H/N—H stretching, other more intense bands (sp^3 C—H and C=O) may be obscured or altered when Beer's Law concentrations are exceeded.

Other differences may be observed in the C=O stretching region. Absorption bands appear near 1700, 1650, 1610, and 1560 cm^{-1} in the dispersed solid phase spectra (Figures 17A to 17D). Curiously, in the more dilute concentrations of dispersed solid (in compressed solid Teflon®, cf. Figure 17B and 17D) the band intensities in the 1700 cm^{-1} region are greatly altered, and a new, intense band appears at 1725 cm^{-1} in Figure 17D. This new band is also found in CCl_4 (Figure 17E) and $CHCl_3$ (ethanol-free, Figure 17F) solution spectra along with weaker bands at 1697 and 1650 cm^{-1}, or 1700 and 1680 cm^{-1}. The sp^3 C—H stretching is clearly represented in the solution spectra, as is the C—O stretching (ca. 1250 cm^{-1}) of the COOH groups.

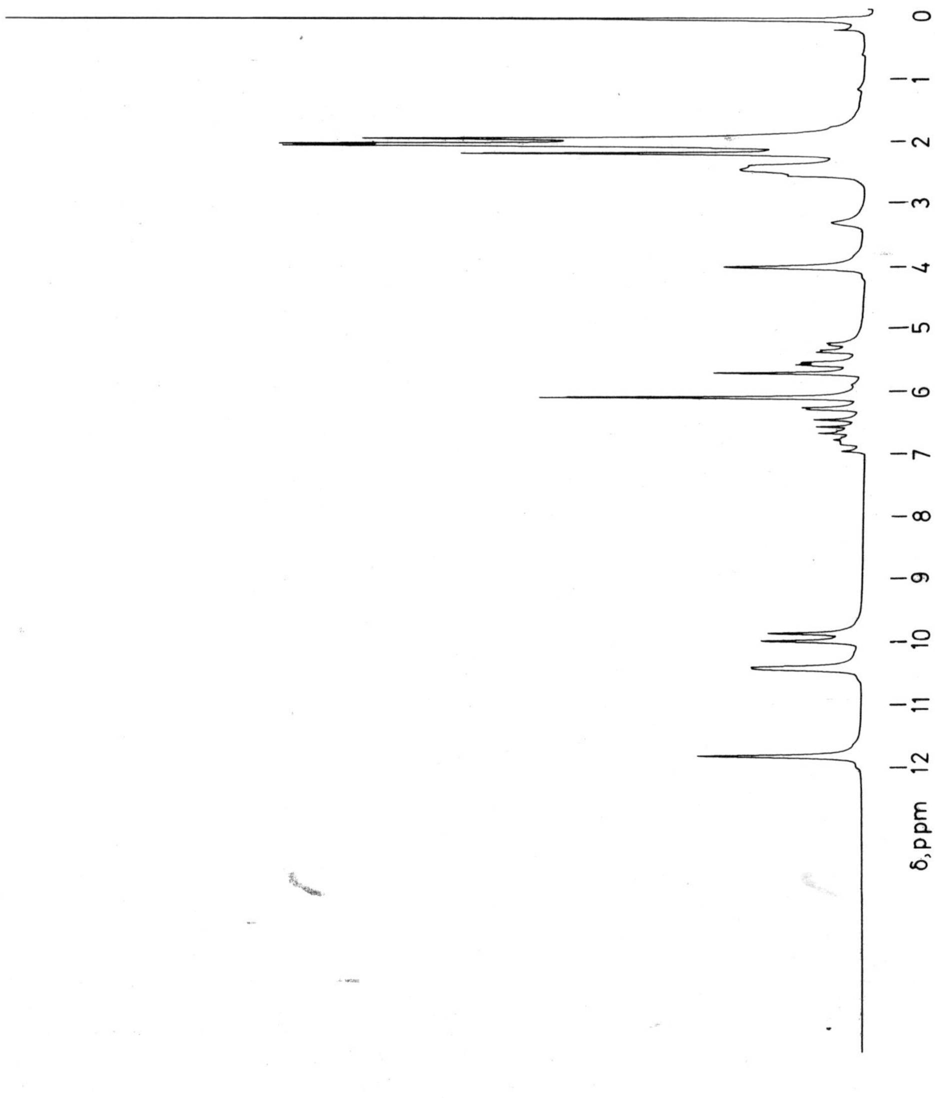
0
1
2
3
4
5
6
7
8
9
10
11
12
δ, ppm

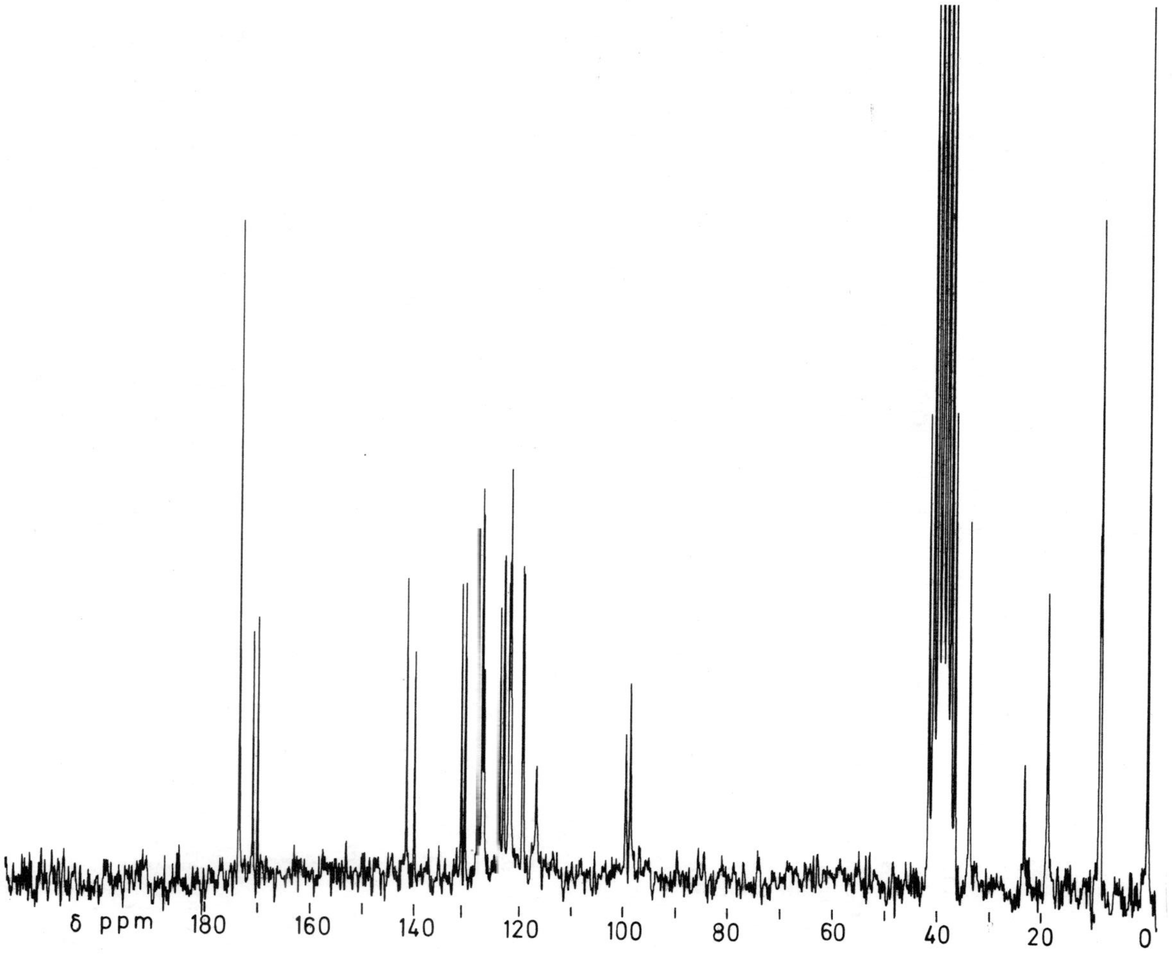

FIGURE 18. (Upper) ^1H-nuclear magnetic resonance spectrum of bilirubin-IXα in d_6-dimethylsulfoxide run at 100 MHz on a JEOL FX-100 instrument. (Lower) ^{13}C-nuclear magnetic resonance spectrum of bilirubin-IXα in d_6-dimethylsulfoxide run at 25.0 MHz on a JEOL FX-100 instrument. All data are reported in δ, ppm downfield from tetramethylsilane and were obtained by G. L. Landen, this laboratory.

c. Nuclear Magnetic Resonance (NMR) Spectroscopy

The possibility that lactam $(-\underset{\underset{O}{\|}}{C}-\underset{H}{N}-)$ and lactim $(-\underset{\underset{OH}{|}}{C}=N-)$ tautomers (Figure 16) of bilirubin in solution might be distinguished on the basis of ^{1}H-NMR and ^{13}C-NMR spectroscopy (Figure 18)[52] proved to be fruitful. However, due to limited solubility, only a few solvents (principally d_6-DMSO) could be used to explore the structure-spectra relationship. Comparatively recently, Nichol and Morell[33] compared the ^{1}H-NMR spectra of bilirubin and bilirubin dimethyl ester and concluded (erroneously) that bilirubin exists predominantly in the lactim form in d_6-DMSO solvent. Shortly thereafter, Kuenzle[16] reported the ^{1}H-NMR spectra of bilirubin, bilirubin dimethyl ester and mesobilirubin and concluded that bilirubin exists largely as a bislactam tautomer in d_6-DMSO. The assignment of the lactam structure rests on the observation that bilirubin and its several derivatives exhibit low field signals near 12 δ ppm (2H, broad singlet, COOH) and near 10 δ ppm (4H, NH) (Figure 19).[40] Because six low-field hydrogen signals (2 COOH, 4 NH) vanish with added D_2O, it can be concluded that COOH to COOD and NH to ND exchange occurs, with the COOH hydrogens exchanging more rapidly than the four NH protons.[32] When the dry NMR solvent is moistened with H_2O, the COOH signals exchange rapidly with H_2O resulting in broading and flattening of the COOH signal.[32] The NH signals are unaffected by added H_2O; thus, one can conclude (logically) that the more acidic COOH protons exchange more rapidly than the NH protons.

The basis for the earlier misassignment of a lactim structure for bilirubin[33] stems from the failure of the authors to find COOH proton signals near 11.9 δ ppm.[16] Apparently the expected COOH signals were flattened due to traces of moisture in the d_6-DMSO in the spectrum run with warmed solvent. The exchange of COOH protons with H_2O slows down at lower temperatures.[36] Failure to locate the 11.9 δ ppm signal led to a misassignment of the NH signals near 10.5 δ ppm as being due to COOH instead of the amide protons.

The assignments of the other hydrogens in bilirubin are given in Figure 19. Several features are worth noting. The *endo*-vinyl group (at C-3) methine signals occur at lower field than those of the *exo*-vinyl group (at C-18). The signals are coupled (ABX) and are found as a complex pattern between 5 and 7 δ ppm. The *meso* olefinic protons (C-5 and C-15) appear as a sharp singlet near 6 δ ppm. All four methyl groups of bilirubin can be seen clearly at 300 MHz, but two of the signals are quite close together and appear unresolved near 2.13 δ ppm at 100 MHz.

Similarly, ^{13}C-NMR (Figure 18[52] and 20) has been used to educe that bilirubin exists in the bislactam rather than the bislactim tautomeric form. Manitto et al.[34,35] first reported on the ^{13}C-NMR spectra of bilirubin and its dimethyl ester and determined that the end ring ^{13}C=O signals (ca. 171 and 174 δ ppm for bilirubin and its dimethyl ester, respectively) were closer to those found in lactam (ca. 176 δ ppm) rather than lactim (167 δ ppm) model compounds. Shortly thereafter, Chedekel and Crist[40] published their ^{13}C-NMR assignments for bilirubin and assumed the bislactam tautomeric form. The observed values for the lactam ^{13}C=O end ring resonances for bilirubin dimethyl ester seem reasonable based on pyrromethenone models,[37] and a complete spectral assignment has been made by Hansen et al.[38] by comparison with bilirubin-XIIIα and mesobilirubin ^{13}C data.

The weight of NMR evidence strongly suggests that bilirubin, mesobilirubin, and their dimethyl esters[53] exist in solution predominantly as lactam tautomers.

2. Z/E Configurational Isomerism

The possibility of *cis* and *trans* (E and Z) geometric isomerism about the meso carbon-carbon double bonds at C_4–C_5 and C_{15}–C_{16} of bilirubin was recognized over 40

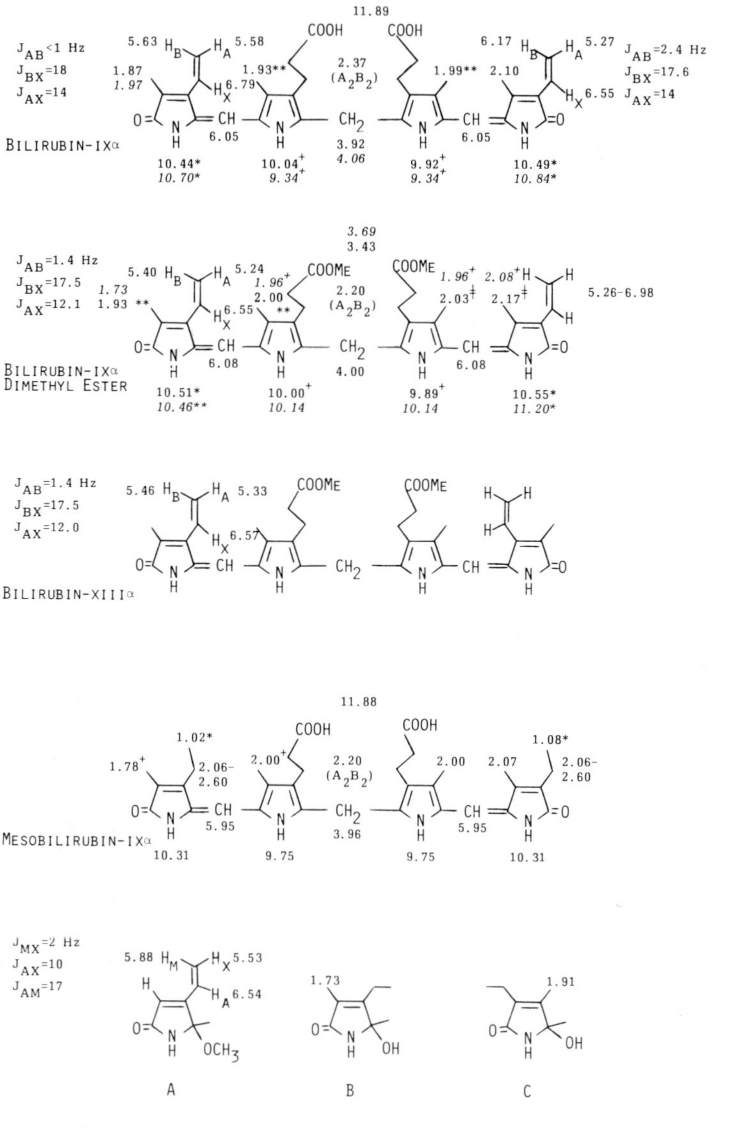

FIGURE 19. ¹H-nuclear magnetic resonance assignments for bilirubin-IXα, its dimethyl ester, mesobilirubin-IXα, bilirubin-XIIIα dimethyl ester, mesobilirubin-IXα and various reference monopyrroles. Assignments with symbols (*, **, +, etc.) may be interchanged within the encompassed designation. The assignments (nonitalicized) for bilirubin-IXα run in d_6-dimethylsulfoxide were determined by Kuenzle[16] and are supported by Navon et al.[39] The vinyl group assignments and coupling constants were determined at 300 MHz: Chedekel, M., Bovey, F. S., Brewster, A. I. R., Petryka, Z. J., Weimer, M., Watson, C. J., Moscowitz, A., and Lightner, D. A., On the Existence of a Mono-Vinyl d-Urobilin, *Proc. Natl. Acad. Sci. (U.S.)*, 71, 1599, 1974. The italicized assignments are due to Manitto et al.[30] For bilirubin dimethyl ester run in deuteriochlorform: (1) The assignments (nonitalicized) are due to Kuenzle.[16] (2) The vinyl group assingments and splittings are due to Manitto et al.[30] (3) The italicized assignments are due to Hutchinson, D. W., Johnson, B., Knell, A. J..[149] The assignments for mesobilirubin-IXα run in d_6-dimethylsulfoxide are due to Kuenzle.[16] The assignments for bilirubin-XIIIα dimethyl ester in dueteriochloroform are due to Manitto.[104] The assignments for the various monopyrroles, run in deuteriochloroform, were determined: *A*, by L. K. Low, this laboratory; *B*, by Lightner, D. A. and Crandall, D. C.[150] and *C* by Lightner, D. A., Norris, R. D., Kirk, D. I., and Key, R. M.[151]

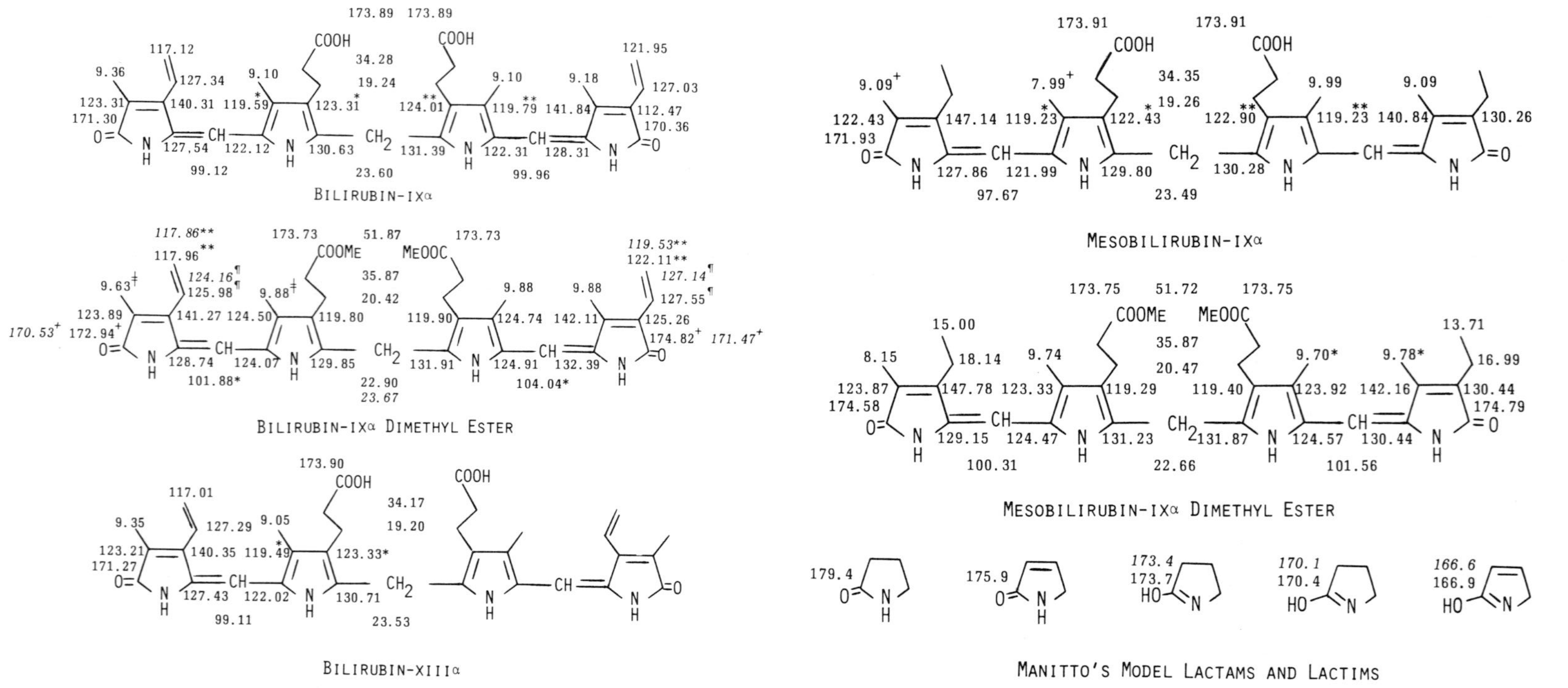

FIGURE 20. ^{13}C-nuclear magnetic resonance assignments are presented for bilirubin-IXα run in d_6-dimethylsulfoxide, bilirubin-IXα dimethyl ester run in deuteriochloroform, bilirubin-XIIIα and mesobilirubin IXα run in d_6-dimethylsulfoxide, mesobilirubin-IXα and mesobilirubin-IXα dimethyl ester run in deuteriochloroform, and model lactams and lactims. Assignments with symbols (*, **, +, etc.) may be interchanged within the encompassed designation. The ^{13}C assignments for bilirubin-IXα are due to Brodersen *et al.*[38] and Gossauer *et al.*[37] and are fairly consistent with those of Navon *et al.*,[39] Chedekel and Crist[40] and Manitto *et al.*[34] The assignments for bilirubin dimethyl ester are due to Gossauer *et al.*[37] Italicized values are due to Manitto *et al.*[34] for the sample run in d_6-dimethylsulfoxide, and the values marked (P) should probably be reversed in view of Gossauer *et al.*[37] For bilirubin-XIIIα, the assignments were made by Brodersen *et al.*[38] but the values marked (*) should probably be reversed in view of the data of Gossauer *et al.*[37] The assignments for mesobilirubin-IXα in d_6-dimethylsulfoxide have been made Brodersen *et al.*[38] and in deuteriochloroform by Gossauer *et al.*[37] In the former, the values marked (*) and (+) should probably be reversed in view of the latter assignments. ^{13}C assignments for various lactams and lactims are due to Manitto *et al.*:[34,35] nonitalicized values are for data obtained in d_6-dimethylsulfoxide; italicized assignments are for data obtained in deuteriochloroform.

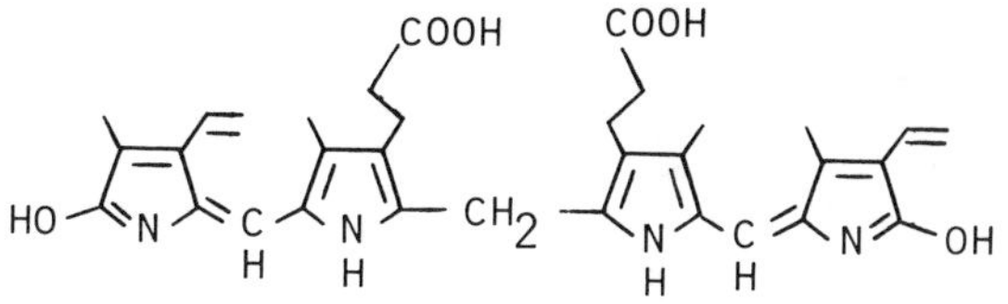

A

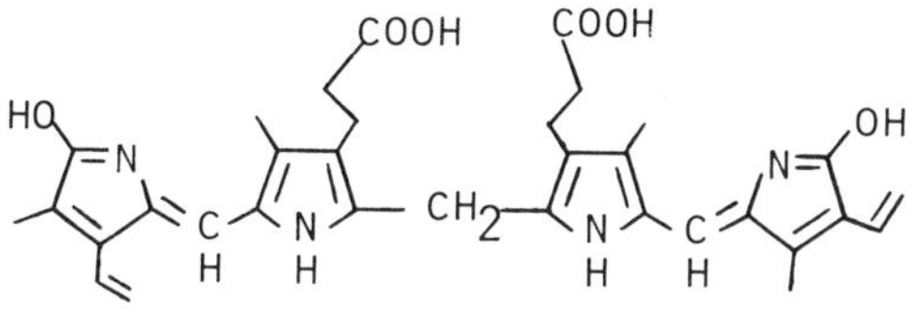

B

FIGURE 21. Lemberg's structures of bilirubin-IXα[54,55] illustrating the 4E,15E (A) and 4Z,15Z (B) geometric isomers. Lemberg preferred structure B on biogenetic grounds.

years ago by Lemberg.[54] He thoughtfully and logically indicated that the usually drawn linear formula of bilirubin (A, Figure 21) has the methene hydrogen *cis* to the pyrrole nitrogen and not *trans* (B, Figure 21) as would be expected from its source of origin: the precursor protoporphyrin-IX has (in Lemberg's nomenclature) all methene H's trans to pyrrole nitrogens. Aside from the fact that Lemberg incorrectly used the bis lactim formulas, his remarkable insight, based on firm logic, has proved to be correct, despite the fact that he and others continued to use the (more easily drawn?) *cis-cis* (4E,15E) configurational representation. More recently Brodersen et al.[49] re-represented a proposed bilirubin structure[56,57] as a 4Z,15Z isomer (see D, Figure 25) in connection with their infrared studies. However, the configurational distinction was not a necessary part of their conclusions, for in the same short work is found represented the 4E,15E isomer (see E, Figure 25) without reference to its being to a differing configurational structure. The 4Z,15Z isomer was also represented by Nichol and Morell[33] in their subsequently discredited[16] ^{1}H-NMR study (see F, Figure 25). Shortly thereafter Blauer and King[58] invoked structures of bilirubin possessing the 4Z,15Z configuration. This was done in order to explain the aqueous albumin-induced circular dichroism of bilirubin, using as a model the intramolecularly H-bonded structure of d-urobilin and ℓ-stercobilin of Moscowitz et al.[59] In their collection of 4Z,15Z conformational structures, Blauer and King[58] clearly represented the subsequently favored conformer, but without intramolecular H-bonding. That particular structure (*syn*-4Z,*syn*-15Z, Figure 22), complete with intramolecular H-bonding, was proposed subsequently, first, by Knell, et al,[60] then by Kuenzle et al.[61] as a novel conformational structure of bilirubin to account for its ground state solubility, and chemical reactivity in addition to its pK, infrared, ultraviolet, and ^{1}H-NMR spectroscopic properties. It should be mentioned, however, that the 4Z,15Z configurational isomer was drawn[61]

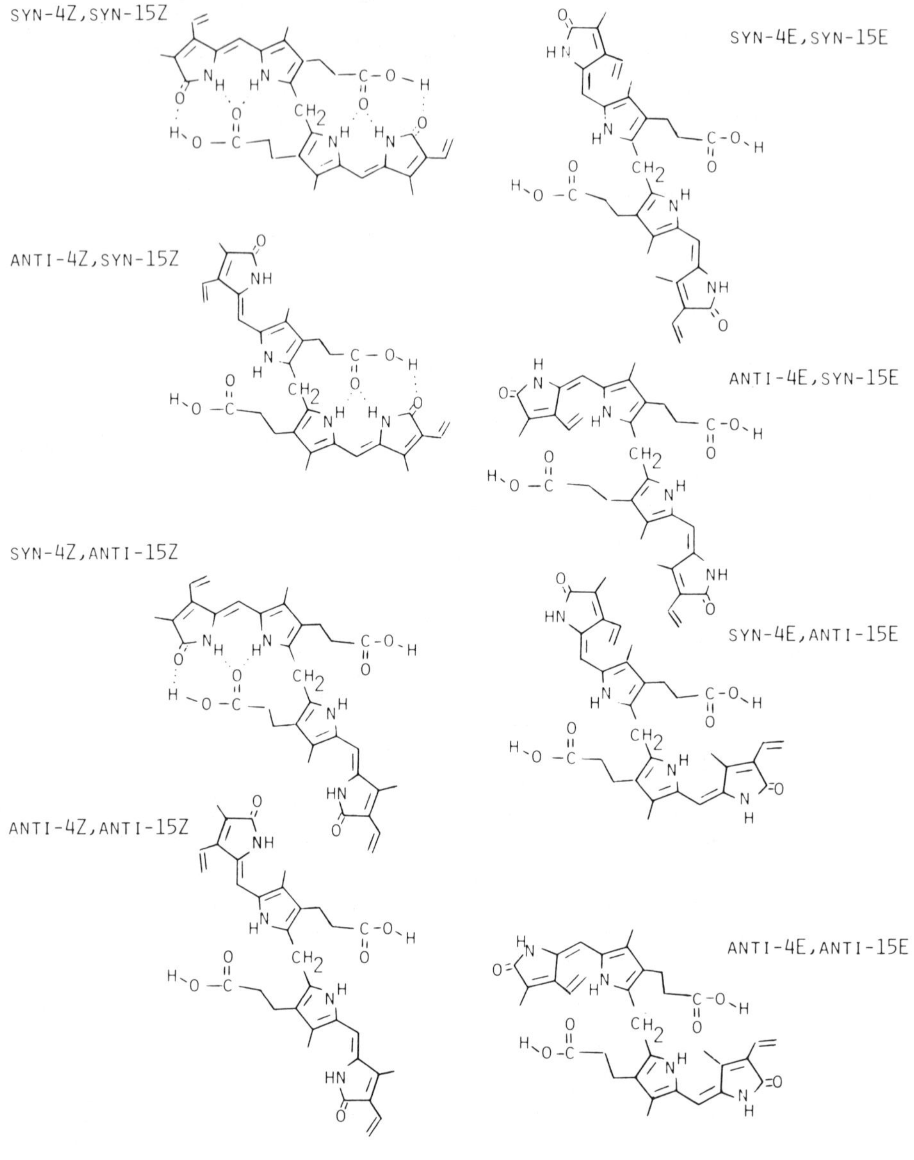

FIGURE 22. Structures of 4Z,15Z-bilirubin-IXα and 4E,15E-biliruin-IXα illustrating various rotational isomers about the C_5-C_6 and C_{14}-C_{15} carbon-carbon single bonds. Not shown are the 4Z,15E- and 4E,15Z-isomers of bilirubin-IXα which have similar rotamers.

without comment on Z/E geometric isomerism. Apparently, the configuration was represented because it was essential to the type of H-bonding marshaled forth.[62]

Direct proof for the 4Z,15Z configuration of solid bilirubin is found in its crystallographic structure.[29] The Z configuration is general and found even in that of diisopropylammonium bilirubinate,[41] mesobilirubin,[42] biliverdin dimethyl ester (4Z,9Z,15Z),[43] and various oxotripyrromethenes[44] and oxodipyrromethenes.[4,45,46] Evidence for distinguishing Z and E geometric isomers in solution was first obtained by Falk et al.[63,64] using ^{1}H-NMR on oxodipyrromethenes (Figure 23) and by Falk et al.[65-67] and by Lightner et al.[68] on benzalpyrrolinones using ^{1}H- and ^{13}C-NMR In all cases examined the Z isomer has its olefinic H at higher field (Figure 23). Similarly, the E-configurational isomers of aetiobiliverdin-IVγ can be distinguished by ^{1}H-NMR[69]

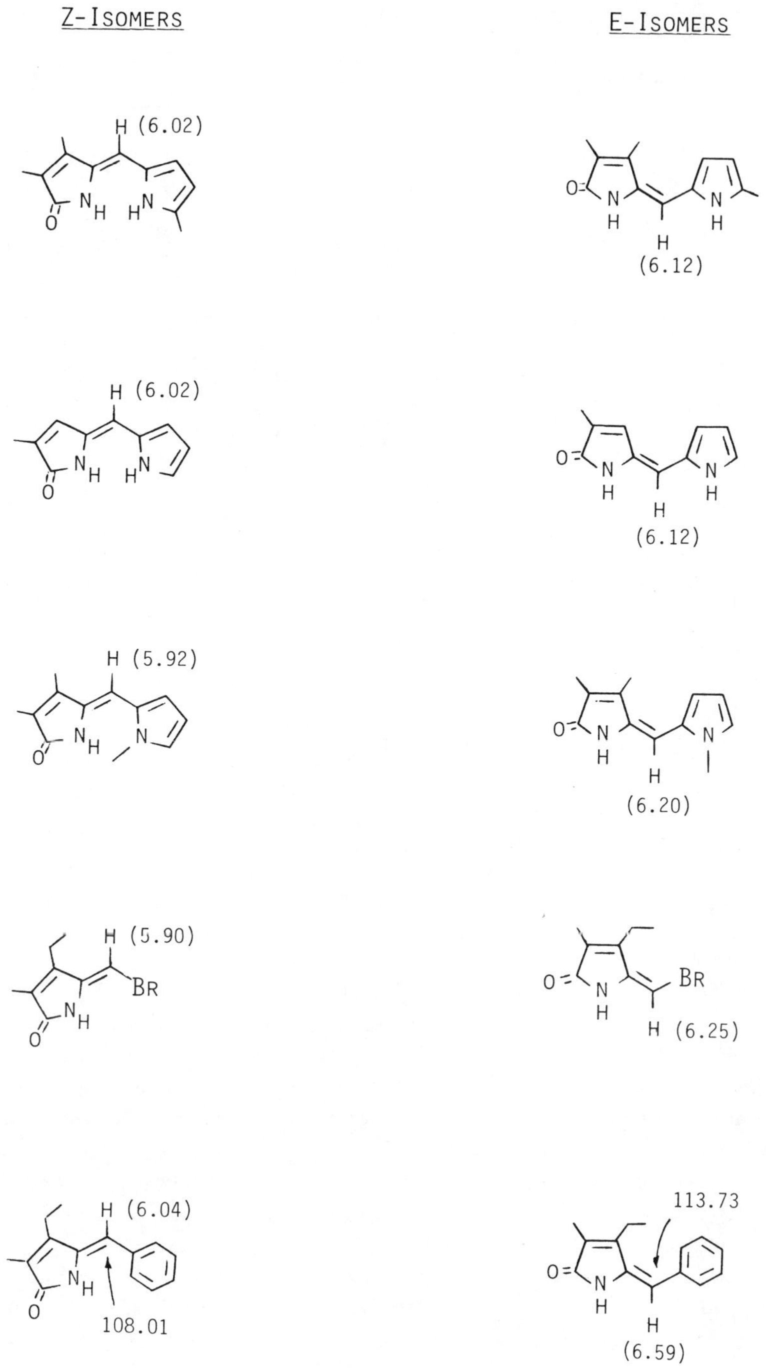

FIGURE 23. Oxopyrromethene and other models for bilirubin-IXα with chemical shift data (downfield, δ ppm for tetramethylsilane) for ^{1}H- and ^{13}C-nuclear magnetic resonance.

and ^{13}C-NMR[70] spectroscopy. Likewise, the Z and E configurational isomers of bilirubin should be distinguishable by ^{1}H- and ^{13}C-NMR. This seems to be borne out in our NMR studies.[71]

As judged from space-filled molecular models, the 4Z,15Z configuration of bilirubin

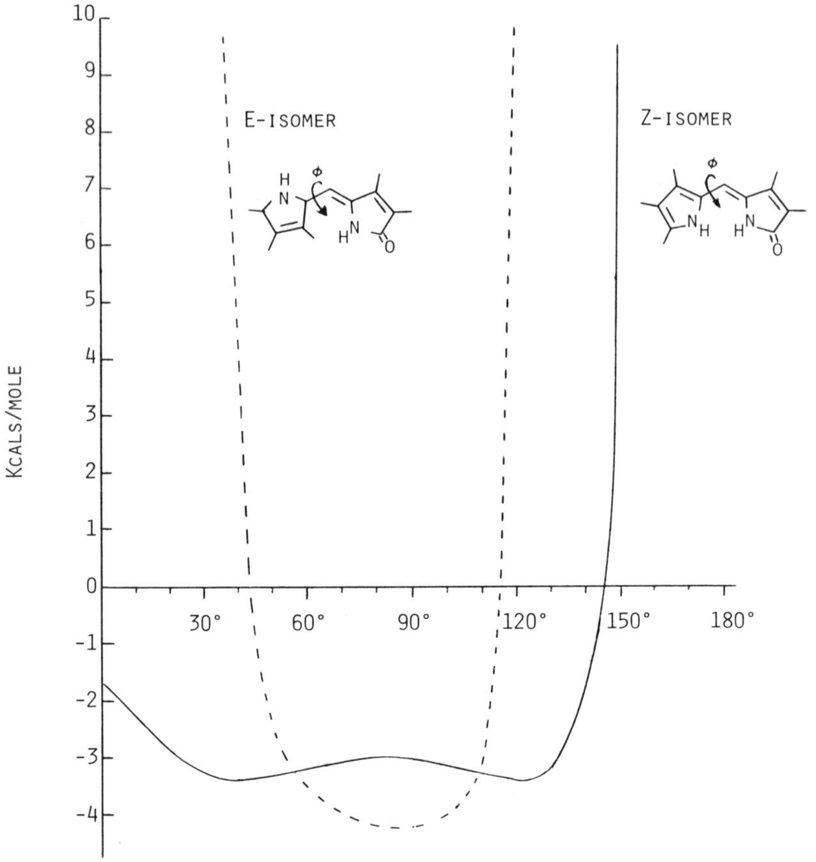

FIGURE 24. Calculated rotational (ϕ) dependence (horizontal axis) of nonbonded interaction energy (vertical axis) according to Geddes, Potterton and Willis.[72]

is less sterically crowded than the 4E,15E isomer and expected to be thermodynamically more stable; even in the absence of intramolecular H-bonding. Rotation about the C-C single bonds between C_5-C_6 and C_{14}-C_{15} of the all Z-isomer produces conformations leading to considerable steric hindrance (Figure 22), especially as the oxodipyrromethene approaches (internal) coplanarity in the *anti* rotameric form. Similar rotation about the corresponding C-C single bonds of the all E-isomer converts the molecule from one severely sterically hindered rotamer to an equally sterically hindered rotamer. An energy profile for the rotational isomerism in an oxodipyrromethene model for bilirubin has been calculated[72] and is shown in Figure 24. Thus, discounting possible added stabilization due to intramolecular H-bonding between the propionic acid group and the lactam ring, only the *syn* Z isomers are stable. This prediction is borne out in experimental work, which finds the E-isomers preferring a nonplanar structure with the pyrrole ring dihedral angle (ϕ, Figure 24) ca 50°[46,65,66] and being thermodynamically less stable than the Z-isomers and easily converted to them under various thermal, photochemical, and catalytic conditions, e.g., acid and iodine.[64,67,68,73-75] It would seem thus that bilirubin and many (most?) other bile pigments with unsaturation at C_4-C_5 and C_{15}-C_{16} possess the Z-configuration at those sites—in the crystal and in solution—as the thermodynamically most favored form, provided steric factors do not intervene, e.g., N-CH_3 and *meso*-CH_3.

C. Tertiary Structure

The biological and chemical consequences of the three-dimensional molecular shape

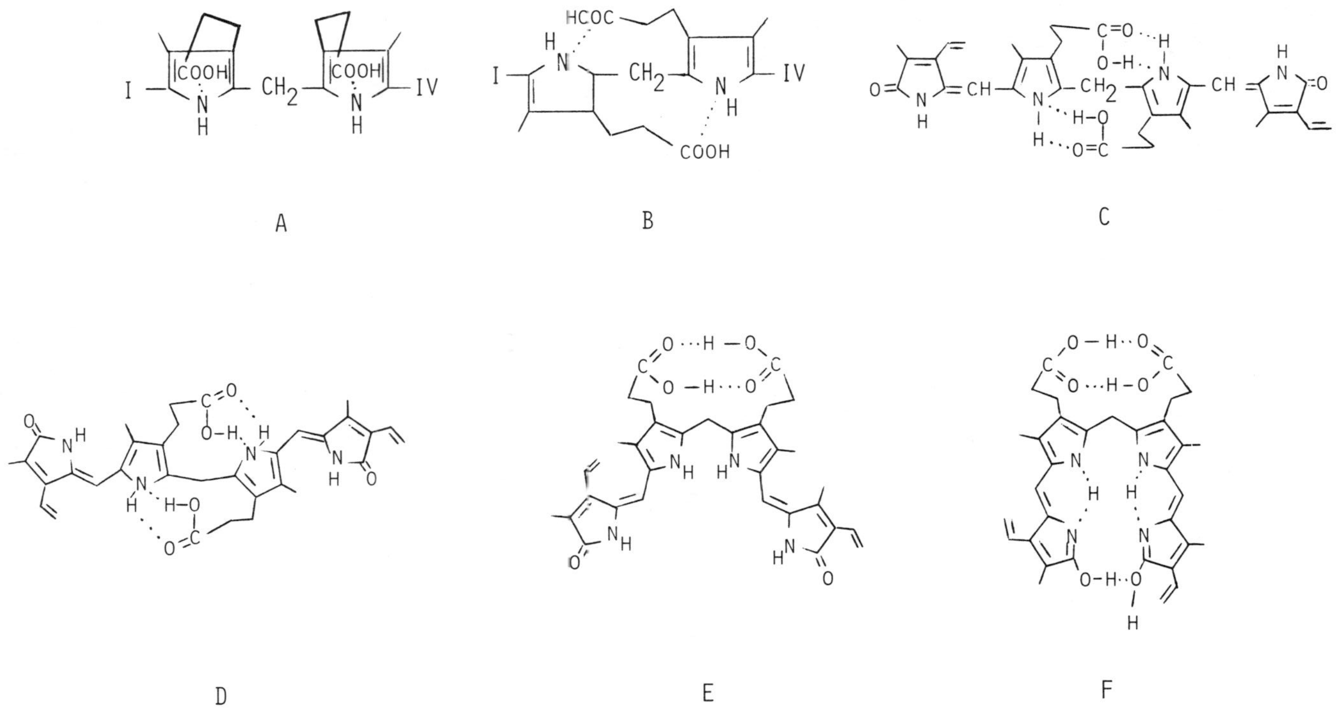

FIGURE 25. Various proposed "early" structures for bilirubin-IXα illustrating intramolecularly hydrogen-bonding. Structures A and B are due to Fog and Jellum.[56] Structure C (redrawn from B) is due to Fog et al.[57] Structures D (redrawn from B) and E are due to Brodersen et al.[49] Structure F is due to Nichol and Morell.[33]

of bilirubin have only recently been addressed. Provided that rotation about C-C single bonds at C_5-C_6, C_9-C_{10}, C_{10}-C_{11} and C_{14}-C_{15} is unhindered, bilirubin is free to assume a wide variety of different tertiary structures (Figure 22). However, as explained in the preceding section, not all rotational isomers are of equal energy, and many involve severe energy-raising steric hindrance problems. Aside from these possibilities, consideration of hydrogen bonding has proved to be of paramount importance.[73-76] Although recognized only recently, it appears to be important in understanding the solubility properties of bilirubin.

One of the more structurally intriguing and biologically significant aspects of bilirubin is its relatively greater lipophilicity as compared with the structurally related (metabolic precursor) biliverdin-IXα (see also Chapter 3). The latter has extended conjugation through both pyrromethenone "halves" by virtue of its sp^2 hydridized C-10. The former has an sp^3 hybridized carbon at C-10, but both have the Z-configurations at the C-4 and C-15 carbon-carbon double bonds. Another aspect of bilirubin chemistry is its relatively greater solution stability (toward autoxidation) than that of its dimethyl ester. To account for the latter observation and differences in the 2500 to 4000 cm^{-1} region of the infrared spectra of bilirubin, mesobilirubin, and mesobilirubin dimethyl ester, Fog and Jellum[56] suggested that intramolecular hydrogen bonding between the COOH groups and pyrrole nitrogen atoms plays an important role in stabilizing bilirubin and proposed structures A and B (Figure 25) to accommodate their hypothesis. Conformational structure A would be expected to be strained on the basis of organic structural principles and hence unlikely. B, although not particularly strained, is an improbable conformational structure in view of the relatively low basicity of the pyrrole N, i.e., the suggested H-bonds would not be expected to be very important. A redrawn version of B appears as C in Figure 25 in a subsequent manuscript by Fog and Bugge-Asperheim[57] It appears, again somewhat revised (the 4Z,15Z configuration is drawn) in D, Figure 25, in the work of Brodersen et al.,[49] who preferred it and a rather different type of H-bonded structure (E in Figure 25) as the structures of bilirubin in chloroform solution and in the solid state, respectively, on the basis of their infrared studies. Curiously, these authors[49] clearly indicate the E-configuration at the 4,5 and 15,16 carbon-carbon double bonds. In one instance (E) the *syn*-E isomer is drawn; in the other case (D) it is the *anti*-Z. The reasons for preferring the different rotamers or even E vs. Z configurations are not discussed. However, the concept of propionic acid-to-propionic acid hydrogen bonding expressed in E[49] was incorporated into yet another structure (F) by Nichol and Morell.[33] Since these authors had concluded in favor of the bislactim tautomeric structure (now known to be relatively unimportant under normal circumstances) on the basis of incomplete ^{1}H-NMR spectral data, they accomodated that structural feature in F.

Knell et al.[60,62] first proposed the strongly intramolecularly H-bonded conformation of bilirubin shown in A (Figure 26) as a structure which would explain its infrared, ^{1}H-NMR circular dichroism and ultraviolet spectra as well as its lipophilicity, reaction with diazomethane (to give lactim methyl ethers) and titration curve. Kuenzle et al.[61] simultaneously proposed the slightly less H—bonded structure B (Figure 26) and its mesomeric partial structures C-E, (Figure 26). Equally important was the recognition that structure B (Figure 26) as drawn represents but one of two enantiomeric (nonsuperimposable mirror image) structures (A and A′, Figure 27) which can be interconverted by breaking all the intramolecular H-bonds followed by rotation about the central -CH_2- group at C_{10}, and reforming the H-bonds. This profound insight proved to be prophetic for the structures of bilirubin in the crystal and is doubtless important for biological reactions of bilirubin.[76] Shortly thereafter, Chedekel and Crist[40] concluded in favor of B in DMSO on the basis of a careful ^{1}H-NMR study and suggested that bilirubin dimethyl ester should also have an intramolecularly H-bonded structure

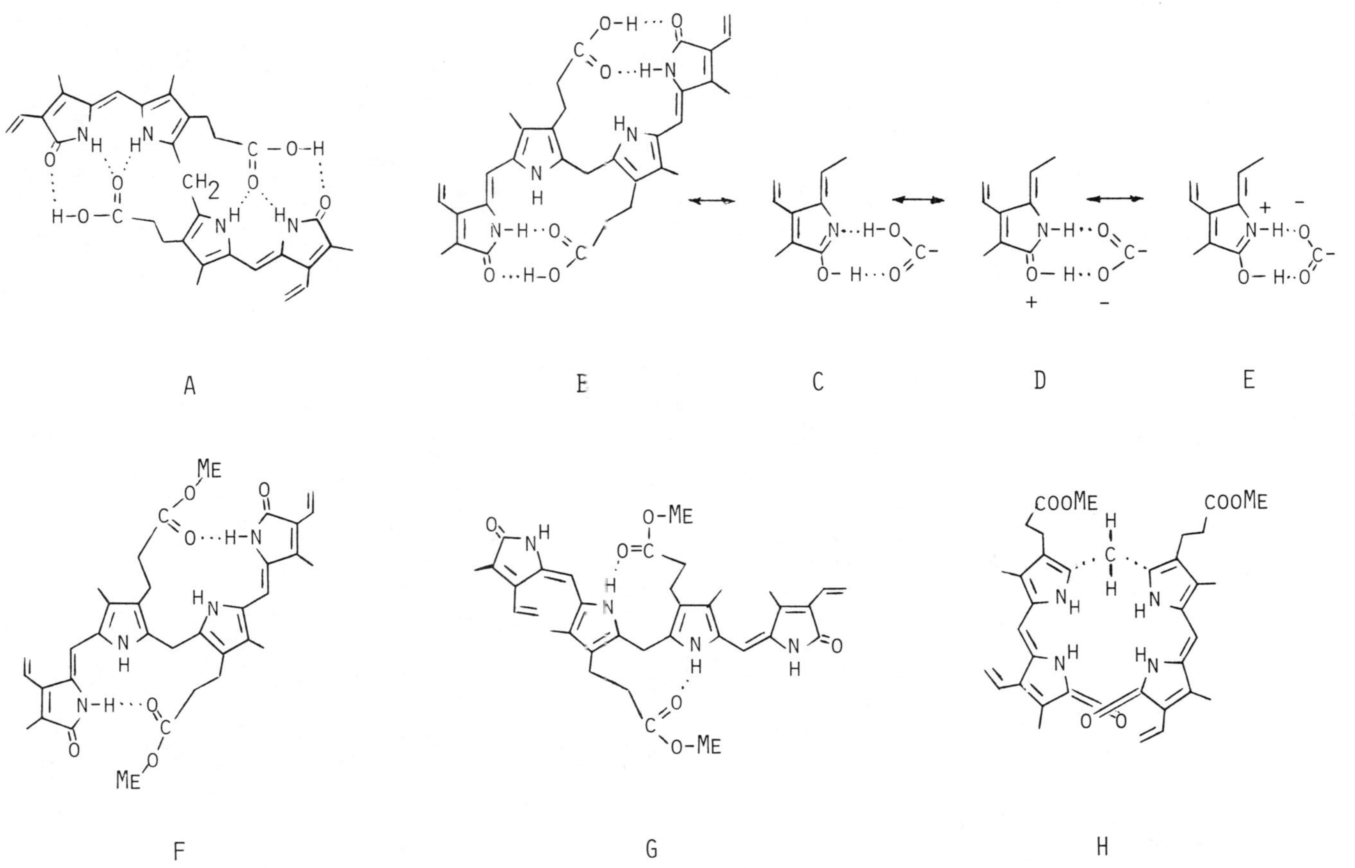

FIGURE 26. Proposed structures for intramolecularly H-bonded bilirubin-IXα. Structure A is due to Knell et al.[60,62] Kuenzle et al.[61] proposed structure B and its mesomeric partial structures C, D and E. Intramolecularly H-bonded structures of bilirubin dimethyl ester have been proposed: F(in chloroform) and G (in dimethylsufoxide) were proposed by Chedekel and Crist;[40] whereas, Manitto et al.[30] favored H in chloroform and in the solid state.

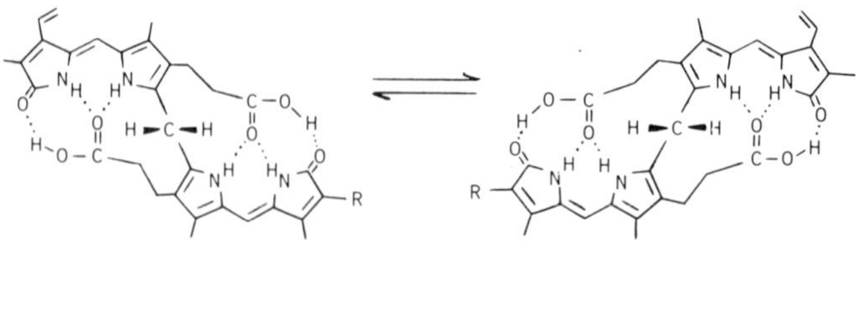

FIGURE 27. Enantiomeric (A,A′) and diastereomeric (B,B′) structures of intramolecularly H-bonded bilirubin-IXα. Interconversion (A ⇌ A′ and B ⇌ B′) involves breaking and reforming all intramolecular H-bonds.

(F Figure 26) in $CDCl_3$ and a slightly different structure (G, Figure 26) in DMSO. Curiously, the latter has the 4E,15E configuration; it is similar to B, Figure 25. Neither F nor G (of Figure 26) was preferred by Manitto et al.[30] On the basis of ¹H-NMR and infrared studies they preferred conformation H (Figure 26) for bilirubin dimethyl ester in $CHCl_3$ solution and in the solid state; conformation B (Figure 26) was preferred for bilirubin itself in $CHCl_3$ and in the solid state.

The deduction that bilirubin in the solid state assumes the intramolecularly H-bonded structure A (Figures 26 and 27) was clearly proved for crystalline bilirubin (crystallized from pyridine-ether) and is shown in Figure 28.[29] This crystallographic proof of molecular structure also confirms the correctness of the chemical structure of bilirubin assigned by Fischer.[9,23] A similarly H-bonded structure obtains for meso-bilirubin[42] and even persists in modified form in its bis-isopropyl-ammonium salt.[41] Of special additional interest is the observation that both enantiomers of bilirubin (represented by A and A′, Figure 27) can be found in the crystal[29] as adjacent "ridge-tile" shaped molecules lying in any one stack (Figure 28). The stacks interleave with similar but inverted stacks, and alternate molecules in any one stack are enantiomeric.

Whether the "ridge-tile" intramolecularly H-bonded conformation of bilirubin persists in solution is as yet incompletely resolved, although it is clearly a reasonable starting point. Evidence supporting such a conformation is educed from the ¹H-NMR studies of Manitto and Monti[77] on the thiolacetic acid adduct to the *exo*-vinyl group of BR to give B and B′ (Figure 27). The methyl groups of the -CH(Me^1)COSMe^2 moiety of B and B′ are seen in the ¹H-NMR spectrum in *dry* $CDCl_3$ at room temperature: (1) as two doublets (δ 1.48 J = 7Hz and δ 1.52 J = 7Hz) representing the diastereotopic (Me^1) groups — one from B and one from B′; and (2) as two lines (δ 2.15 and δ 2.21) representing the diastereotopic (Me^2) groups—one from B and one from B′. At slightly elevated temperatures (53 ± 3°C) the Me^1 signals coalesce into one doublet (δ 1.50, J = 7 Hz) and the Me^2 signals coalesce into a broad singlet. This corresponds to a more rapid interconversion of B and B′ on the NMR time scale. The activation energy for the B ⇌ B′ conformational inversion is determined from the coalescence temperature (53 ± 3°C) to be $\Delta G^{\neq}$ = 17.9 ± 0.5 kcal/mole[77]—the approximate energy required to break six hydrogen bonds.

D. Aggregation

The state of aggregation of bilirubin in solution is of relatively recent interest, especially in connection with understanding its aqueous insolubility near physiological pH.

Although it has been known for some time[78] that aqueous buffered solutions of

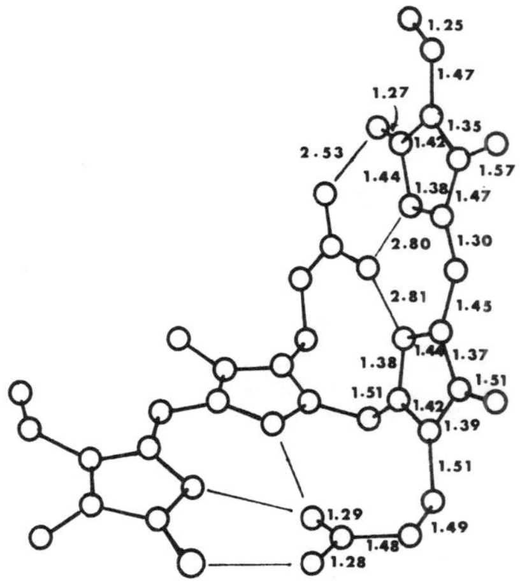

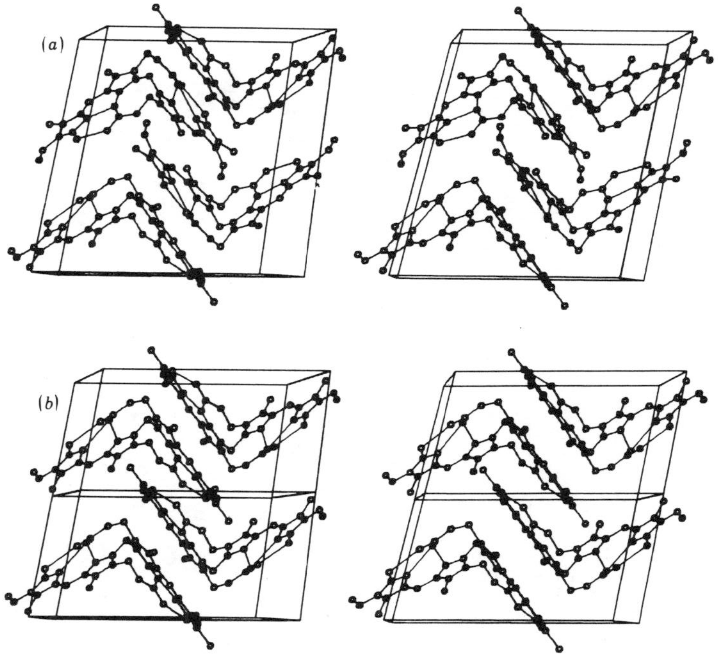

FIGURE 28. (Left) Diagram of bilirubin-IXα with bond distances (Å) determined by Bonnett et al.[29] (Right) Figure 6 of Bonnett et al.[29] (a) Bilirubin: stereoscopic view of the four molecules in the unit cell. (b) Hypothetical structure with a = 9.720 Å ($P\bar{1}$). In both diagrams, the b axis is approximately perpendicular to the page and the c axis is horizontal. (Right part reproduced with permission.)

Table 5
PARTIAL SPECIFIC VOLUMES ($\bar{v}$) AND WEIGHT-AVERAGE MOLECULAR WEIGHTS FOR BILIRUBIN-IXα IN SOLUTION (2×10^{-5} *M*)[82]

Solvent	$\bar{v}_{exp}$[a]	Mol. wt. (Da)	No. of bilirubin units
Chloroform	0.755	570.7	0.97
Tris buffer[b]	0.720	4195.4	7.17
60% EtOH	0.669	2448.9	4.18
80% EtOH	0.651	482.7	0.82

[a] T = 25.004 ± 0.004°C.
[b] pH = 8.5.

bilirubin became colloidal, there have been few, relatively recent studies of the state of aggregation of bilirubin in solution. In 1966, Brodersen[79] studied what he saw as the reversible dimerization of bilirubin in aqueous buffers, pH 7.5 to 9.0. Brodersen and Theilgaard[80] shortly thereafter observed and reported on colloidal bilirubin formation in aqueous buffer between pH 7.4 and 8. More recently Carey and Koretsky[81] observed the reversible formation of dimeric bilirubin and higher self aggregates in pH 10 aqueous buffer. The first direct measurements of the state of aggregation of bilirubin in solution were performed in our laboratories[82] using standard ultracentrifugation sedimentation equilibrium analysis.[83] Bilirubin is found to be monomeric in chloroform solution and aggregated in pH 8.5 aqueous buffer, as indicated in Table 5.

III. PHOTOCHEMISTRY

A. Electronic Excited States

The ultraviolet-visible (electronic) absorption spectrum of bilirubin-IXα in solution (Figure 29) exhibits an intense ($\varepsilon \sim 60{,}000$) absorbance in the visible centered near 450 nm with relatively little variation in the position of the long wavelength λ_{max} (Table 6) in organic solvents. Shorter wavelength maxima can also be recognized near 280 nm (and 220 nm in methanolic ammonia). Excitation with visible light, narrowly energetic at ca 450 nm, should lead, in principle, to the lowest lying excited state, one different, in principle, from those directly accessible by excitation near 300 or 220 nm. One might expect different chemical reactivity from the differing excited states. Radiative decay from the lowest lying excited state, accessible by visible (blue) light irradiation has been of considerable photophysical interest relative to the now widely used phototherapy for jaundiced newborn babies.[76,84] Although bilirubin has not been observed to phosphoresce from its lowest triplet state,[85] it fluoresces from its lowest singlet excited state under a variety of conditions.[1,53,86] Bilirubin fluoresces weakly in chloroform (Figure 30), with enhanced fluorescence in chloroform-amines, and other selected organic solvents[82] (contrary to what is commonly believed) as well as from low temperature glasses with emission near 525 nm.[1,85-88] Curiously, the fluorescence excitation spectrum of bilirubin (Figure 30) does not coincide with its absorption spectrum. One is tempted to conclude that only certain more conformationally restrained conformations of bilirubin (probably A, Figure 26) fluoresce sufficiently to be observed; whereas, conformationally mobile structures, (e.g., the non or less H-bonded structures of Figure 22) dissipate energy more efficiently by molecular motion and do not fluoresce as well or at all. The quantum yield for fluorescence is about 0.05 in 77 K glasses with a half-life of $< 5 \times 10^{-9}$ sec.[87,88]

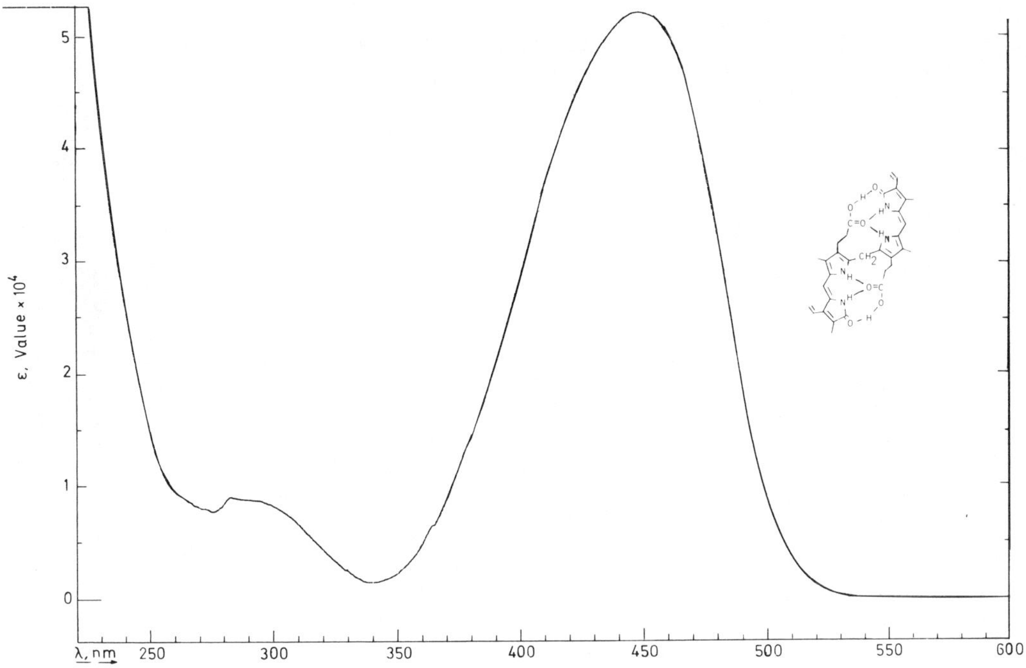

FIGURE 29. Visible-ultraviolet spectrum of bilirubin-IXα (9.0×10^{-6} *M*) in acetonitrile at 25°C. Data from W. P. Linnane, this laboratory.

The lowest lying singlet excited state of bilirubin lies ca. 63 kcal/mole (450 nm) above its ground state. The lowest lying triplet state (T_1) of bilirubin was determined to be ca. 36 kcal/mole above the ground state with a half-life in benzene of 9×10^{-6} sec.[89] Intersystem crossing from S_1 to T_1 bilirubin is small, <0.1;[89] consequently, the formation of T_1 is not readily accessible by direct irradiation.[90] Measurements of triplet state properties of bilirubin by Land[89] were achieved by direct excitation to T_1 using the pulse radiolysis technique and by anthracene-sensitized energy transfer. Recently, direct irradiation by a 347 nm ruby laser source has been reported to yield bilirubin triplets (quantum yield <0.005 in aqueous and methanolic basified solution and ca. 0.01 in benzene).[90]

B. Reactions of Excited States

1. Geometric Configurational Isomerization

Aside from the (correct) recognition by Lemberg[54,55] that bilirubin should exist most likely in the 4Z,15Z configuration rather than the commonly written 4E,15E configuration, the question of dynamic geometric isomerization about these double bonds was raised first by McDonagh et al.[91-95] and by Lightner et al.[96-97] and then only in connection with jaundice phototherapy for newborn babies. Light-mediated *cis-trans* (E-Z) isomerization about carbon-carbon double bonds is a well-studied phenomenon and it may be approached from either the E or Z isomer (Figure 31).[98] It involves: (1) absorption of a photon with the right energy, to give a π-π* excited state with planar geometry; (2) relaxation of the excited state to a lower energy metastable and C=C twisted conformation; and decay of the C=C twisted conformation either back to starting planar olefin or to geometrically isomerized planar olefin. Application of these principles (shown in Figure 31) to bilirubin should lead to a photoequilibrium mixture of the original 4Z,15Z isomer in addition to the three possible remaining configurational isomers: 4E,15Z, 4Z,15E and 4E,15E (Figure 2). The latter three isomers, taken collec-

Table 6
VISIBLE ABSORPTION SPECTRAL CHARACTERISTICS OF BILIRUBIN-IXα

Solvent	λ_{max}(nm)	ε ($M^{-1}\cdot cm^{-1}$)
Chloroform	454	60,700
Carbon tetrachloride	453	58,900
Benzene	450	60,000
Acetonitrile	448	52,000
Carbon disulfide	468	45,600
Pyridine	452	50,900
Dimethylsulfoxide	458	63,400
Methanol — NaOH, pH 8.8	450	48,000
Methanol — 1% NH_4OH	451	60,700
N,N-Dimethylformamide	449	25,300
N-Methylformamide	451	51,100
H_2O, pH 7.4 (0.1 *M* phosphate)	440	46,700
H_2O, pH 8.8 (0.1 *M* borate)	435	43,000
0.002 *M* aqueous NaOH	438	52,000
0.1 *M* NH_4OH, pH 11.0	435	46,000
0.1 *M* NaOH, pH 13.0	420	46,000
Conc. NH_4OH, pH 13.2	442	59,000
Aqueous human serum albumin, pH 7.4	460	47,000
Aqueous bovine serum albumin, pH 7.4	460	54,000

Note: Data were determined on 1-2 × 10^{-5} *M* solutions by W. P. Linnane[51] or taken from References 1 and 78.

tively, have been called photobilirubin and are obtained by direct irradiation of bilirubin with blue light in a photochemical isomerization[73-75] proceeding mainly through excited singlet states.[99,100] Ample precedent for the Z⇌E photoisomerization may be found in the structurally related oxodipyrromethenes and benzalpyrrolinones, whose Z⇌E photoisomerizations are well documented.[63-69]

As explained earlier (II.C), one of the crucially imporant biological consequences of the photochemical conversion of bilirubin to photobilirubin is altered aqueous solubility: 4Z,15Z-bilirubin is converted to the less intramolecularly H-bonded and more hydrophilic photobilirubin (4E,15Z + 4Z,15E + 4E,15E bilirubin) (Figure 32). The enhanced excretion of unconjugated bilirubin into bile during phototherapy of jaundiced babies or Gunn rats is thereby explained.[76]

2. Constitutional Isomerization[101]

Bilirubin-IXα has been observed to rearrange in solution, under a variety of catalytic conditions, to a mixture of the IIIα, IXα, and XIIIα isomers (Figure 33). Thus, short treatment (1 min) with strong acids such as HCl and *p*-toluenesulfonic acid catalyze the rapid isomerization in DMSO solvent to a nearly 1:2:1 mixture of the pIIIα:IXα:XIIIα isomers. This is an ionic reaction; with weaker acids, e.g., hot acetic acid, the reaction is slower. Isomerization can also be accomplished in aqueous pH 7.4-12 buffer by warming in the dark in the presence of oxygen. This is a free radical reaction and does not occur when oxygen is excluded. It can, however, be catalyzed by NO, I_2, or benzoylperoxide. Slow isomerization of bilirubin-IXα in *deoxygenated* pH 8.0 or 8.5 aqueous buffer is accomplished by visible light irradiation. The photochemical isomerization is solvent sensitive short-term irradiation of solutions of bilirubin-IXα in 0.1 *M* NaOH, pH 8.5 aq. bovine serum albumin, or DMSO does not lead to significant isomer formation. In chloroform solution there is a small degree of isomerization.

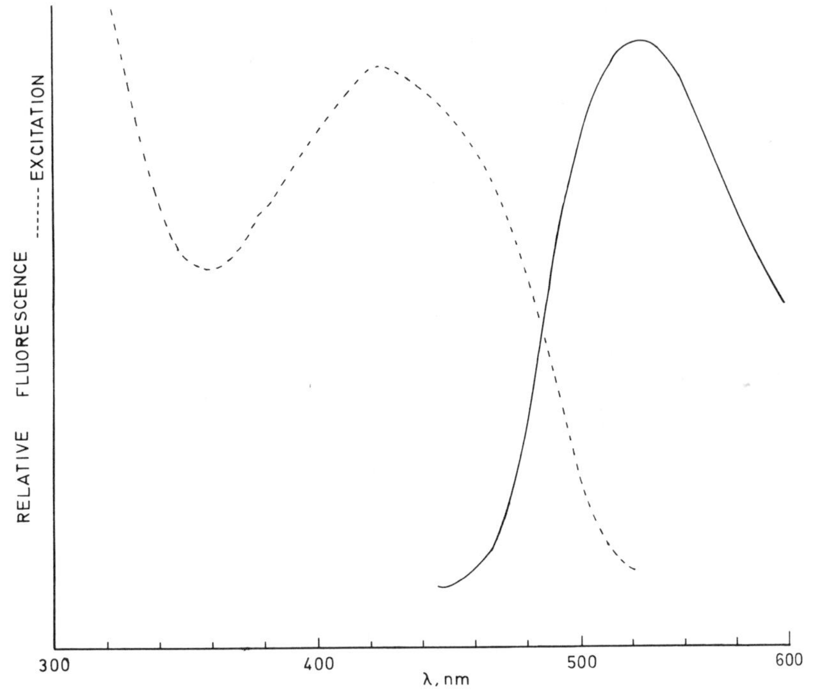

FIGURE 30. Fluorescence emission and excitation spectra of bilirubin-IXα (1.36 × 10^{-5} *M*) in chloroform at 25°C, with exciting λ = 450 nm. Data from T. A. Wooldridge and S. Wolf, this laboratory.

The constitutional isomerization is not merely the interchanging of the end ring vinyl and methyl groups, since neither the symmetrical IIIα or XIIIα isomers alone responds to the isomerization conditions. It is, rather, the exchange of "halves" of bilirubin molecules, and it is concentration dependent. Thus, even a mixture of the IIIα and XIIIα isomers can be isomerized to give some IXα isomer. The reaction must involve breaking and re-forming the 9-10 and/or 10-11 carbon-carbon bonds. Thus, two IXα isomers are capable of providing one IIIα and one XIIIα (and vice-versa), and the statistical equilibrium should be 1:2:1 of IIIα:IXα:XIIIα, barring differing rates of decomposition (to other products) under the reaction conditions. The acid-catalyzed and free-radical reaction mechanisms appear to involve attack by an electrophile or radical at C-9 or C-10 as outlined in Figures 34 and 35 respectively. The photochemical mechanism is less clear but probably involves ion-radical reactions (Type I) with C-C bond dissociation-recombination in a bilirubin aggregate as illustrated in Figure 36. It must be stressed that the available evidence for this photochemical constitutional isomerization indicates it to be a slow reaction and one requiring anaerobic conditions. Anaerobic conditions are required presumably because oxygen quenches the proposed intermediate bilirubin ion-radical, as has been noted previously.[99,102] In view of these reaction characteristics, photochemical constitutional isomerization would appear to have no important role in jaundice phototherapy, as has been stated.[101]

3. Photoaddition to Vinyl Groups

Photoirradiation of bilirubin-IXα in the presence of alcohols or thiols results in slow formation of Markownikov adducts to the *exo*-vinyl group only.[1] Thus, for example, 30 hr of irradiation of a O_2-free, Ar-blanketed solution of bilirubin in chloroform-10% methanol with a 125 W high pressure Hg lamp led to a 20% yield of methanol adduct,[103,104] as shown in Figure 37. Sulfhydryl-groups add more rapidly. Thiols and

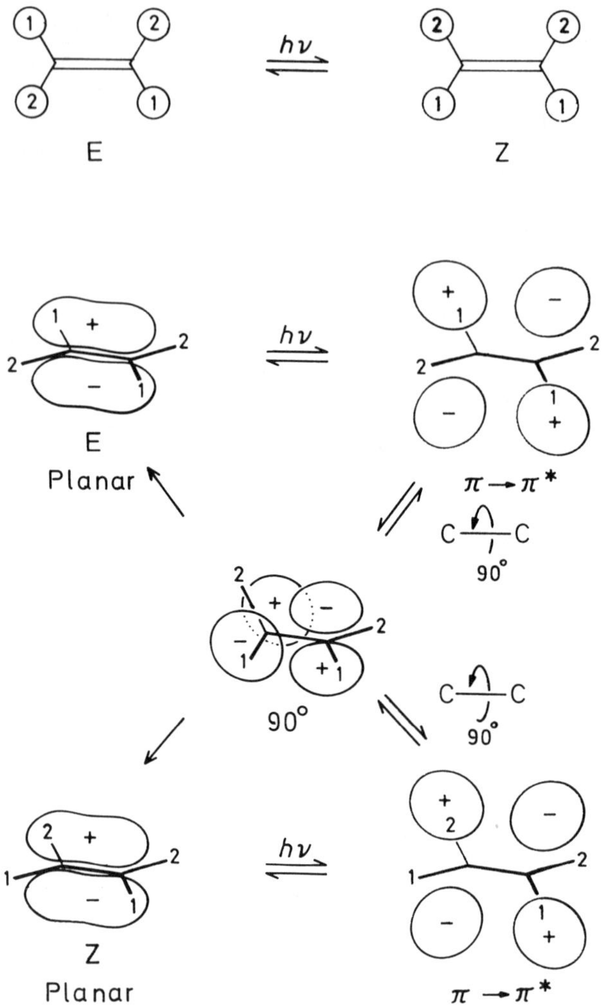

FIGURE 31. (Upper) Diagrammatic representation for E ⇌ Z carbon-carbon double bond isomerization. The E isomer is determined by its having two higher priority atoms (or groups), labeled (1), on opposite sides (entgegen, *trans*). The Z-isomer is determined by its having the two higher priority groups on the same side (zusammen, *cis*-). (Lower) Diagrammatic orbital representation for photochemical breaking of the olefinic π-bond, first by excitation to a π-π* excited state (antibonding π orbital), then rotation about the carbon-carbon single bond to give a 90° twisted intermediate. The intermediate can collapse by rotation to starting planar olefin or to the planar isomer.

alcohols can also be added in Markownikov fashion under acid-catalyzed conditions.[103,105] Whether the photochemical addition results from a spurious acid-catalyzed process from trace amounts of acid formed during photoirradiation,[101] or whether a reactive form of bilirubin is produced[103] is still uncertain. As a simple photoaddition, the regiospecific reaction is not easy to rationalize.

4. Photooxidation and Singlet Oxygen

Photooxidation reactions of bilirubin proceed through an electronically excited state, either the singlet, $S_1(BR)$ or the triplet, $T_1(BR)$. Absorption of light, e.g., at 450

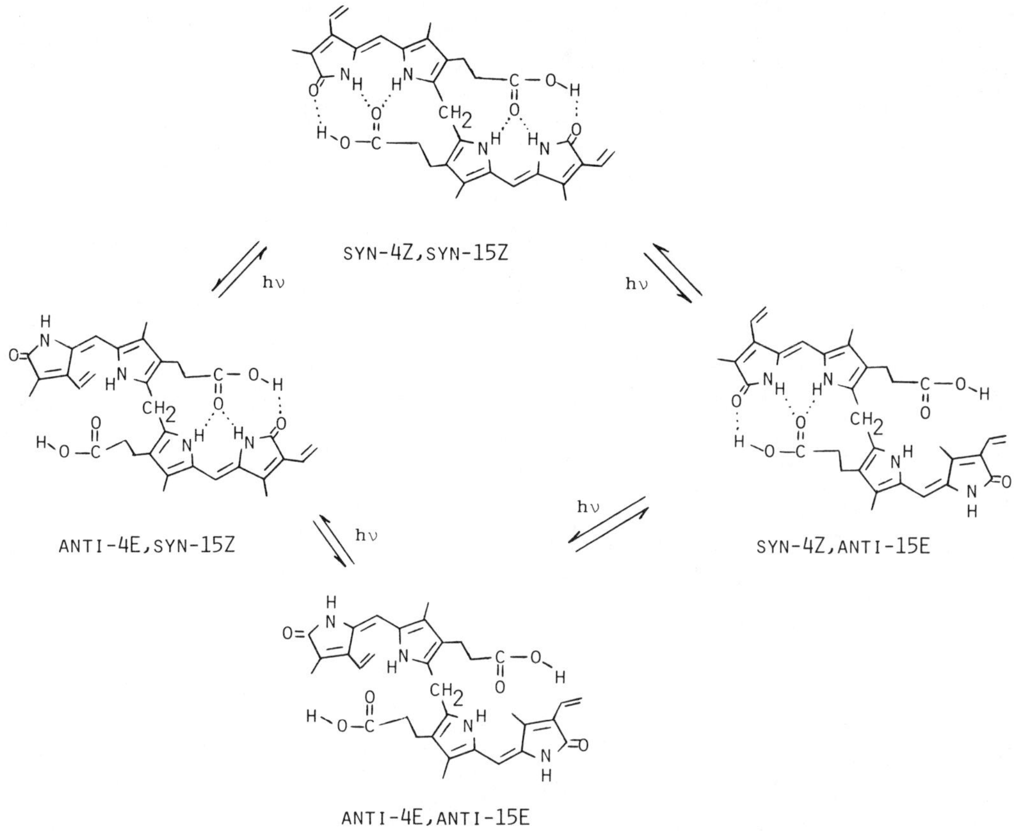

FIGURE 32. Photochemical reaction cycle for bilirubin-IXα depicting Z $\rightleftharpoons$ E isomerization and concomitant disruption (or formation) of intramolecular H-bonds. Photobilirubin is a mixture of the 4Z,15E; 4E,15Z and 4E,15E isomers.

nm, promotes a ground state, S_0(BR), electron to a higher energy orbital without change of spin; consequently, the first excited state, S_1(BR) is a singlet in which there are no unpaired spins, but one with two singly occupied orbitals. Under the proper conditions, a nonspin-paired electron of the excited singlet, S_1(BR), may undergo spin inversion to give the triplet state, T_1(BR), which has two unpaired spins and two singly occupied orbitals. The single electron found in the high energy orbital of S_1(BR) and T_1(BR) is less strongly bound, hence more easily removed by oxidizing agents than in S_0(BR). Moreover, the "hole" left in the formerly doubly occupied orbital of S_0(BR) when the electron was promoted is in an orbital which would be expected to bond electrons comparatively strongly, with the effect that both S_1(BR) and T_1(BR) would be more readily reduced than S_0(BR). Consequently, excited states are expected to be both oxidized and reduced more easily than the ground state. Oxidizing behavior is particularly common, and with only a few exceptions photosensitized oxidations proceed via the longer lived triplet excited state.[106]

Properties of the bilirubin excited states are summarized in Figure 38. The extremely short-lived singlet excited state would not be expected to participate as effectively in bimolecular reactions as the longer-lived (but curiously much shorter-lived than most triplets) triplet excited state, T_1(BR). However, in reactions requiring long periods of photoirradiation, e.g., those described in Sections III.B.2, III.B.3, and III.B.5., S_1(BR) may be implicated.

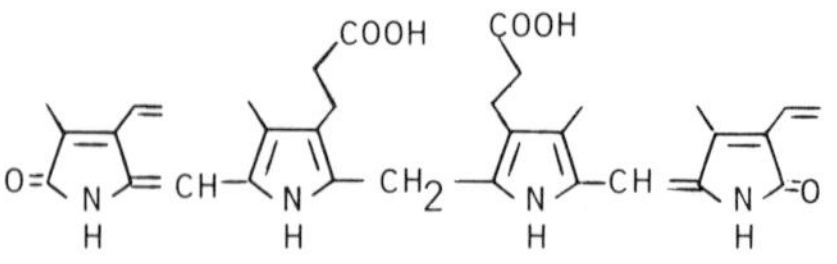

BILIRUBIN-IXα

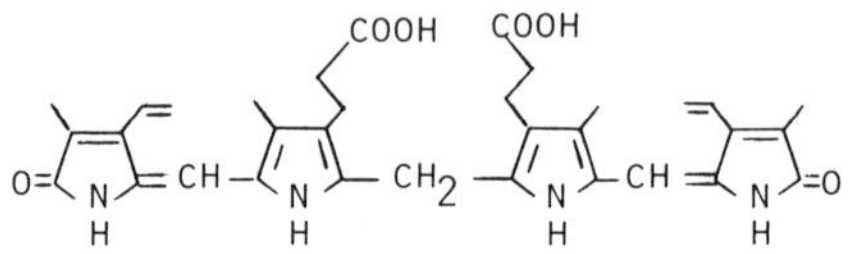

BILIRUBIN-XIIIα

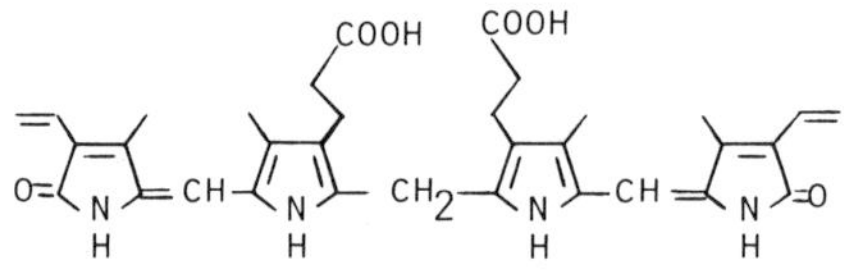

BILIRUBIN-IIIα

FIGURE 33. Constitutional isomers of bilirubin obtained by acid-catalyzed, radical-catalyzed or photochemical processes on bilirubin-IXα. The IIIα and XIIIα isomers have a symmetric ordering of the pyrrole β-substituents.

Photooxidation reactions of bilirubin may go through S_1(BR) or through T_1(BR). The latter fall into two broad mechanistic classes: Type I or Type II[106] (Figure 39). Singlet and Type I photooxidations of bilirubin would involve interaction of excited bilirubin with another molecule (A or X) directly, usually with electron or hydrogen atom transfer, to give bilirubin radical ions ($BR^{+\cdot}$) or radicals ($BRH^{\cdot}$) which might undergo the reactions illustrated in Figure 39. Type II photooxidation of bilirubin (Figure 39) involves quenching of T_1(BR) to give singlet excited oxygen [$^1O_2$] and ground state bilirubin, S_0(BR). In view of its poor intersystem crossing quantum yield ($\Phi < 0.1$) and short T_1(BR) lifetime, bilirubin is expected to be an inefficient sensitizer for $^1O_2$, and this is observed.[1,107] Type I photooxidation of bilirubin is probably the mechanism followed in the self-sensitized formation of biliverdin, especially since the yields of biliverdin are considerably enhanced in aprotic and deoxygenated solvents, and the reaction is promoted by radical quenchers or electron-transfer acceptors.[102,107] It may well turn out that most self-sensitized photooxidation reactions of bilirubin

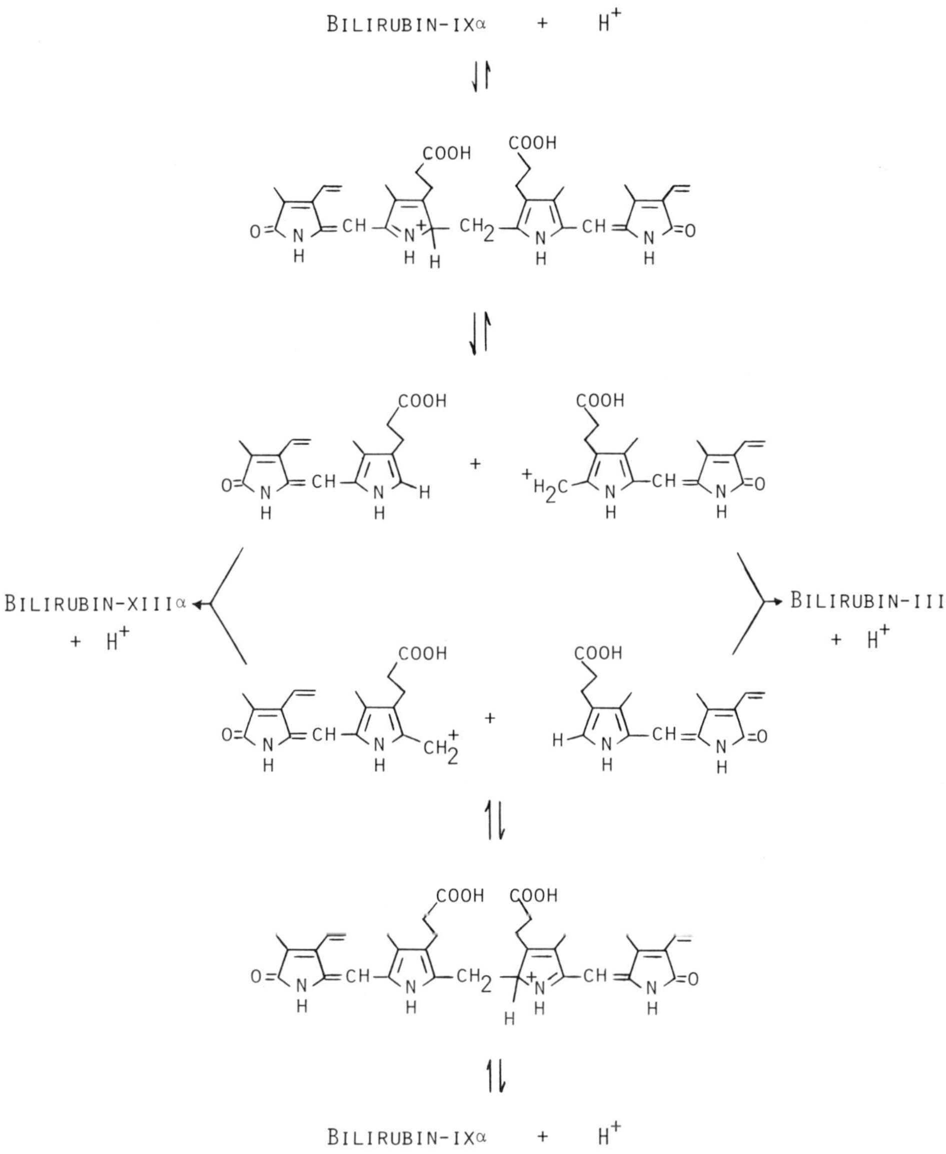

FIGURE 34. Reaction mechanisms for the acid-catalyzed constitutional isomerization of bilirubin-IXα to the IIIα and XIIIα isomers.

follow singlet or a Type I mechanism, *including even self-sensitized photooxygenation,*[108] which has generally been ascribed to a Type II $^1O_2$ mechanism.[107] For example, in Figure 39, Type I, when X is ordinary (triplet) oxygen (X = $^3O_2$), formation of reactive superoxide ion ($O_2^{-\cdot}$) by electron transfer from T_1(BR) is possible, and the course of reaction of the superoxide ion-bilirubin radical ion pair [$BR^{+\cdot}$ $O_2^{-\cdot}$] could well lead to the same products as reaction of $^1O_2$ with bilirubin[107] either directly or indirectly by the radical ion-pair (see under Type II, Figure 39).[68,100,107-110] To distinguish between the various types of photooxygenation mechanisms is very difficult, especially because [$BR^{+\cdot}$ − $O_2^{-\cdot}$] is expected to give $^1O_2$-type products, and the various kinetic and competitive quenching reactions do not allow for facile distinction between $^1O_2$ as a reactant vs. $O_2^{-\cdot}$.[110] Bilirubin is known to react chemically with $^1O_2$ but at a rate k_R = 0.1 − 0.4 × 10^9 $M^{-1}s^{-1}$) which is approximately an order of magnitude less

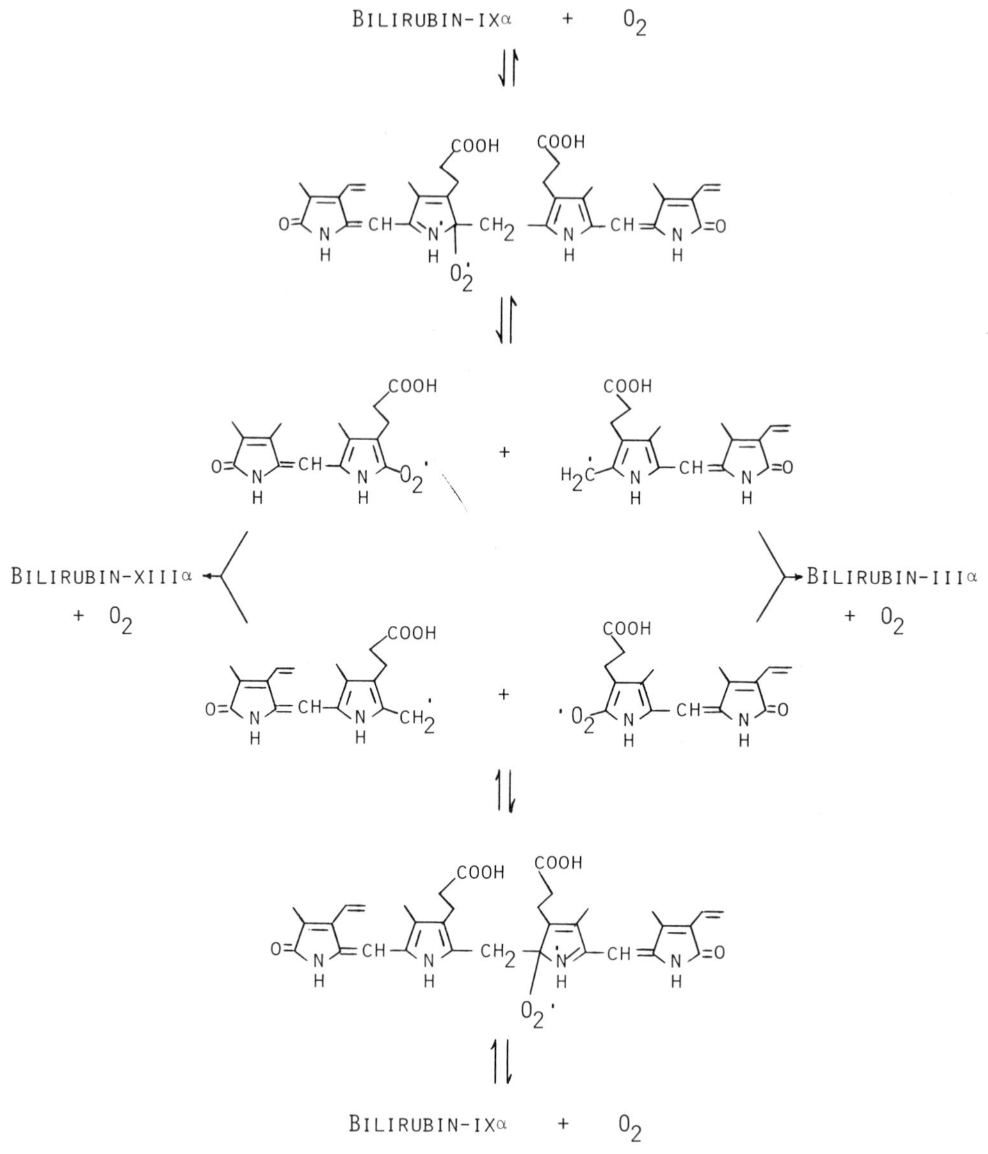

FIGURE 35. Reaction mechanism for the free radical (O_2) catalyzed isomerization of bilirubin-IX*α* to the XIII*α* and III*α* isomers.

than the quenching rate ($k_Q = 2.1 - 2.8 \times 10^9\ M^{-1}s^{-1}$).[110] Since the $^1O_2$ quenching reaction probably involves electron transfer (see under Type II, Figure 39), radical ion pair [$BR^{+\cdot} - O_2^{-\cdot}$] formation is probably the first process with [$BR^{+\cdot} - O_2^{-\cdot}$] partitioning into the chemically reactive (k_R) and physically quenching (k_Q) pathways. In view of this evidence, spin-trapping data[108] and comparative ion-radical reactions in other systems,[111] we favor an electron transfer component in both the self-sensitized and the dye-sensitized photooxygenation reactions of bilirubin. Whether $^1O_2$ is formed at all, or to what extent it participates in the self-sensitized photooxygenation of bilirubin has not been unequivocally ascertained, for the various procedures employed in recognizing $^1O_2$, e.g., competitive reaction, quenching[112,113] and rate effects in deuterated solvents[113] respond in a similar way to $O_2^{-\cdot}$ and thus cannot be used to exclude its intermediacy.[111]

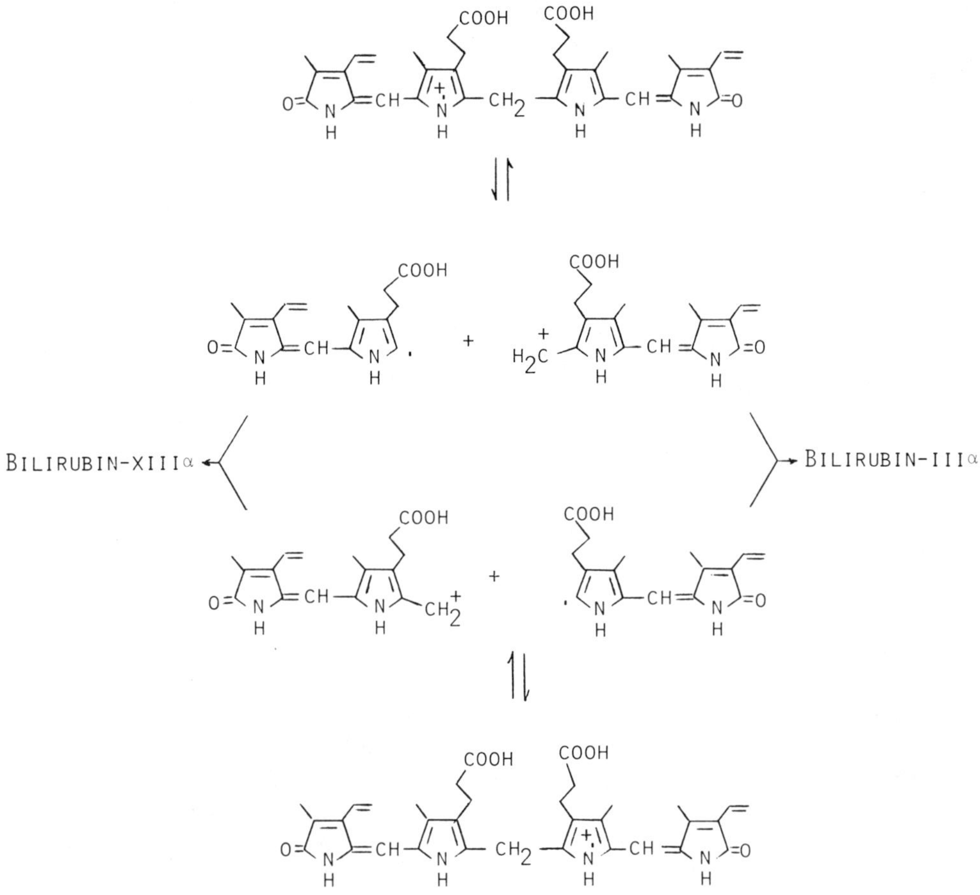

FIGURE 36. Reaction mechanism for the photochemical route (via radical cations) for isomerization of bilirubin-IXα to the IIIα and XIIIα isomers.

If the photooxygenation reaction mechanism is in doubt, the structures of the reaction products are more clearly established and have been reviewed by Lightner.[107] The product distribution and type vary somewhat from protic (methanolic or ethanolic ammonia or aqueous ammonia) to aprotic (chloroform) solvents. Bilirubin photodecomposition products found in protic solvents include biliverdin-IXα[1,107,114] (Figure 12), methylvinylmaleimide[1,107,115-120] (Figures 9 and 40), hematinic acid imide[1,107,117-119] (Figures 9 and 40), the acyclic hydrolysis products[119] of the cyclic imides (Figure 40), the dipyrrole dialdehyde[1,107,115,116,118] (Figure 40), and various propentdyopents[1,107,115-119] (Figure 40). Of these products, the major type is the propentdyopent which accounts for 60% (by weight) of the total photoproducts.[107,115] However, only three of the propentdyopents (Figure 40) are actually isolated since a sterically hindered isomer (not shown) rearranges to the left-hand structure of Figure 40 under the reaction conditions.

In chloroform, a different set of bilirubin photooxygenation products is thought to arise. In one case, various monopyrrole and dipyrrole compounds have been detected by paper chromatography following exposure of a chloroform solution of bilirubin to air and diffuse daylight for up to 500 days (!) at room temperature.[121] In that work and earlier work[114,122] it was deduced that biliverdin is also a photooxidation product from bilirubin. Subsequently, Lightner et al.[123] isolated biliverdin (as its dimethyl ester) in high yield, and Bonnett and Stewart[124] detected biliverdin, its dimethyl ester and

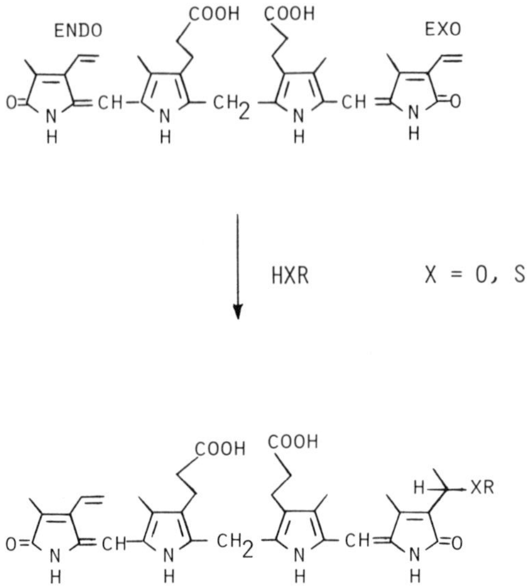

FIGURE 37. Scheme showing *exo* vs. *endo* vinyl group regioselective addition (acid-catalyzed or photochemical) of alcohols and thiols to bilirubin-IXα.

two other minor verdins by TLC. The yield of biliverdin appears to increase with increasing bilirubin concentration in methanolic ammonia or chloroform.

Bilirubin has been photooxidized in a wide variety of solvents with apparently differing rates.[1,107] The product type and distribution are also solvent-dependent. Thus, propentdyopents are formed in relatively greater amounts in protic solvents than in aprotic solvents, whereas, the reverse is true for biliverdin formation. The more widely studied conditions involve broad spectrum visible light or sunlight and aerated solvents such as chloroform, methanolic ammonia, aqueous ammonia and pH 7.2-9.0 buffers, with or without added albumin. However, McDonagh[1] has also examined the photoreactivity of bilirubin-IXα in pyridine, benzene, DMSO, in pH 7.4 aqueous Triton® X-100, in pH 7.4 aqueous cetyl trimethylammonium bromide, in liposome suspensions of lecithin, in 2% gelatin, and even adsorbed on silica gel, polyamide, or fabrics. Under all of these aerobic conditions, photobleaching is the major fate. Bilirubin photooxidation is also influenced by additives to aqueous, buffered solutions. In connection with its effect on bilirubin photochemistry, the most widely studied additive is albumin, which binds bilirubin. Most authors generally agree that albumin-bound bilirubin undergoes photooxidation at a slower rate than unbound bilirubin.[1,107] Albumin has been shown to be important in inhibiting bilirubin IX$\alpha \rightleftharpoons$ XIII$\alpha \rightleftharpoons$ IIIα isomerization, and it is apparently important in bilirubin photochemistry leading to the "443", "420", or other pigment(s).

Some work has been done on the influence of wavelength and radiant energy flux on bilirubin photoreactivity in buffered albumin solutions and in plasma.[125] As might be anticipated, the most effective wavelengths of visible light are those in the vicinity of the intense absorption band of bilirubin near 450 nm. Lightner and Cu[102] have examined bilirubin photoreactivity in the presence and absence of oxygen at 280, 340, or 440 nm excitation wavelengths in chloroform and methanolic ammonia solvents. Bilirubin undergoes photobleaching most rapidly with 280 nm light in either solvent.

To account for the stepwise formation of the bilirubin photoproducts, methylvinylmaleimide and the dipyrroledialdehyde may be viewed as originating from an unstable intermediate 1,2-adduct of $^1O_2$ or $O_2^{-\cdot}$ such as the dioxetane[1,107,116,119] (Figure 41), as

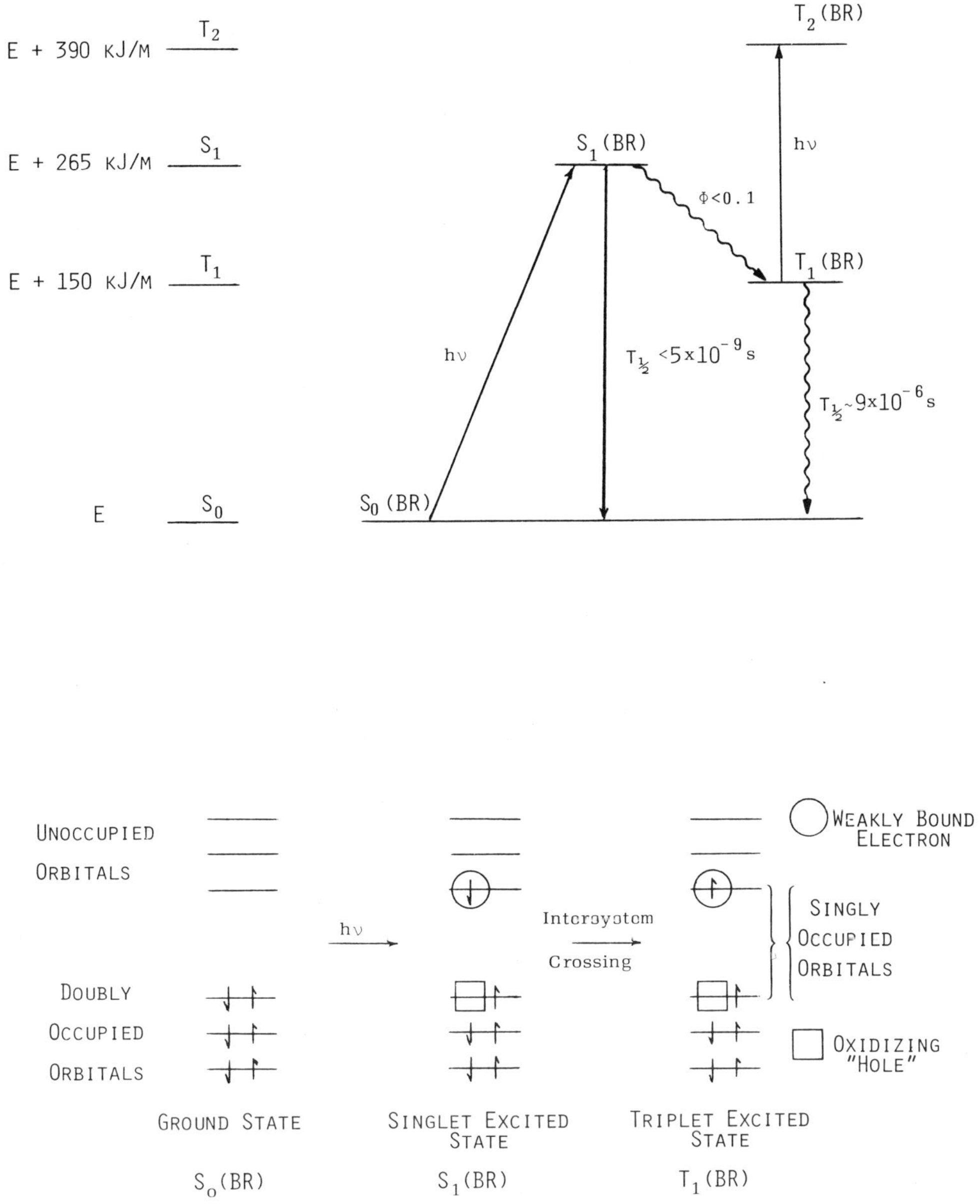

FIGURE 38. (Upper) Photochemical reaction cycle for electronic excitation of ground state bilirubin-IXα [S_o(BR)] to its first excited singlet [S_1(BR)], which can decay to S_o(BR) with fluorescence or undergo intersystem crossing to the lowest lying triplet excited state [T_1(BR)]. T_1(BR) can be excited to T_2(BR) and it can decay back to the ground state [S_o (BR)] by nonradiative intersystem crossing as shown or by phosphorescence (not shown). Phosphorescence of T_1(BR) has not been detected, but the half-life of T_1(BR) is ∿ 9 us. The data are taken from Land[89] and Bonnett et al.[85] (Lower) Schematic diagram illustrating electron excitation in bilirubin and oxidizing and reducing properties of the excited states, according to Foote, page 21 in the book of Ref. 119.

predicted by McDonagh.[112] Hematinic acid imide and the propentdyopents can similarly be seen as originating from an unstable intermediate ($^1O_2$ or $O_2^{-\cdot}$) adduct,[1,107] such as the *endo*peroxide (Figure 41) as predicted by Bonnett[115,116,124] and Lightner[118,119] based on the observed photooxygenation of monopyrroles by Lightner et al.[126,127] Neither of the postulated intermediates have yet been observed directly; however, NMR evidence has confirmed the existence of pyrrole *endo*peroxides.[127]

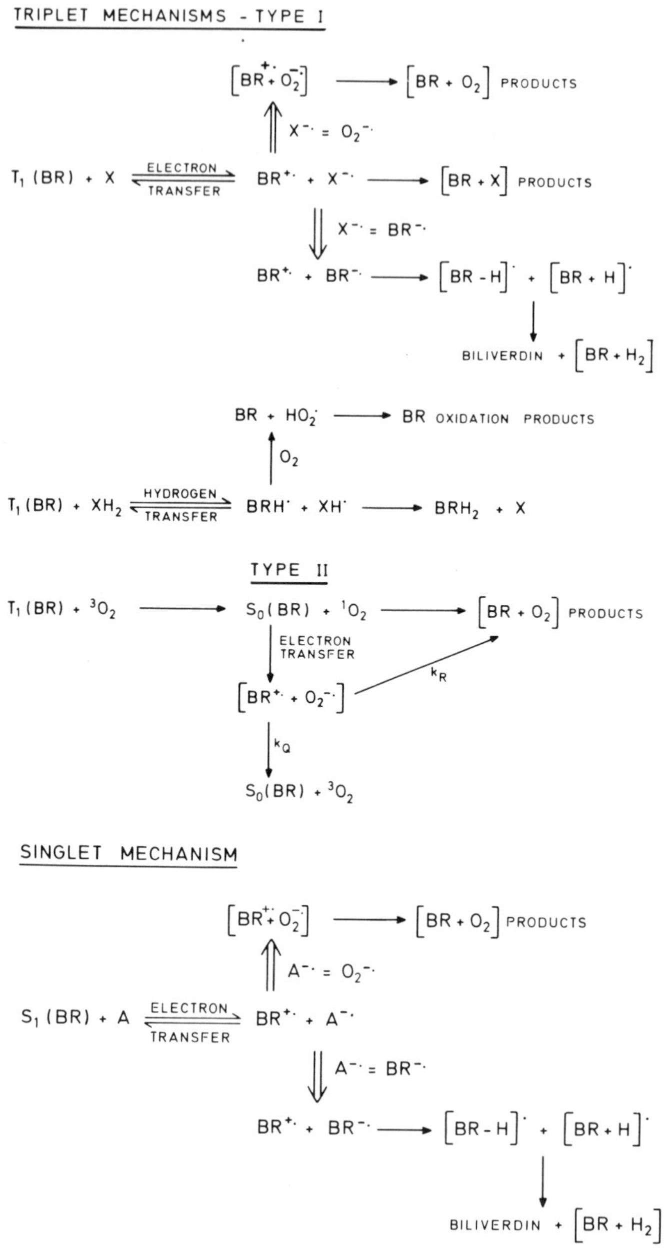

FIGURE 39. Reaction schemes for the fate of singlet excited [S_1(BR)] and triplet [T_1(BR)] excited bilirubin, involving electron transfer, hydrogen transfer and energy transfer photooxidation mechanisms.

5. Other Photochemical Reactions

Photoirradiation of bilirubin in oxygenated aqueous albumin solutions leads to alteration of the protein with destruction of histidyl residues in addition to a slowed photodestruction of bilirubin[1,128,129] and covalent binding of bilirubin to albumin.[130] In the absence of oxygen, visible light irradiation of aqueous bilirubin-albumin solutions leads to the formation of small amounts of a new pigment(s) absorbing at 443 nm[92,131] and 430 nm.[132,133]

McDonagh[92,131] has found that irradiation (400 Watt high-pressure Hg with UV filter) of anaerobic 43 μM bilirubin-IXα solutions in pH 7.4 or 8.5 buffer, aqueous al-

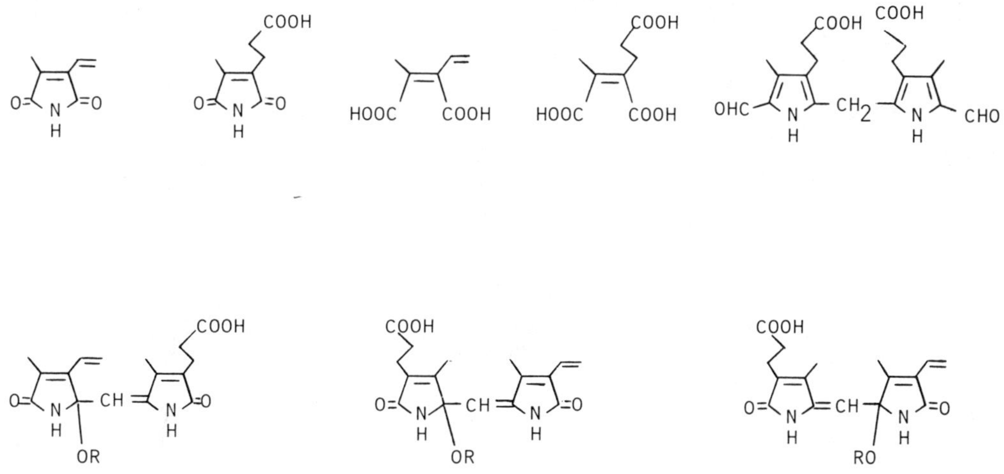

FIGURE 40. Photodegradation (via photooxidation) products of bilirubin-IXα. The upper line of products supposedly obtains from a dioxetane intermediate. The lower line of propentdyopent products apparently arises from an endoperoxide intermediate (Figure 41). The 11,14-endoperoxide shown in Figure 41 would be expected to give the right-most propentdyopent structure, which can undergo allylic rearrangement to the middle structure. The propentdyopent expected to arise from bilirubin-IXα 6,9-endoperoxide is not isolated, only the allylically rearranged structure is found.[102] R = alkyl or hydrogen.

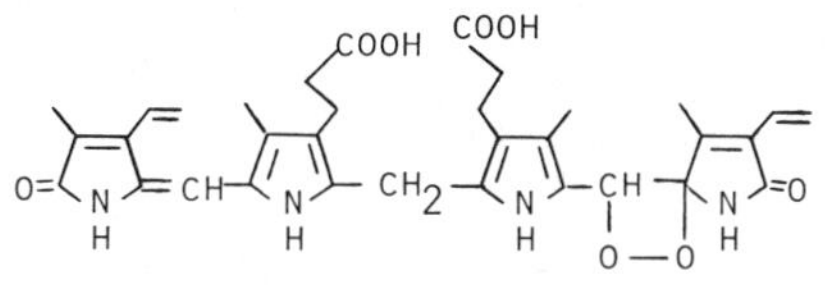

BILIRUBIN-IXα 15,16-DIOXETANE

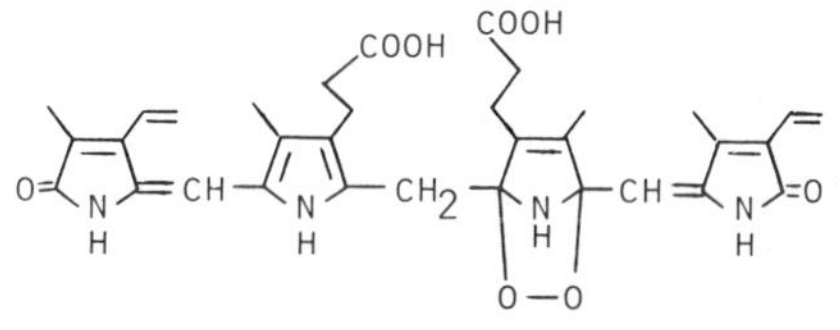

BILIRUBIN-IXα 11,14-ENDOPEROXIDE

FIGURE 41. Bilirubin-dioxetane (upper) and bilirubin-endoperoxide (lower), supposed intermediates in the photooxidation of bilirubin-IXα to the products listed in Figure 40.

bumin, or rat serum leads to a low yield (13% under optimal conditions) of a new pigment (compound X) with an absorption maximum at 442 to 444 nm (in chloroform). Kapitulnik et al.[131,132] isolated a new pigment with an absorption maximum at 430 to 435 nm (veronal buffer) following illuminations of bilirubin-albumin solutions. The two pigments may be the same compound.[92] When the reaction is investigated carefully compound X as well as two other new pigments (compounds Y and Z) having

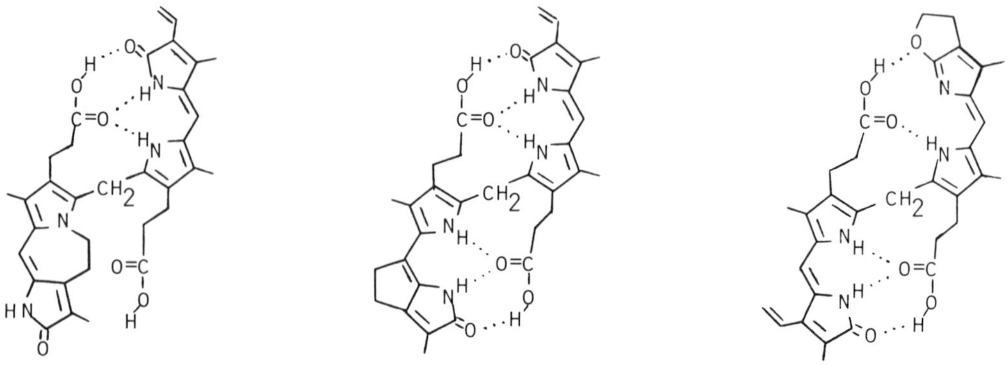

FIGURE 42. Possible structures for Compounds X, Y, and Z without reference to order. Where Z isomers are drawn, E isomers might obtain as well. The left structure is a variation on the intramolecular vinyl group addition found in photolysis of pterobiline and biliverdin-IX.[152] The middle structure is a variation of the acid-catalyzed intramolecular cyclization involving a vinyl group of bacteriochlorophylls c.[153] The right-most structure is an H-bonded variation of the old Fischer structure for bilirubin.[6] It was proposed as a photoproduct of bilirubin[136] and was considered by Ostrow et al.[135]

similar visible absorption characteristics can be found.[134] They appear to have the same molecular weight (584 amu) as bilirubin, as determined by field desorption mass spectrometry. Possible structures for X,Y, and Z are shown in Figure 42.

Anaerobic irradiation of 2.5×10^{-4} *M* bilirubin in DMSO with an unfiltered 100 W high pressure Hg lamp gave two new pigments, called stable photobilirubin IIA and IIB, in <3% total yield.[135] These are alleged to be different conformers of 4E,15E-bilirubin-IXα.[135] However, in view of their stability, that is scarcely possible. They are, in fact, identical to compounds Y and Z[134] (Figure 42) isolated following anaerobic photoirradiation of aqueous albumin-bilirubin solutions. Irradiation of bilirubin in dimethylformamide solution with blue fluorescent light is argued to give an even different pigment (Figure 42),[136] whose structure is that proposed originally by Fischer for bilirubin-IXα.

C. Phototherapy

Newborn babies develop hyperbilirubinemia, and often jaundice, because the hepatic system for conjugating and excreting bilirubin is functionally immature at birth and shortly afterward.[138] Consequently neurotoxic bilirubin accumulates in the circulation and extravascular tissues until the excretory apparatus becomes fully functional, which usually occurs within the first postnatal week. Neonatal jaundice may lead to retarded motor development, cerebral palsy, or death; thus, some form of treatment is in order. Each year thousands of newborn babies with neonatal jaundice are treated with phototherapy, i.e., prolonged irradiation with bright blue or white light.[76] This is done to prevent brain damage caused by the cytotoxic yellow metabolite bilirubin. Phototherapy works because it reduces the concentration of bilirubin in the circulation and diminishes the risk that the pigment will diffuse into the brain where it can exert its toxic effect. How phototherapy works was not at all clear.[76] A widely held notion was that light therapy causes photooxidation or photodegradation of bilirubin to other compounds that are easily excreted.[138] But, in fact, there is no reliable, convincing scientific evidence to back up this view.

The key observation, made originally by Ostrow,[139,140] is that phototherapy appears to stimulate excretion of unconjugated bilirubin by the liver into bile. This observation is particularly intriguing because normally bilirubin cannot be excreted significantly by the liver unless it is first metabolized to so-named conjugates with glucuronic acid and other sugars[137] (see Chapter 2, and Chapter 3, Volume II). The most consistent

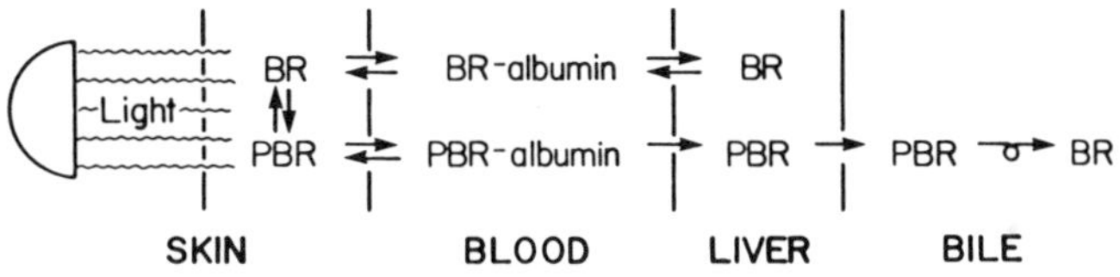

FIGURE 43. Figure 6 of McDonagh et al.[76] The mechanism of bilirubin excretion during phototherapy of neonatal jaundice. (BR, 4Z,15Z-bilirubin-IXα; PBR, photobilirubin). (From McDonagh, A. F., Palma, L. A., and Lightner, D. A., *Science,* 208, 145, 1980. With permission.)

and well-documented rationale for how light therapy induces excretion of unconjugated bilirubin by the liver has been provided by McDonagh et al.[76] in their work with Gunn rats. The mechanism involves light-induced conversion of bilirubin to unstable intermediates (photobilirubin, Figure 32) that can be excreted by the liver into bile and that can subsequently revert to natural bilirubin. Photobilirubin was detected and identified spectroscopically in the serum of photoirradiated Gunn rats and was also shown to be excreted rapidly from their liver into bile.[76] Formation and excretion of photobilirubin is now believed to be the major mechanism of phototherapy[76,84,142] (Figure 43); however, there is also evidence for bilirubin (photo)oxidation products appearing in bile and urine.[139]

The biological importance of the Z→E photoisomerization of 4Z,15Z-bilirubin to photobilirubin (mixture of 4Z,15E, 4E,15Z and 4E,15E-bilirubin) was first expressed by McDonagh as early as 1974.[91,92] The photoisomerization rationale for phototherapy, stated by McDonagh et al.[91-95] and Lightner et al.,[96,97,107] emerged during a period when it was widely believed that photooxidation was an important mechanism. The idea had clearly occurred independently to others.[29,128] It was at first rejected by Ostrow,[141] then subsequently advanced by Ostrow et al.[84,135] as well as Brodersen et al.[128,142] The source of confusion regarding priorities for the rationale might originate in the chemical term, photoisomerization, which had been used even earlier in connection with the light-induced constitutional isomerization of bilirubin-IXα to a mixture of the IIIα, IXα, and XIIIα isomers (see Section III.B.2).[101] However, the term photoisomerization is a general one and applies equally well to other light-induced isomerizations, e.g., geometric or configurational, and that is the sense as first conveyed by McDonagh, either implicitly[91,95] or explicitly[92,93] and explicitly by Lightner.[96,97,133]

The notion that bilirubin undergoes Z → E photoisomerization to more polar isomers (photobilirubin) was invoked by Pedersen et al.[128] to explain the detection of minute amounts of a new pigment following blue light irradiation of aqueous bilirubin-albumin solutions under anaerobic conditions. The evidence is insufficient to conclude that the new pigment is photobilirubin,[73-76] although it is likely. Ostrow et al.[143,144] also incorporated the notion of Z → E isomerization in showing that three new pigments[143] of a yellow, polar photoproduct,[144] all isolated following anaerobic photoirradiation of bilirubin in chloroform with intense visible light, could be excreted into Gunn rat bile. Details of the work were reported,[135] subsequent to the first reports of photobilirubin,[73-75] which explain that only two photoproducts are obtained following anaerobic irradiation of 1.7×10^{-4} *M* bilirubin in chloroform for > 3 hr with unfiltered light from a 100 W high-pressure Hg lamp. Those products were assigned as 4E,15Z- and 4Z,15E-bilirubin-IXα. Similar irradiation of 2.5×10^{-4} *M* bilirubin in DMSO for 5 hr gave two new but different and even more stable pigments. Their structures were assigned as two rotamers (*anti*-4E, *syn*-15E and *syn*-4E, *anti*-15E, Figure 22) of 4E,15E-bilirubin-IXα.[135] The evidence[84,135] for the structure assignments is tenuous, and the arguments[84,135] in their support are specious. For example, *inter alia,* if the

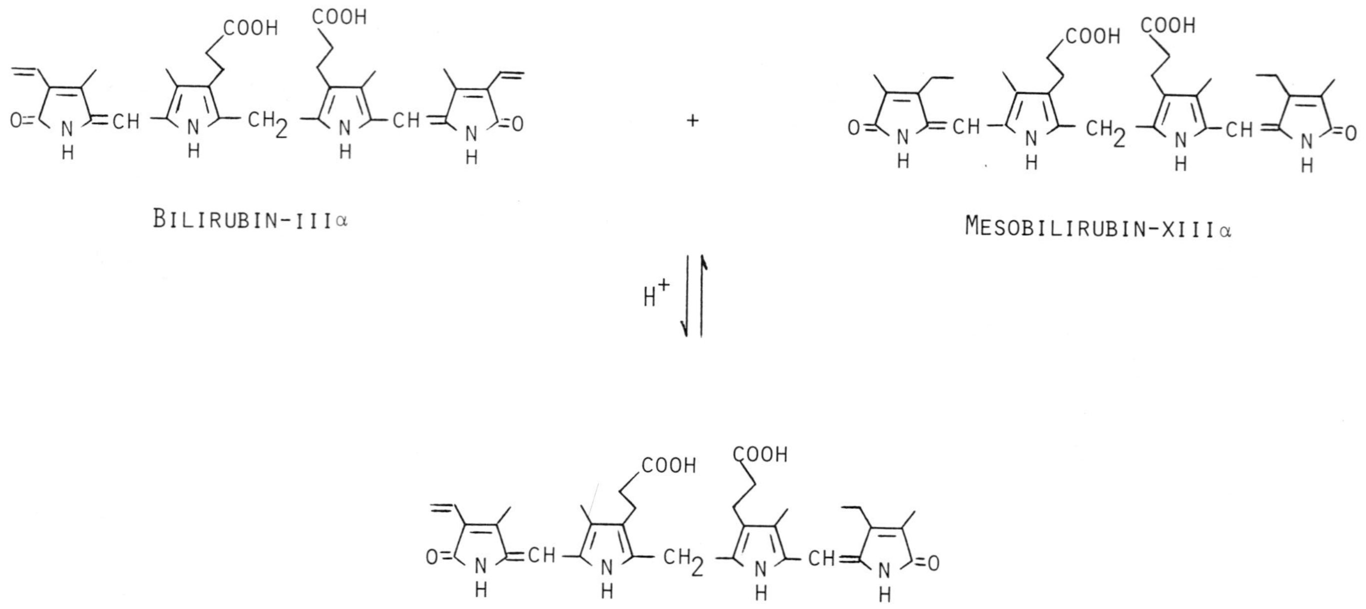

FIGURE 44. Reaction scheme showing the synthetic utility of the acid-catalyzed constitutional isomerization of McDonagh et al.[117] to make the mono-exo-vinyl, mono-endo-ethylbilirubin-IXα.

E,E isomer is indeed more stable thermodynamically, one must question why the photochemical process, which is purported to lead to Z → E isomerization in chloroform, would not go on to give the more stable E,E isomer in that solvent. And, to ascribe a greater thermodynamic stability to an E,E isomer vs. a Z,E isomer violates fundamental principles. The stable pigments from DMSO are almost surely not 4E,15E-bilirubin (see Section III.B.5).

IV. SYNTHETIC PROCEDURES

A. From Heme and Verdins

Bilirubin-IXα, β, γ and δ may be obtained from the corresponding biliverdins following coupled oxidation of hemin in aqueous pyridine — O_2/ascorbic acid. The procedure for coupled oxidation of hemin on a 25 mg scale has been published by Bonnett and McDonagh.[1,145] A nearly statistical (1:1:1:1) ratio of the four isomeric biliverdins is obtained as found by separation of dimethylesters by TLC (32% IXα, 22% IXβ, 18% IXγ, 22% IXδ) Bilirubin-IXα, IXβ, IXγ, and IXδ were prepared from reduction of the corresponding biliverdins with sodium borohydride followed by alkaline hydrolysis.[20] Another method of reduction of biliverdin to bilirubin uses zinc-acetic acid.[1]

B. Partial Synthesis by Left-Half — Right-Half Scrambling

The constitutional isomerization discovered by McDonagh[101] offers a simple, direct method for preparing the symmetrical bilirubin-IIIα and XIIIα isomers using acid catalysis in DMSO. Since the IXα isomers can also be prepared in this way from a mixture of IIIα and XIIIα isomers, the procedure may be viewed as a general one for making "mixed" or nonsymmetrical bilirubin isomers, as illustrated in Figure 44. The remaining problem is one of separation; however, this obstacle should not be insurmountable because HPLC[1,146] or TLC[1] have worked in related instances.

C. Total Synthesis

The total synthesis of bilirubin has been worked out by Fischer and Plieninger[23] (Section II.A.2); however, improved syntheses have been developed by Gossauer and Plieninger[25] using modern synthetic methods and reagents.[147]

D. Labeled Biladienes

^{14}C-Labeled bilirubin [2, 4, 6, 8, 14, 17, 19-^{14}C] may be prepared biosynthetically using rats infused with 5-amino-[4-^{14}C]levulinic acid and isolated from the rat's bile.[1] Administration of [2-^{14}C]glycine or 5-amino[5-^{14}C]levulinic acid leads to formation of [1, 5, 9, 10, 11, 15, 16-^{14}C]-bilirubin.[1] [5-^{14}C]-Bilirubin has been prepared by total synthesis.[25] Various tritium-labeled bilirubin-IXα's have been prepared biosynthetically, as above, using 5-amino[2,2-^{3}H]levulinic acid (to give [2,17-[1′, 2′-^{3}H]-3, 7, 13, 18-[1′-^{3}H]-8,12-[1′,2′-^{3}H]bilirubin-IXα) and 5-amino[3,5-^{3}H]levulinic acid (to give [5, 10, 15-^{3}H]- 2,17-[1′-^{3}H]-8,12-[1′-^{3}H]bilirubin-IXα).[1] Direct tritiation of bilirubin-IXα has also been employed (sodium methoxide + $^{3}H_2O$ + bilirubin dimethyl ester) to give 8,12-[2′-^{3}H]bilirubin-IXα,[1] bilirubin labeled in the propionic acid groups.[1] Tritium labeling of the *exo*-vinyl group of bilirubin was achieved by tritiation of its thiolacetic acid adduct.[1]

ACKNOWLEDGMENTS

The author thanks the National Institute of Child Health and Human Development (U.S. Public Health Service) and the National Science Foundation. Thanks, too, to his many co-workers, especially Drs. Quistad, Wooldridge, Low, Crandall, Norris,

Pak, Park, Cu, Bisacchi, Kirk, Landen, and Crist; and Mssrs. Linnane, Wolf, and Rodgers.

REFERENCES

1. **McDonagh, A. F.,** Bile pigments: bilatrienes and 5,15-biladienes, in *The Porphyrins,* Vol. VIA, Dolphin, D., Eds., Academic Press, New York, 1979, chap. 6.
2. **Merritt, J. E. and Loening, K. L.,** Nomenclature of tetrapyrroles, *Pure and Applied Chem.,* 51, 2251, 1979.
3. IUPAC Commission on Nomenclature of Organic Chemistry. Rules for the nomenclature of organic chemistry, Section E: stereochemistry, *Pure and Applied Chem.,* 45, 13, 1976.
4. **Cullen, D. L., Black, P. S., Meyer, E. F., Jr., Lightner, D. A., Quistad, G. B., and Pak, C. S.,** The crystal and molecular structure of an oxodipyrromethene related to bilirubin, *Tetrahedron,* 33, 477, 1977.
5. **Bergstrom, D. E. and Blumenthal, S. G.,** Abbreviations and Symbols for Bile Pigments and Their Azopyrromethene Derivatives, submitted to the IUPAC-IUB Joint Commission on Biochemical Nomenclature.
6. **Fischer, H. and Orth, H.,** *Die Chemie des Pyrrols,* Vol. II, First half, Akademische Verlagsgesellschaft, M. B. H., Leipzig, 1937, 622.
7. **Fischer, H. and Orth, H.,** *Die Chemie des Pyrrols,* Vol. II, First half, Akademische Verlagsgesellschaft, M. B. H., Leipzig, 1937, 650.
8. **Fischer, H. and Hess, R.,** Neo- and xanthobilirubinic acid and partial synthesis of mesobilirubin and mesobilirubinogen (urobilinogen), *Hoppe-Seyler's Z. Physiol. Chem.,* 194, 193, 1931.
9. **Fischer, H. and Siedel, W.,** On the constitution of bilirubin, syntheses of neo- and isoneoxanthobilirubinic acids, *Hoppe-Seyler's Z. Physiol. Chem.,* 214, 145, 1933.
10. **Fischer, H. and Orth, H.,** *Die Chemie des Pyrrols,* Vol. II, First half, Akademische Verlagsgesellschaft, M. B. H., Leipzig, 1937, 121.
11. **Rüdiger, W.,** Gallenfarbstoffe und Biliproteide, *Fortschr. Chem. Org. Naturst.,* 29, 60, 1971.
12. **Hudson, M. F. and Smith, K. M.,** Bile pigments, *Chem. Soc. Rev.,* 4, 363, 1975.
13. **Petryka, Z., Nicholson, D. C., and Gray, C. H.,** Isomeric bile pigments as products of the fission of hemin, *Nature (London),* 194, 1047, 1962.
14. **Tipton, G. and Gray, C. H.,** Gas chromatographic analysis of pyrrolic acid esters from the potassium permanganate oxidation of bile pigments, *J. Chromatog.,* 59, 29, 1971.
15. **Fatiadi, A. J. and Schaffer, R.,** Periodic acid as a new oxidant for the degradation of bile pigments. Isolation of a biliverdin type of reaction intermediate on oxidation of bilirubin with periodic acid, *Experientia,* 27, 1139, 1971.
16. **Kuenzle, C. C.,** Bilirubin conjugates of human bile, *Biochem J.,* 119, 395, 1970.
17. **Heirwegh, K. P. M., Van Hees, G. P., LeRoy, P., Van Roy, F. P., and Jansen, F. H.,** Heterogeneity of bile pigment conjugates as revealed by chromatography of their ethyl anthranilate azopigments, *Biochem. J.,* 120, 877, 1970; Blanckaert, N., Fevery, J., Heirwegh, K. P. M., and Compernolle, F., Characterization of the major diazo-positive pigments in bile of homozygous Gunn rats, *Biochem. J.,* 164, 237, 1977.
18. **Compernolle, F., Jansen, F. H., and Heirwegh, K. P. M.,** Mass-spectrometric study of the azopigments obtained from bile pigments with diazotized ethyl anthanilate, *Biochem. J.,* 120, 891, 1970.
19. **Jansen, F. H. and Stoll, M. S.,** Separation and structural analysis of vinyl- and isovinyl-azobilirubin derivatives, *Biochem. J.,* 125, 585, 1971.
20. **Blanckaert, N., Heirwegh, K. P. M., and Compernolle, F.,** Synthesis and separation by thin-layer chromatography of bilirubin- IX Isomers, *Biochem. J.,* 155, 405, 1976.
21. **Hutchinson, D. W., Johnson, B., and Knell, A. J.,** The reaction between bilirubin and aromatic diazo compounds, *Biochem. J.,* 127, 907, 1972.
22. **van den Bergh, A. A. H. and Müller, P.,** Direct and indirect diazo-reaction with bilirubin, *Biochem. Z.,* 77, 90, 1916.
23. **Fischer, H. and Plieninger, H.,** Synthese des Biliverdins (uteroverdins) und Bilirubins, der Biliverdine XIIIα und IIIα sowie der Vinylneoxanthosaüre, *Hoppe-Seyler's Z. Physiol. Chem.,* 274, 231, 1942; Fischer, H. and Plieninger, H., Synthese des Biliverdins (Uteroverdins) und Bilirubins, *Naturwissenschaften,* 30, 382, 1942.
24. **Stoll, M. S. and Gray, C. H.,** The preparation and characterization of bile pigments, *Biochem. J.,* 163, 59, 1977.

25. **Gossauer, A. and Plieninger, H.**, Synthesis, purification and characterization of bile pigments and related compounds, in *The Porphyrins,* Vol. VIA, Dolphin, D., Ed., Academic Press, New York, 1979, 586.
26. **Kuster, W.**, *Handbuch Biol. Arbeitsmeth.,* Section I, part 8, Abderhaldens, 1922, 321.
27. **Falk, H. Gergely, S., and Grubmayr, K.**, Das Tautomere Gleichgewicht des Bilirubins, *Monatsh.,* 107, 827, 1977.
28. **Birch, A. J.**, personal communication; Birch, A. J., The structure of stercobilin, *Chemistry and Industry (Brit.),*652, 1955; Gray, C. H. and Nicholson, D. C., Structure of d-urobilin, *Nature (London),* 180, 336, 1957; and Plieninger, H. and Decker, M., Eine Neue Synthese für Pyrrolone, Insbesondere für "Isooxyopsopyrrol" und "Isooxyopsopyrrolcarbonsaüre", *Liebigs Annalen,* 598, 198, 1956.
29. **Bonnett, R., Davis, J. E., Hursthouse, M. B., and Sheldrick, G. M.**, The structure of bilirubin, *Proc. R. Soc. Lond. B,*202, 249, 1978.
30. **Manitto, P., Ricca, G. S., and Monti, D.**, The conformations of bilirubin and its esters, *Gazz. Chim. Ital.,* 104, 633, 1974.
31. **Kuenzle, C. C., Weibel, M. H., and Pelloni, R. R.**, The reaction of bilirubin with diazomethane, *Biochem. J.,* 133, 357, 1973.
32. **Hutchinson, D. W., Johnson, B., and Knell, A. J.**, Tautomerism and hydrogen bonding in bilirubin, *Biochem J.,* 123, 483, 1971.
33. **Nichol, A. W. and Morell, D. B.**, Bilirubin and biliverdin structure, *Biochim. Biophys. Acta,* 177, 599, 1969.
34. **Ricca, G. S., Manitto P., Monti, D., and Randall, E. W.**, The carbon-13 nuclear magnetic resonance spectra of bilirubin and its derivatives, *Gazz. Chim. Ital.,* 105, 1273, 1975.
35. **Ricca, G. S., Manitto, P., Monti, D., and Randall, E.**, The Carbon-13 Nuclear Magnetic Resonance Spectra of Bilirubin and its Derivatives. A Conformation of the Bis-Lactam Form for These Biladienes, presented at a Meeting on Metabolism and Chemistry of Bilirubin and Related Tetra pyrroles in Hemsedal, Norway, September 1974; *Bilirubin and Related Tetra-pyrroles,* Bakken, A. F. and Fog, J., Eds., Pediatr. Res. Institute, Rikshospitalet, Oslo l, Norway, 1975, 230.
36. **Navon, G.**, The nuclear magnetic resonance spectrum of bilirubin, in *Bilirubin Metabolism in the Newborn (II),* Bergsma, D. and Blondheim, S. H., Eds., Elsevier, New York, 1974, 141.
37. **Wray, W., Gossauer, A., Grüning, B., Reifenstahl, G., and Zilch, H.**, A study of the bile pigments and related compounds in solution by ^{13}C nuclear magnetic resonance spectroscopy, *J. Chem. Soc. Perkin I,* 1558, 1978.
38. **Hansen, P. E., Thiessen, H. and Brodersen, R.**, Bilirubin acidity. titrimetric and ^{13}C NMR studies, *Acta Chem. Scand.,* B 33, 281, 1979.
39. **Kaplan, D. and Navon, G.**, On the assignment of the carbon-13 NMR spectrum of bilirubin, *Spectroscopy Lett.,* 13, 59, 1980.
40. **Chedekel, M. R. and Crist, B. V.**, Bilirubin: intramolecular bonding and conformation, in *Chemistry and Physiology of Bile Pigments,* Berk, P. D. and Berlin, N. I., Eds., DHEW Publication No. (NIH) 77-1100, U.S. Dept. of Health, Education and Welfare, Public Health Service, National Institutes of Health, Bethesda, Md., 1977, 493
41. **Mugnoli, A., Manitto, P., and Monti, D.**, Structure of di-isopropyl-ammonium bilirubinate, *Nature (London),* 273, 568, 1978.
42. **Becker, W. and Sheldrick, W. S.**, Bile pigment structures II. The crystal structure of mesobilirubin-IXα-bis(chloroform), *Acta Cryst.,* B 34, 1298, 1978; Sheldrick, W. S. and Becker, W., Bile pigment structures. III. Crystal and molecular structure of dimethoxybilirubin dimethyl ester, *Z. Naturforsch.,* 34b, 1542, 1979.
43. **Sheldrick, W. S.**, Crystal and molecular structure of biliverdin dimethyl ester, *J. Chem. Soc. Perkin II,* 1457, 1976.
44. **Cullen, D. L., Meyer, E. F., Jr., Eivazi, F., and Smith, K. M.**, Crystal and molecular structure of 3,8,12-triethyl-14-formyl-2,7,13-trimethyl-l(15H)-tripyrrinone, a tripyrrolic aldehyde derived from aetiobiliverdin-IVγ, *J. Chem Soc. Perkin II,* 259, 1978.
45. **Cullen, D. L., Pèpe, G., and Meyer, E. F., Jr.**, *syn-* and *anti-* Conformation in oxodipyrromethenes: crystal and molecular structure of 3,4-dimethyl-2,2′-pyrromethen-5(1H)-one and its N-methyl derivative, *J. Chem. Soc. Perkin II,* 999, 1979.
46. **Sheldrick, W. S., Borkenstein, A., Blacha-Puller, M., and Gossauer, A.**, Stereoisomerism in partial bile pigment structures. The crystal structures of the Z and E isomers of 5′-ethoxycarbonyl-3,4-dighdro-3,4′-dimethyl-5(1H)-2,2′-pyrromethenone and their reaction products with $Et_2O^+BF_4^-$, *Acta Cryst.,* B 33, 3625, 1977.
47. **Henry, R. J., Jacobs, S. L., and Chiamori, N.**, Determination of bile pigments. I. Standard of purity for bilirubin, *Clin. Chem.,* 6, 529, 1960.
48. **Newbold, B. T. and LeBlanc, G.**, Physical properties of commercial bilirubins, *Can. J. Biochem.,* 42, 1697, 1964.

49. **Brodersen, R., Flodgaard, H., and Hansen, J. K.**, Intramolecular hydrogen bonding in bilibubin, *Acta Chem. Scand.*, 21, 2284, 1967.
50. **Schram, B. L. and Kroes, H. H.**, Structure of phycocyanobilin, *Eur. J. Biochem.*, 19, 581, 1971.
51. **Linnane, W. P., III and Lightner, D. A.**, unpublished data.
52. **Landen, G. L. and Lightner, D. A.**, unpublished data.
53. **Holzwarth, A. R., Langer, E., Lehner, H., and Schaffner, K.**, Absorption, luminescence, solvent-induced circular dichroism and ^{1}H-NMR study of bilirubin dimethyl ester: observation of different forms in solution, *Photochem. Photobiol.*, 32, 17, 1980.
54. **Lemberg, R.**, The physiological disintegration of haemoglobin, *Austral. Chem. Inst. J. and Proc.*, 6, 170, 1939.
55. **Lemberg, R. and Legge, J. W.**, *Hematin Compounds and Bile Pigments*, Interscience, New York, 1949, 103.
56. **Fog, J. and Jellum, E.**, Structure of bilirubin, *Nature (London)*, 198, 88, 1963.
57. **Fog, J. and Bugge-Asperheim, B.**, Stability of bilirubin, *Nature (London)*, 203, 756, 1964.
58. **Blauer, G. and King, T. E.**, Interactions of bilirubin with bovine serum albumin in aqueous solution, *J. Biol. Chem.*, 245, 372, 1970.
59. **Moscowitz, A., Krueger, W. C., Kay, I. T., Skewes, G., and Bruckenstein, S.**, On the origin of the optical activity in the urobilins, *Proc. Natl. Acad. Sci. (U.S.)*, 52. 1190, 1964; Lightner, D. A., Docks, E. L., Horwitz, J., and Moscowitz, A., Urobilinoid conformation from temperature dependent circular dichroism measurements, *Proc. Natl. Acad. Sci (U.S.)*, 67, 1361, 1970.
60. **Knell, A. J., Johnson, B., and Hutchinson, D. W.**, Intramolecular hydrogen bonds in bilirubin, *Digestion*, 6, 288, 1972.
61. **Kuenzle, C. C., Weibel, M. H., Pelloni, R. R., and Hemmerich, P.**, Structure and conformation of bilirubin, *Biochem J.*, 133, 364, 1973.
62. **Knell, A. J., Hancock, F., and Hutchinson, D. W.**, Bilirubin Revisited, presented at a Meeting on Metabolism and Chemistry of Bilirubin and Related Tetrapyrroles, Hemsedal, Norway, September 1974.
63. **Falk, H., Grubmayr, K., Herzig, U., and Hofer, O.**, The configurations of the isomeric 3,4-dimethyl-5-(1H)-2,2′-pyrromethenones, *Tetrahedron Lett.*, 559, 1975.
64. **Falk, H., Grubmayr, K., Höllbacher, G., Hofer, U., Leodolter, A., Neufingerl, F., and Ribó, J. M.**, Pyrromethenone—Partialstrukturen von Gallenpigmenten Struktur und Eigenschaften in Lösung, *Monatsh.*, 108, 1113, 1977.
65. **Falk, H. and Grubmayr, K.**, 5-[5-Methyliden-(5H-pyrrolyl-2-methyliden)]-3-pyrrolin-2-on — eine Partial Struktur von Gallenpigmenten, *Monatsh.*, 108, 625, 1977.
66. **Falk, H., Grubmayr, K., Hofer, O., and Neufingerl, F.**, Die Lichtabsorption Geometrische Isomeren Arylmethylidenpyrrolinone — Konformationsanalytische Studien, *Monatsh.*, 106, 991, 1975.
67. **Falk, H., Grubmayr, K., Hofer, O., Neufingerl, F., and Ribó, J. M.**, Die Thermische Stabilität der Geometrischen Isomeren von Arylmethyliden-pyrrolinonen, *Monatsh.*, 107, 831, 1976.
68. **Lightner, D. A. and Park, Y. T.**, Synthesis, photooxidation and $Z \rightleftharpoons E$ isomerization of benzalpyrrolinones, *J. Heterocyclic Chem.*, 14, 514, 1978; Lightner, D. A. and Landen, G. L., unpublished work.
69. **Falk, H., Grubmayr, K., Haslinger, E., Schlederer, T., and Thirring, K.**, Die Diastereomeren (Geometrische Isomeren) Biliverdindimethylester — Struktur, Konfiguration und Conformation, *Monatsh.*, 109, 1451, 1978.
70. **Falk H., Grubmayr, K., and Haslinger, E.**, Zum Diagnostischen Wert der ^{13}C-Kernresonanzspektroskopie bei Diastereomeren Bilatrienen-abc, *Monatsh.*, 110, 1429, 1979.
71. **Lightner, D. A., Landen, G. L., and Wooldridge, T. A.**, unpublished data.
72. **Geddes, A. J., Potterton, E., and Willis, G.**, Steric hindrance in proposed photoisomers of bilirubin, *Photochem. Photobiol.*, 34, 337, 1980.
73. **Lightner, D. A., Wooldridge, T. A., and McDonagh, A. F.**, Photobilirubin: an early bilirubin photoproduct detected by absorbance difference spectroscopy, *Proc. Natl. Acad. Sci. (U.S.)*, 76, 29, 1979.
74. **McDonagh, A. F., Lightner, D. A. and Wooldridge, T. A.**, Geometric isomerization of bilirubin-IXα and its dimethyl ester, *J. Chem. Soc. Chem. Commun.*, 110, 1979.
75. **Lightner, D. A., Wooldridge, T. A., and McDonagh, A. F.**, Configurational isomerization of bilirubin and the mechanism of jaundice phototherapy, *Biochem. Biophys. Res. Comm.*, 86, 235, 1979.
76. **McDonagh, A. F., Palma, L. A., and Lightner, D. A.**, Blue light and bilirubin excretion, *Science*, 208, 145, 1980.
77. **Manitto, P. and Monti, D.**, Free energy barrier of conformational inversion in bilirubin, *J. Chem. Soc. Chem. Comm.*, 122, 1976.
78. **Lightner, D. A., Cu, A., McDonagh, A. F., and Palma, L. A.**, On the autoxidation of bilirubin, *Biochem. Biophys. Res. Commun.*, 69, 648, 1976.

79. **Brodersen, R.**, Dimerisation of bilirubin anion in aqueous solution, *Acta Chem. Scand.*, 20, 2895, 1966.
80. **Brodersen, R. and Theilgaard, J.**, Bilirubin colloid formation in neutral aqueous solution, *Scand. J. Clin. Lab. Invest.*, 24, 395, 1969.
81. **Carey, M. C. and Koretsky, A. P.**, Self-association of unconjugated bilirubin-IXα in aqueous solution at pH 10.0 and physical-chemical interactions with bile salt monomers and micelles, *Biochem J.*, 179, 675, 1979.
82. **Wolf, S.**, The Structure of Bilirubin in Solution, M. S. thesis, University of Nevada, Reno, 1980.
83. **Hagen, U.**, Ultracentrifugation, in *Experimental Methods in Biophysical Chemistry,* Nicolau, Ed., John Wiley & Sons, New York, 1973, chap. 5.
84. **Cohen, A. N. and Ostrow, J. D.**, New concepts in phototherapy: photoisomerization of bilirubin IXα and potential toxic effects of light, *Pediatrics,* 65, 740, 1980.
85. **Dalton, J., Milgrom, L. R., and Bonnett, R.**, Luminescence of bilirubin, *Chem. Phys. Lett.*, 61, 242, 1979.
86. **Cu, A., Bellah, G. G., and Lightner, D. A.**, On the fluorescence of bilirubin, *J. Am. Chem. Soc.*, 97, 2579, 1975.
87. **Bonnett, R., Dalton, J., and Hamilton, D. E.**, Luminescence of bilirubin, *J. Chem. Soc. Chem. Comm.*, 639, 1975.
88. **Matheson, I. B. C., Faini, G. F., and Lee, J.**, Low temperature absorption and fluorescence spectra and quantum yields of bilirubin, *Photochem. Photobiol.*, 21, 135, 1975.
89. **Land, E. J.**, The triplet excited state of bilirubin, *Photochem. Photobiol.*, 24, 475, 1976.
90. **Sloper, R. W. and Truscott, T. G.**, Excited states of bilirubin, *Photochem. Photobiol.*, 31, 445, 1980.
91. **McDonagh, A. F.**, Photochemistry and photometabolism of bilirubin, in *Phototherapy for Neonatal Hyperbilirubinemia,* Brown, A. K. and Showacre, J., Eds., Dept. of Health, Education and Welfare, Washington, D.C., Public No. NIH 76-1075, 1974, 185: "These observations suggest a fourth explanation for the enhanced biliary output of bilirubin during phototherapy. Perhaps photodissociation, or *photoisomerization reactions,* or even photothermal effects cause the release of bilirubin from tissue binding sites and lead to an increase in the unbound fraction of bilirubin in the serum."
92. **McDonagh, A. F.**, Photochemistry and Photometabolism of Bilirubin IXα, in the book of Reference 36, p. 37: "This suggests that the phenomenon is due either to a photothermal effect, in which light is converted to thermal energy within the skin, or to photodissociation of bilirubin from binding sites by a process which could involve either isomerization or conformational changes of the pigment molecule."
93. **McDonagh, A. F. and Palma, L. A.**, Mechanism of Bilirubin Photodegradation: Role of Singlet Oxygen, in the book of reference 40, p. 90: "A more plausible hypothesis is that bilirubin in subcutaneous lipid (where unsaturated fats would inhibit singlet-oxygen photodegradation) undergoes photochemical conversion to a stable conformational or geometric isomer that can be excreted without conjugation."
94. **McDonagh, A. F.**, Jaundice Phototherapy: Photochemical Aspects, Paper WAM-B2, *Proc. 4th Ann. Meet. Am. Soc. Photobiol.*, Denver, Colo., 1976, 59: "How phototherapy causes hepatic excretion of bilirubin remains an unanswered and intriguing conundrum. Several theories have been proposed and some ruled out experimentally. Perhaps the simplest and most appealing is that bilirubin IX-α can be converted photochemically into a more polar, but less thermodynamically stable, geometrical isomer that can be excreted rapidly."
95. **McDonagh, A. F.**, Phototherapy of neonatal jaundice, *Biochem. Soc. Trans.*, 4, 219, 1976. "One appealing, yet entirely speculative, theory is that bilirubin can be converted photochemically into a more polar, but less thermodynamically stable, isomer that does not need to be conjugated to be excreted. Cis-trans photo-isomerization of a model dipyrrolylmethene has been demonstrated and the individual isomers isolated (Falk et al., Reference 63), but analogous reactions of bilirubin have not been reported."
96. **Lightner, D. A. and Park, Y. T.**, Dye-sensitized photooxygenation of oxopyrromethenes related to bilirubin, *Tetrahedron Lett.*, 2209, 1976: Footnote 20. "(Photo)isomerizations of BR involving the various *syn* and *anti* Z and E configurations at *a* and *c* are possible and would require the breaking of intramolecular H-bonds [Kuenzle, C. C. Weible, M. H. Pelloni, R. R., and Hemmerich, P., *Biochem. J.*, 133, 304, 1973] between the P groups and opposite end rings A and D. Such photo-induced H-bond breaking would be expected to alter the solubility of BR, perhaps make it more H_2O soluble and thus explain the excretion of unconjugated BR during phototherapy."

97. Reference 68a, page 420: "Furthermore, the observations that Z ⇌ E isomerization of the ene-amide carbon-carbon double bonds of 5-10 can occur may provide an understanding for the recognized excretion of unconjugated bilirubin in the bile of jaundiced infants or Gunn rats undergoing light treatment (22). For a change in configuration in bilirubin from Z → E at its ene-amide carbon-carbon double bonds would necessarily expose its polar parts and render it more water soluble (hence more excretable into the bile) than form 1."
98. **Cowan, D. O. and Drisko, R. L.** *Elements of Organic Chemistry,* Plenum Press, New York, 1976, chap. 9.
99. **Falk, H. and Neufingerl, F.,** Zur Anaeroben Photochemie von Gallenpigmenten: Zum Mechanismus der Photochemischen Isomerisierung an Exo-cyclische Doppelbindungen, *Monatsh.,* 110, 1243, 1979.
100. **Park, Y. T.,** The Synthesis and Photochemistry of Oxomono- and Oxodipyrro-methene Models for Bilirubin, Ph.D. Dissertation, University of Nevada, Reno, 1977.
101. **McDonagh, A. F.,** Thermal and photochemical reactions of bilirubin-IXα, *Ann. N.Y. Acad. Sci.,* 244, 553, 1975.
102. **Lightner, D. A. and Cu, A.,** Wavelength dependence of bilirubin photoreactivity, *Life Sci.,* 20, 723, 1977.
103. **Manitto, P. and Monti, D.,** Photochemistry of bilirubin in the absence of oxygen, in Meeting on Metabolism and Chemistry of Bilirubin and Related Tetrapyrroles, Hemsedal, Norway, September 1974.
104. **Manitto, P.,** Photochemistry of bilirubin, *Experientia,* 27, 1147, 1971.
105. **Manitto, P. and Monti, D.,** Acid-catalyzed addition of alcohols and thiols to bilirubin, *Experientia,* 29, 137, 1973.
106. **Foote, C. S.,** Photosensitized oxidation and singlet oxygen: consequences in biological systems, in *Free Radicals in Biology,* Vol. II, Pryor, W. A., Ed., Academic Press, 1976, chap. 3.
107. **Lightner, D. A.,** The photoreactivity of bilirubin and related pyrroles, *Photochem. Photobiol.,* 26, 427, 1977.
108. **Lightner, D. A., Landen, G. L., and Rodgers, S. L.,** Photooxidation of Bilirubin and Model Dipyrroles, Paper MAM-B1, *Proc. 7th Ann. Meet. Am. Soc. Photobiol.,* Asilomar, Calif., 1979, 59.
109. **Lightner, D. A. and Park, Y. T.,** On the syntheses and singlet oxygen reactivity of oxopyrromethene models for bilirubin, *Tetrahedron,* 35, 463, 1979.
110. **Lightner, D. A. and Park, Y. T.,** Singlet oxygen reactivity of bilirubin and related tetrapyrroles, *Experientia,* 34, 555, 1978.
111. **Erikson, J., Foote, C. S., and Parker, T. L.,** Photosensitized oxygenation of alkenes and sulfides via a non-singlet oxygen mechanism, *J. Am. Chem. Soc.,* 99, 6455, 1977; Manring, L. E., Eriksen, J., and Foote, C. S., Electron-transfer photooxygenation. 4. Photooxygenation of *trans* stilbene sensitized by methylene blue, *J. Am. Chem. Soc.,* 102, 4275, 1980.
112. **McDonagh, A. F.,** The role of singlet oxygen in bilirubin photo-oxidation, *Biochem. Biophys. Res. Commun.,* 44, 1306, 1971.
113. **Bonnett, R. and Stewart, J. C. M.,** Singlet oxygen in the photo-oxidation of bilirubin in hydroxylic solvents, *Biochem. J.,* 130, 895, 1972.
114. **Ostrow, J. D., Hammaker, L., and Schmid, R.,** The preparation of crystalline bilirubin-^{14}C, *J. Clin. Invest.,* 40, 1442, 1961.
115. **Bonnett, R. and Stewart, J. C. M.,** Photo-oxidation of bilirubin in hydroxylic solvents, *J. Chem. Soc. Perkin I,* 224, 1975.
116. **Bonnett, R.,** Mechanisms of the photodegradation of bilirubin, *Biochem. Soc. Trans.,* 4, 222, 1976.
117. **Lightner, D. A. and Quistad, G. B.,** Hematinic acid and propentdyopents from bilirubin photooxidation in vitro, *FEBS Lett.,* 25, 94, 1972.
118. **Lightner, D. A.,** Products of bilirubin photodegradation, in *Chemistry and Physiology of Bile Pigments,* Berk, P. D. and Berlin, N. I., Eds., National Institutes of Health, Bethesda, Md., 1977, 93.
119. **Lightner, D. A.,** In vitro photoxidation products of bilirubin, in *Phototherapy in the Newborn: An Overview,* Odell, G. B., Schaffer, R., and Simopoulos, A. P., Eds., National Academy of Sciences, Washington, D.C., 1974, 35.
120. **Lightner, D. A. and Quistad, G. B.,** Methylvinylmaleimide from bilirubin photooxidation, *Science,* 175, 324, 1972.
121. **Gray, C. H., Kulczyka, A., and Nicholson, D. C.,** The photodecomposition of bilirubin and other bile pigments, *J. Chem. Soc. Perkin I,* 228, 1972.
122. **Velapoldi, R. A. and Menis, O.,** Formation and stabilities of free bilirubin and bilirubin complexes with transition and rare-earth elements, *Clin. Chem.,* 17, 1165, 1971.
123. **Lightner, D. A., Crandall, D. C., Gertler, S., and Quistad, G. B.,** On the formation of biliverdin during photooxygenation of bilirubin in vitro, *FEBS Lett.,* 30, 309, 1973.
124. **Bonnett, R. and Stewart, J. C. M.,** Photo-oxidation of bilirubin in hydroxylic solvents: propentdyopent adducts as major products, *J. Chem. Soc. Chem. Comm.,* 596, 1972.

125. **Lightner, D. A. Wooldridge, T. A., Rodgers, S. L., and Norris, R. D.,** Action spectra for bilirubin photo-disappearance, *Experientia,* 36, 380, 1980.
126. **Lightner, D. A.,** Photochemistry of Pyrroles, Bile Pigments and Porphyrins, *Photochem. Photobiol.,* 19, 457, 1974.
127. **Lightner, D. A., Bisacchi, G. S., and Norris, R. D.,** On the mechanism of the sensitized photooxygenation of pyrroles, *J. Am. Chem. Soc.,* 98, 802, 1976.
128. **Pedersen, A. O., Schønheyder, F., and Brodersen, R.,** Photooxidation of human serum albumin and its complex with bilirubin, *Eur. J. Biochem.,* 72, 213, 1977.
129. **Rubaltelli, F. F. and Jori, G.,** Visible light irradiation of human and bovine serum albumin-bilirubin complex, *Photochem. Photobiol.,* 29, 991, 1979.
130. **Jori, G., Rossi, E., and Rubaltelli, F. F.,** Evidence for Visible Light-Induced Covalent Binding Between Bilirubin and Serum Albumin "In Vitro" and "In Vivo", Paper THAM-B6, *Proc. 7th Ann. Meet. Am. Soc. Photobiol.,* Asilomar, Calif., 1979, 176.
131. **McDonagh, A. F.,** Photochemistry and photometabolism of bilirubin, in *Phototherapy in the Newborn: An Overview,* Odell, G. B., Schaffer, R., and Simopoulos, A. P., Eds., National Academy of Sciences, Washington, D.C., 1974, 56.
132. **Kapitulnik, J., Kaufmann, N. A., Alayoff, A., and Blondheim, S. H.,** Characteristics of a photoproduct of bilirubin found in vitro and in vivo, and its effect on the bilirubin binding affinity of serum, in *Bilirubin Metabolism in the Newborn,* Bergsma, D. and Blondheim, S. H., Eds., Elsevier, New York, 1974, 53.
133. **Lightner, D. A., Wooldridge, T. A., and Park, Y-T.,** Reversible Photochemistry of Bilirubin and Its Relevance to Jaundice Phototherapy, Abstr. No. 121 in Photochemistry Symposium of the 1977 Pacific Conference on Chemistry and Spectroscopy, Anaheim, CA, 1977, 63.
134. **Ehler, K. W. and Lightner, D. A.,** unpublished data.
135. **Stoll, M. S., Zenone, E. A., Ostrow, J. D., and Zarembo, J. E.,** Preparation and properties of bilirubin photoisomers, *Biochem J.,* 183, 139, 1979.
136. **Roos, W. T., Wieger, H. H., Windler, S. C. H., and Jones, C. O.,** Bilirubin isomers and phototherapy, *Gastroenterol.,* Abstr., A-132, 73, A-45/1243, 1977.
137. **Schmid, R. and McDonagh, A. F.,** Hyperbilirubinemia in *The Metabolic Basis of Inherited Disease,* 4th ed., Stanbury, J. B., Wyngaarden, J. B., and Frederickson, D. S., Eds., McGraw-Hill, New York, 1978, 1221.
138. **Ostrow, J. D.,** Photochemical and biochemical basis of the treatment of neonatal jaundice in *Progress in Liver Diseases,* Vol. 4, Popper, H. and Schaffner, F., Eds., Grune and Stratton, New York, 1972, chap. 27.
139. **Ostrow, J. D.,** Photocatabolism of labeled bilirubin in the congenitally jaundiced (Gunn) rat, *J. Clin. Invest.,* 50, 707, 1971.
140. **Lund, H. T. and Jacobsen, J.,** Influence of phototherapy on the biliary bilirubin excretion pattern in newborn infants with hyperbilirubinemia, *J. Pediatrics,* 85, 262, 1974.
141. **Ostrow, J. D.,** Effects of Phototherapy on Organic Ion Excretion, Abstract WAM-B3, in *Proc. 4th Ann. Meet. Am. Soc. Photobiol.,* Denver, Colo., 1976, 60. "This precludes the possibility that photoisomerization of the pigment, to a form incapable of internal hydrogen bonding, accounts for excretion of unconjugated bilirubin in bile during phototherapy."
142. **Brodersen, R.,** Bilirubin transport in the newborn, reviewed with relation to kernicterus, *J. Pediatrics,* 96, 349, 1980.
143. **Stoll, M. S., Zenone, E. A., Ostrow, J. D., and Zarembo, J. E.,** Photoisomers of bilirubin and their excretion by the Gunn rat, Abstr. No. SAM-D7 in *Proc. 5th Ann. Meeting Am. Soc. Photobiol.,* San Juan, P. R., 1977, 97.
144. **Zenone, E. A., Stoll, M. S., and Ostrow, J. D.,** Mechanism of excretion of unconjugated bilirubin (UCB) during phototherapy, Abstract, *Gastroenterol.,* 72, A-157/1180, 1977.
145. **Bonnett, R. and McDonagh, A. F.,** The *meso* reactivity of porphyrins and related compounds. VI. Oxidative cleavage of the haem system. The four isomeric biliverdins of the IX series, *J. Chem. Soc. Perkin I,* 881, 1973.
146. **Wooldridge, T. A. and Lightner, D. A.,** Separation of the IIIα, IXα and XIIIα isomers of bilirubin and bilirubin dimethyl ester by high performance liquid chromatography, *J. Liq. Chromat.,* 1, 653, 1978.
147. **Plieninger, H., El-Barkawi, F., Ehl, K., Kohler, R., and McDonagh, A. F.,** Neve Synthese und ^{14}C-Markierung von Bilirubin-IXα, *Liebigs Ann.,* 758, 195, 1972.
148. **Fischer, H., Plieninger, H., and Weissbarth, X.,** Uber die Konstitution des Bilirubins und uber Bilirubinoide Farbstoffe, *Hoppe Seyler's Z. Physiol. Chem.,* 268, 197, 1941.
149. **Hutchinson, D. W., Johnson, B., and Knell, A. J.,** The synthesis of esters of bilirubin, *Biochem. J.,* 133, 493, 1973.

150. **Lightner, D. A. and Crandall, D. C.**, The dye-sensitized Photooxygenation of Kryptopyrrole, *Experientia*, 29, 262, 1973.
151. **Lightner, D. A., Norris, R. D., Kirk, D. I., and Key, R. M.**, The dye-sensitized photooxygenation of hemopyrrole, *Experientia*, 30, 587, 1974.
152. **Choussy, M. and Barbier, M. M.**, Transformations photochimique de pigments biliaires des series IXγ et IXδ, *C. R. Acad. Sci. Paris, Serie C*, 619, 1976.
153. **Kenner, G. W., Rimmer, J., Smith, K. M., and Unsworth, J. F.**, Pyrroles and related compounds. Part 39. Structural and biosynthetic studies of the *Chlorobium* Chlorophylls-660. Incorporation of methionine and porphobilinogen, *J. Chem. Soc. Perkin I*, 845, 1978.
154. **Roos, W. T., Wieger, H. H., Windler, S. C. H., and Jones, C. O.**, Bilirubin isomers and phototherapy, Abstract A-137, *Gastroenterology*, A-45, 1243, 1977.

Chapter 2

BILIRUBIN CONJUGATES: ISOLATION, STRUCTURE ANALYSIS AND SYNTHESIS

Frans Compernolle

TABLE OF CONTENTS

I. HISTORICAL OVERVIEW OF MAJOR STRUCTURAL ISSUES

In mammals, bilirubin-IXα is excreted by liver cells as carbohydrate conjugates.[1-7] Initial evidence, indicating an ester glucuronoside structure for a conjugated azo pigment fraction (Figure 1), was based on its hydrolysis with β-glucuronidase and with dilute alkali.[8-10]

Using reverse phase column chromatography, Billing et al.[8] separated unmodified tetrapyrrole bile pigments into three fractions, apparently consisting of diconjugated, monoconjugated, and free bilirubin. However, evaporation and rechromatography of the monoconjugated fraction reproduced the original three-component mixture, and the hypothesis of a 1:1 complex between bilirubin and bilirubin diglucuronide was advanced to explain these findings.[11] The existence of truly monoconjugated bilirubin was proven only recently,[5] when it was shown that the ester function of bilirubin monoconjugates reacts with ammonia[12] or alkaline methanol[13,14] yielding bilirubin monoamide or monomethyl ester respectively (Figure 1, R^1 or R^2 = NH_2 or OCH_3). Formation of bilirubin and diconjugated bilirubin from the monoconjugated fraction was accounted for by the easy disproportionation of bilirubins to form a mixture of IXα-, XIIIα- and IIIα- isomers (Figure 1).[6]

Heterogeneity of carbohydrate conjugates was demonstrated for dog bile azo pigments by several workers,[15-18] who in addition to glucuronosyl esters also isolated and identified xylosyl and glucosyl ester conjugates. Quite generally, the β-1-*o*-acyl pyranoside structure was assigned to the sugar moieties.[16,19,20] TLC separation of the native bilirubin conjugates from dog bile, followed by diazonium cleavage of individual bile pigments, showed the presence of monoconjugates and of homogeneous and mixed diconjugates,* involving the three sugars (Figure 1).[18,21-25] Although glucose and xylose are minor components only for rat,[26] rhesus monkey,[24,25] and human bile,[18,24-26] chromatographic evidence suggests that these conjugates constitute an important fraction of bile pigments in some other animal species.[26-27]

In 1970, Kuenzle[28,29] questioned the notion that carbohydrate conjugates of bilirubin in human bile are simple glucuronides, and proposed various disaccharidic structures for a series of azo pigments isolated by reverse phase column chromatography. However, the evidence presented in favor of disaccharidic conjugates was mainly indirect and has been discounted recently.[20,30] It appears that Kuenzle's analysis of carbohydrates was hampered by the presence of glucose-containing compounds and other impurities. Moreover, a series of unknown hexuronic acid derivatives detected during gas-liquid chromatography (GLC) mass spectrometry analysis have now been identified as incompletely silylated glucuronic acid and glucuronolactone.[30]

The chromatographic heterogeneity of conjugated azo pigments, that was observed by Kuenzle[28] for human bile originated from the same cause as that found by Heirwegh et al.[31] and Fevery et al.[32] for postobstructive biles of man and rat. At the pH of bile (about 7.8), the native bilirubin 1—*O* -acylglucuronides are transformed into 2-, 3- and 4-*O*-acyl positional isomers (Figure 2).[20,30,33] This base-catalyzed, sequential migration of the bilirubin acyl group can be detected in several ways for older and postobstructive bile samples. First, partial separation of glucuronide azo pigments occurs during reverse phase chromatography[20,28,30] or TLC on silicone-treated silica gel plates.[20,33] Complete separation of the 1-, 2-, 3- and 4-*O*-acyl positional isomers can be obtained for the methyl esters of the azo pigments.[20,33] Finally, when an excess of aniline or ethyl anthranilate is used in the diazonium cleavage reaction, performed at pH 2.7, the free glycosidic function of 2-, 3- and 4-*O*-acylglucuronides reacts with the amine yielding aniline or ethyl anthranilate *N*-glucuronides (Figure 2).[20,34] These *N*-

* Homogeneous and mixed diconjugates refer to the presence of two identical and two different sugars, respectively.

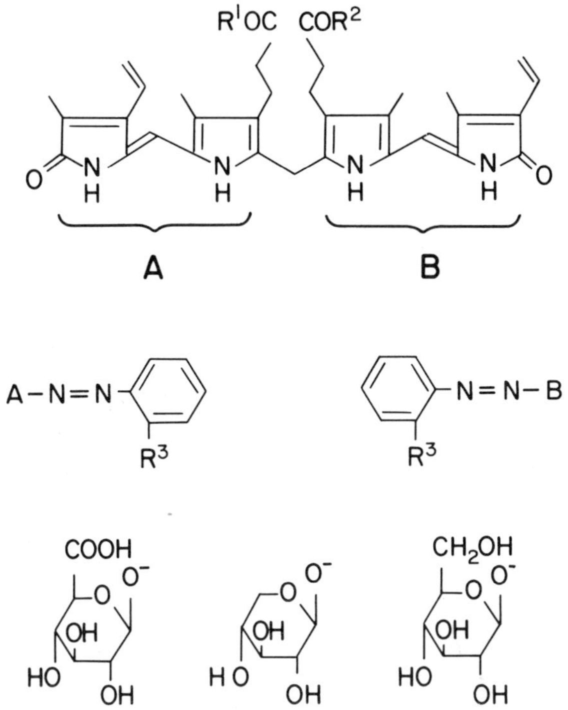

FIGURE 1. (a)Bilirubin-IXα (A-CH_2-B), -XIIIα (A-CH_2-A), and -IIIα (B-CH_2-B) (R^1 = R^2 = OH). (b)Dipyrrolic azo derivatives: phenylazo (R^3 = H); ethyl anthranilylazo (R^3 = CO_2Et). (c) Bilirubin-IXα mono- and di-β-slycosidic conjugates: R^1 and/or R^2 = one or two of sugar moieties shown. Azodipyrrole conjugates are formed by diazonium cleavage of tetrapyrrole conjugates.

glucuronides constitute the major part of compounds previously denoted as azo pigments β and γ.[31,32]

The presence in bile of "alkali-stable" noncarbohydrate conjugates of bilirubin remains controversial. Evidence adduced[35-37] in favor of the existence of a sulfate conjugate includes (1) chromatographic and optical-spectrum similarities between azo pigments supposedly derived from a natural bilirubin sulfate and those prepared from a synthetic bilirubin sulfate of unknown structure, and (2) observation of a 1:1 molar ratio between purified azo pigment and sulfate liberated from it by acid. However, final confirmation of bilirubin sulfate as a genuine conjugate still requires isolation at the tetrapyrrole stage and structure elucidation (mono- or diconjugate, site of attachment of sulfate group) of both synthetic and natural compounds.

Alkali-stability and, hence, covalent binding was demonstrated for an azodipyrrolic polypeptide conjugate isolated in trace amounts.[38] However, an amide bond may have been formed by aminolysis of sugar ester conjugates (e.g. by lysine ε-amino groups), occurring at the slightly alkaline pH of bile. This aminolysis reaction with proteins is suggested also by the increased proportion of "alkali-stable" bilirubin conjugates, observed when serum protein is added to bile or even to purified bilirubin glucuronides before alkaline hydrolysis.[39]

In summary, bilirubin occurs in bile as mono- and diester conjugates with various sugars. For rat and human bile, glucuronic acid is the main carbohydrate constituent, whereas bile of dogs and some other animal species also contains important quantities of glucose and xylose conjugates.

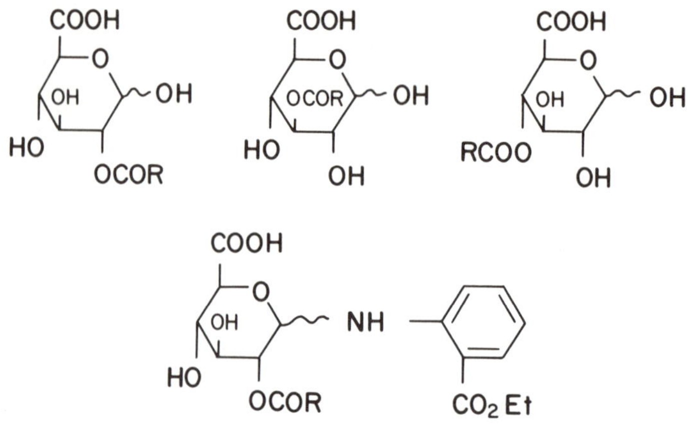

FIGURE 2. Bilirubin and azodipyrrole 2-, 3- and 4-*O*-acylglucuronides produced by sequential migration of 1-*O*-acyl group to positions 2, 3, and 4 of glucuronic acid (R = bilirubin or azodipyrrole moiety). The structure of an ethyl anthranilate *N*-glucuronide (azo pigment γ, R = azodipyrrole moiety) is also shown.

The following deals with the isolation and structural characterization of bilirubin carbohydrate conjugates, either as the native tetrapyrroles or as their dipyrrolic azo derivatives. Finally, various approaches to the chemical synthesis of bilirubin glucuronides are described.

II. ISOLATION OF BILIRUBIN CONJUGATES

A. General Conditions and Requirements for Isolation

In view of the heterogeneity and labile nature of bilirubin conjugates, several criteria should be satisfied for their successful analytical and preparative separation. Mineral acids, oxygen, and light must be excluded to prevent free-radical and acid-catalyzed disproportionation of bilirubin (Figure 1) and oxidative breakdown.[6] Protection against oxidation and disproportionation in neutral media is provided by low temperatures, ascorbic acid, and albumin.[6] Alkaline conditions (pH 7-9) promote rearrangement of 1-*O*-acyl *β*-glycosidic esters to positional isomers (Figure 2).[20,33] A pH region 4-6 appears to be optimal for storage of bile and for separations involving aqueous buffers.

Chromatographic techniques must provide adequate resolution for separation of xylose, glucose, and glucuronic acid conjugates of bilirubin, occurring as monoesters and as homogeneous and mixed diesters (Figure 1). An ideal system also would resolve the C-8 and C-12 positional isomers of monoconjugates. Obviously, other constituents of bile, e.g., bile acids and their conjugates, can interfere seriously with the separation of bilirubin conjugates and, for preparative purposes, are best removed in a preliminary step.

Older methods for separation of bilirubin conjugates have been reviewed by Brodersen and Jacobsen.[40]

B. Extraction and Precipitation Procedures

Partitioning between organic solvents, e.g., chloroform-methanol and ethyl acetate, and various aqueous buffers can be used to remove bile salts and to effect a partial separation of bilirubin mono- and diglucuronide.[41] Efficient extraction of bilirubin conjugates from acidified aqueous solutions (NaCl-saturated glycine buffer, pH 1.8, containing ascorbic acid) is obtained with chloroform-ethanol,[42] chloroform-isopropyl alcohol,[43,44] and butanol.[25] Ion pairs formed from bilirubin glucuronides and tetraheptylammonium chloride can be extracted with chloroform.[18]

Precipitation of bilirubin glucuronides is obtained (1) as the acids by acidifying bile with oxalic acid or as the sodium salt from acetone solution;[40,45] (2) by adding acetone[46] or acetone and $MgCl_2$[18,21] to bile; (3) as a cinchonidine adsorbate[46] and strychnine salt,[47] and (4) as Pb^{2+}, Ca^{2+}, Ba^{2+}, and Zn^{2+} salts from whole bile and as Pb^{2+} salts from aqueous solutions of purified bilirubin glucuronides.[41] Precipitation procedures are suitable for preliminary purification of large quantities of natural and synthetic bilirubin glucuronides while solvent partitioning is more convenient for small-scale prepurification.[41]

C. Chromatography: Reverse Phase, Gel Filtration, Gel Affinity, Thin-Layer and High-Performance Liquid Chromatography

Reverse phase column chromatography separates mono- and diconjugates of bilirubin[8,48] but does not remove bile salts completely. Disproportionation of bilirubins occurs during rotary evaporation of eluates and possibly also during rotary evaporation of ethanol-deproteinized bile before application to the column.

Gel chromatography on columns of Sephadex® LH-20 effects a partial separation of bilirubin mono- and diglucuronides[41,47] and is valuable for prepurification of bilirubin conjugates.[49] Bile salts, phospholipids, and cholesterol can also be removed by utilizing albumin-agarose gel affinity chromatography, yielding relatively large quantities of conjugated bilirubins.[50]

Speed and high resolving power validate TLC as a method of choice for analytical and semipreparative separation of bilirubin conjugates.[18,21-25,51] While whole bile can be applied directly to the plate,[23,52,53] prior removal of bile salts and phospholipids by extraction, precipitation, or column techniques (see above) gives rise to cleaner separations of the various mono- and homogeneous and mixed diconjugates of bilirubin. Remaining problems are associated with (1) the difficult elution of polar pigments from silica gel layers, necessitating use of methanol which also elutes part of the chromatographic support, and (2) partial disproportionation of bilirubins during chromatographic manipulations, particularly when the pigments are adsorbed to dry silica gel or when water-containing eluates are evaporated.

Impressive analytical separations were obtained recently by using HPLC, for xylose, glucose, and glucuronic acid conjugates of bilirubin including C-8 and C-12 positional isomers of the monoconjugates.[54,55] Reverse phase columns were utilized[55] with a linear gradient of aqueous buffer (pH 4.0) and acetonitrile as the mobile phase. It remains to be seen whether HPLC can be adapted to a preparative procedure and if so, whether pure bilirubin conjugates can be isolated from the aqueous eluates.

III. STRUCTURE ANALYSIS OF BILIRUBIN CONJUGATES

Structure analysis of conjugates as the azodipyrrole derivatives circumvents difficulties associated with the lability of bilirubin tetrapyrroles. Especially useful analytical results are provided by diazo treatment of individual bile pigment fractions,[18,21-25] since well-characterized azodipyrrolic conjugates, i.e., xylose, glucose and glucuronic acid esters, are readily available.[15,19,20]

A. Analysis of Free Sugars

Glucuronic acid, glucose and xylose are liberated by treatment of the conjugates with ammonia,[1,8,15,20] and by alkaline methanolysis.[13,14,17,18,21] The sugars were identified by using paper[8] and thin-layer chromatography,[1,15,20] anion-exchange chromatography of boric acid complexes,[15] proton nuclear magnetic resonance (NMR) spectrom-

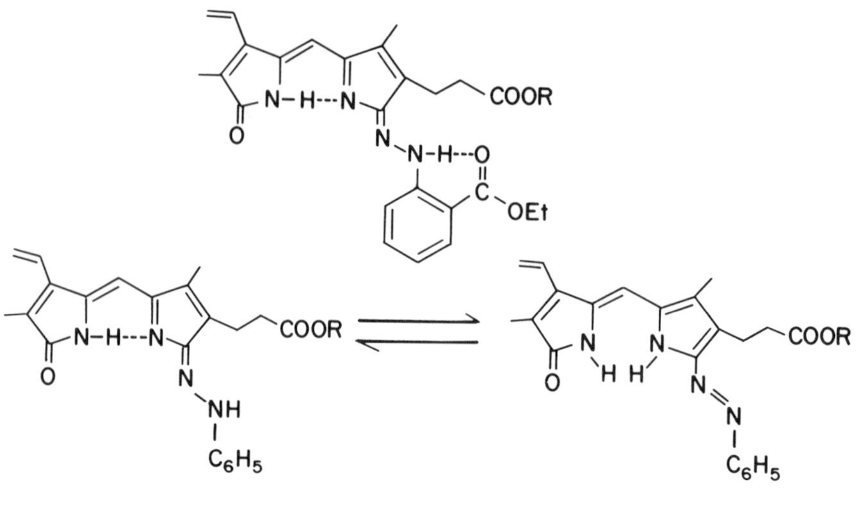

FIGURE 3. Hydrazone tautomeric structure for ethyl anthranilate azopigments, stabilized by internal hydrogen bridges. Tautomeric equilibrium between hydrazone and azobenzene forms is shown for aniline azopigments. Only the endo-vinyl isomers are shown. R = H, CH_3 or carbohydrate moiety.

etry[17,18,21] and gas chromatography and mass spectrometry of various derivatives, e.g., trimethylsilyl ethers.[17,18,20,21]

B. Analysis of Dipyrrolic Azo Derivatives

Diazo cleavage of the dissymmetric bilirubin-IXα molecule yields a pair of dipyrrolic azo pigments, i.e., the endo-vinyl and exo-vinyl isomers (Figure 1). As shown by ^{13}C NMR spectrometry,[56] the actual structure of ethyl anthranilate azo pigments corresponds to the hydrazone tautomer depicted in Figure 3. For aniline azo pigments, the chemical shift for C-9 indicated the existence of a 3:1 equilibrium mixture of hydrazone and azobenzene tautomers. The hydrogen-bridged structure (Figure 3) provides a rationale for chemical stability of ethyl anthranilate azo pigments, for decreased dependence[57] of the electronic spectrum on solvent and pH, and for lack of reactivity of the lactam function, e.g., towards silylation, when compared to aniline azo pigments.[34,56]

Four azo pigments are produced from bilirubin monoconjugates, which occur as a mixture of positional isomers with the carbohydrate ester moiety located at either the C-8 or C-12 propionic side chain. They correspond to the endo- and exo-vinyl isomeric pairs of unconjugated and conjugated azodipyrroles. Likewise, two isomers are formed from homogeneous diconjugates, and two pairs of isomers from mixed diconjugates.

While at first sight diazo cleavage of bilirubin conjugates merely multiplies the complexity of the analytical problem, in actual practice TLC pictures are much simplified. For instance, TLC of the native bilirubin conjugates from dog bile shows a multitude of yellow pigments, corresponding to various monoconjugates and homogeneous and mixed diconjugates.[18,21-25] By contrast, only four major azo pigments are observed, i.e., unconjugated azodipyrrole and the glucuronoside, glucoside, and xyloside. No separation of endo- and exo-vinyl isomers occurs at this stage.

For structural characterization by mass spectrometry, the isolated azodipyrrolic conjugates were converted to volatile derivatives, i.e., methyl esters (glucuronides only), acetates or trimethylsilyl ethers (Figure 4).[16,19,20] Charge stabilization by the azodipyrrole moiety gave rise to generally abundant molecular ions and characteristic electron-impact mass spectra.[16,19,20,34] Table 1 lists molecular ions for various derivatives.

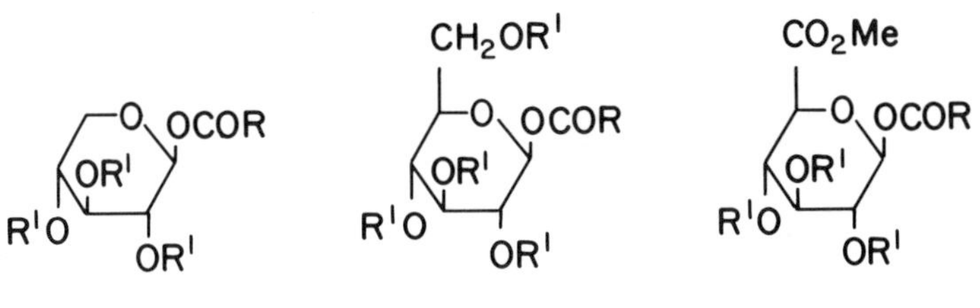

FIGURE 4. Derivatives of xylose, glucose and glucuronic acid conjugates of dipyrrolic azo pigments. R = azodipyrrole moiety, R^1 = Ac or Me_3Si.

Table 1
MOLECULAR IONS IN THE ELECTRON-IMPACT MASS SPECTRA OF AZODIPYRROLE CONJUGATES

	Acetates	Trimethylsilyl ethers
Azodipyrrole conjugates	M^+	M^+
Xyloside	720	810
Glucoside	792	912
Gluduronide methyl ester	778	868

The 1-*O*-acylglucuronide methyl ester also was characterized by field-desorption mass spectrometry and proton NMR spectrometry.[20] The field-desorption spectrum showed the molecular ion at m/e 652 and further $[M + K]^+$ and $[M + Na]^+$ ions resulting from cationization. The NMR-spectrum revealed the β-configuration for the glycosidic ester linkage, with $\delta = 5.45$ and $J_{1,2} = 7$ Hz for the anomeric proton.

Methyl ester formation and acetylation are also useful for further purification of azo pigments and for their identification on TLC by comparison with structurally known azo pigments at each stage of derivatization.[1] Methyl esters of the 1-, 2-, 3- and 4-*O*-acylglucuronides were separated completely, and observation of the same set of molecular ions after further acetylation (M^+ 778) or silylation (M^+ 868) provided a first clue to their structure elucidation as positional isomers.[20] Separation of endo- and exo-vinyl isomers was generally accomplished after acetylation,[1,16,20] and the isomeric azodipyrrole aglycones were identified as the previously[58] characterized methyl esters after alkaline methanolysis.

C. Site of Attachment of Sugar and Nature of Attaching Bond

Enzymic hydrolysis of azodipyrrole derivatives shows the β-C-1 attachment of the bilirubin ester group to the various carbohydrates.[1,15] Thus, the glucuronoside is hydrolyzed with β-glucuronidase, the glucoside with β-glucosidase (emulsin or Mylase-P) and the xyloside with Mylase-P. The β-glycosidic linkage was confirmed by NMR for the glucuronoside (see above).[20]

The C-1 attachment and the pyranose ring structure were demonstrated chemically by conversion of the acetates of conjugated azodipyrroles (Figure 4) to the known α-1-bromo derivatives and β-methyl glycosides by consecutive treatments with HBr-acetic acid and methanol-Ag_2CO_3.[1,16,20] No interconversion of furanoses and pyranoses was observed when suitable model compounds, i.e., acetylated pyranose and furanose derivatives of glucuronic acid, glucose, and xylose, were subjected to the same treatments.

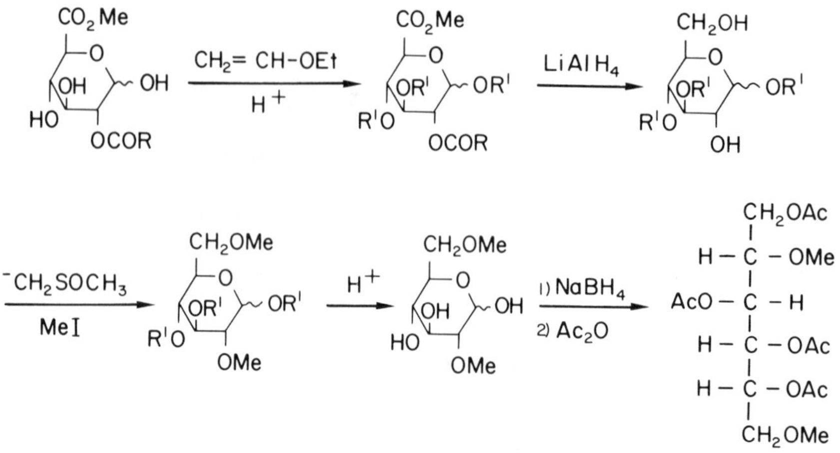

FIGURE 5. Procedure for replacement of labile azodipyrrole acyl group with stable methyl ether group, exemplified for 2-*O*-acylglucuronide. The final product, a 2,6-dimethyl alditol acetate, is suitable for mass spectral analysis (see Figure 6). R = azodipyrrole moiety, R_1 = CHMeOEt.

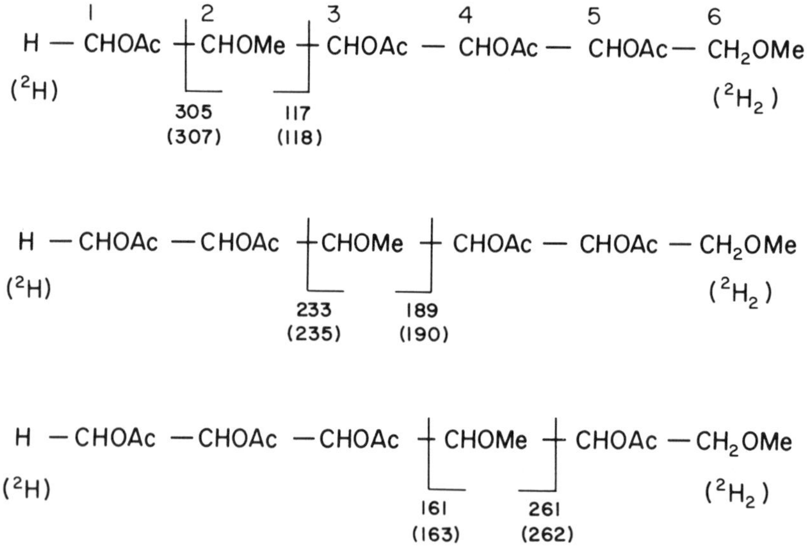

FIGURE 6. 2,6-Dimethyl, 3,6-dimethyl and 4,6-dimethyl alditol acetates produced from methyl esters of 2-, 3- and 4-*O*-acylglucuronides (see Figure 5). C-1 bears either ^1H or ^2H ($NaBH_4$ or NaB^2H_4), while C-6 bears either $^1H_2$ or $^2H_2$ ($LiAlH_4$ or $LiAl^2H_4$), removing any ambiguity in the assignment of structures from the mass spectral fragmentation.

Determining the site of attachment of the acyl group in rearranged azodipyrrole glucuronides represented a difficult analytical problem. The basic approach, exemplified for the 2-*O*-acylglucuronide in Figure 5, consisted of replacement of the labile acyl group with a stable methyl group and further chemical modification to derivatives suitable for mass spectral analysis.[20] Free hydroxyl groups were protected as the acetals with ethyl vinyl ether. Treatment with $LiAlH_4$ or $LiAl^2H_4$ removed the acyl group and reduced the C-6 carboxymethyl group. Methylation of the newly formed hydroxyl groups with dimsyl anion and MeI was followed by deprotection in acid medium, reduction with $NaBH_4$ or NaB^2H_4 to the alditols and acetylation.

In this way, 2,6-dimethyl-, 3,6-dimethyl-, and 4,6-dimethylalditol acetates were formed respectively from methyl esters of azodipyrrole 2-, 3-, and 4-*O*-acylglucuronides (Figure 6). Mass spectral analysis of the alditols was straightforward, as preferential cleavage occurs at carbon atoms bearing the charge stabilizing methoxy groups (Figure 6).

Although complex, this analytical procedure probably will find broader application, since a host of carboxylic acids, both endemic and drugs, are excreted as glucuronides. Not all of these are hydrolyzed with β-glucuronidase, as migration of the acyl group already can occur at the pH of biologic fluids.

D. Tetrapyrrole Analysis

Methods involving structure analysis at the tetrapyrrole stage of intact or sugar-protected bilirubin conjugates so far are not common practice. The usual procedure, as pointed out above, consists of their conversion to a pair of dipyrrolic azo pigments, following separation by TLC[18,21-25] or HPLC.[54,55] As structures of azodipyrrolic conjugates can be analyzed completely, including their isomeric status (see above), this method is acceptable, provided that no chromatographic overlap occurs between various bilirubin conjugates, which unfortunately is not always the case.

Another approach consists of methanolysis of bilirubin conjugates under mild alkaline conditions, followed by TLC or HPLC and structural analysis of bilirubin methyl esters.[14,59] An inherent advantage of this method, as compared to diazo cleavage, is a more certain differentiation between mono- and diconjugates of bilirubin, indentified as mono- and dimethyl esters, respectively. Further, conjugates of bilirubin-IXα, -IIIα and -XIIIα, resulting from disproportionation of bilirubin-IXα conjugates, can be detected and estimated as separate mono- and dimethyl esters. The methanolysis method has been used both for characterization of purified bilirubin conjugates[14,49] and for quantitation of mono and diester conjugates in whole bile and serum.[14,59]

IV. CHEMICAL SYNTHESIS OF BILIRUBIN CONJUGATES

A. Taurine, 1-Aminosugar, 2-, 3- and 4-*O*-Acylglucuronide, and Allyl-Protected 1-*O*-Acylglucuronide Conjugates of Bilirubin

Taurine conjugates of bilirubin were prepared by activation of the carboxyl groups with ethyl chloroformate and further reaction with taurine.[60]

$$R(COOH)_2 \xrightarrow[ClCO_2Et]{} R(COOCO_2Et)_2 \xrightarrow[H_2NCH_2SO_3^-Na^+]{} R(CONHCH_2SO_3^-Na^+)_2$$

The chromatographic and chemical properties were found to be similar to those of natural bilirubin conjugates.

Esterification of unprotected glucuronic acid with bilirubin di-imidazole yielded a mixture of positional isomers of bilirubin mono- and diglucuronides.[61] Probably 2-, 3- and 4-*O*-acylglucuronides were present, as no hydrolysis was observed with β-glucuronidase. The presence of α-1-*O*-acylglucuronides can be excluded on the basis that, if formed, they would undergo quick rearrangement to 2-*O*-acylglucuronides under the basic reaction conditions (see below).

1-Aminosugar conjugates of bilirubin were prepared by selective reaction of the amino group of 1-aminoxylose and 1-aminoglucose with bilirubin activated with diphenyl phosphorylazide.[62]

Allyl-protected glucuronides of bilirubin were prepared by esterification of allyl 2,3,4-tri-*O*-allyl D-glucopyranuronate with bilirubin di-imidazole.[63] However, removal

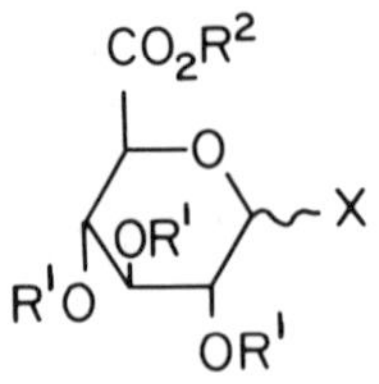

FIGURE 7. Synthesis of compound 6, an acetal protected derivative of glucuronic acid, as a mixture of diastereoisomers. *1*, R^1 = Ac, R^2 = Me, X = OAc *2*, R^1 = Ac, R^2 = Me, X = α-Br *3*, R^1 = Ac, R^2 = Me, X = β-$OCH_2C_6H_5$ *4*, R^1 = R^2 = H, X = β-$OCH_2C_6H_5$ *5*, R^1 = R^2 = -CHMeOEt, X = β-$OCH_2C_6H_5$ *6*, R^1 = R^2 = -CHMeOEt, X = OH.

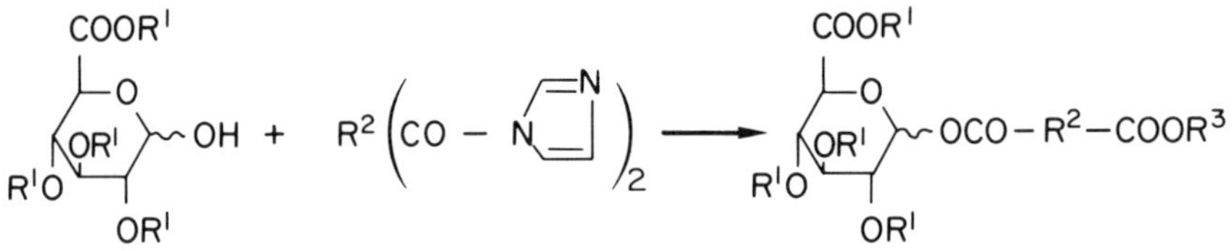

FIGURE 8. Esterification of bilirubin di-imidazole (R^2 = bilirubin residue) with compound *6* (R^1 = CHMeOEt) to form monoesters (R^3 = H) and diesters (R^3 = acetal protected glucuronic acid residue). Bilirubin esters are oxidized to biliverdins (R^2 = biliverdin residue), deprotected (R^1 = H, R^2 = biliverdin residue, R^3 = H or deprotected glucuronic acid residue) and reduced to the corresponding bilirubin glucuronides.

of the allyl protecting groups of either bilirubin or biliverdin esters [obtained by oxidation of bilirubin esters with 2,3-dichloro-5,6-dicyano-1,4-benzoquinone (DDQ)] with palladium on charcoal and dilute acid (0.02 *M* HCl in methanol-water) gave rise to degradation of the tetrapyrrole chromophore and/or adsorption of pigments to charcoal.

B. Synthesis of αβ-Glucuronides of Bilirubin[43,64]

An acetal-protected derivative of glucuronic acid (compound *6*, Figure 7) was prepared[64] from methyl tetra-*O*-acetyl-α or β-D-glucopyranuronate *1* via the α-1-bromosugar *2* and the β-benzyl glycoside *3*. Alkaline hydrolysis of ester groups, acetal protection with ethyl vinyl ether, and hydrogenolysis yielded compound 6 as a mixture of diastereoisomers (R^1 = CHMeOEt contains a chiral carbon atom).

Esterification of the 1-hydroxy acetal *6* with bilirubin di-imidazole gave a mixture of mono- and diesters (Figure 8).

Bilirubin di-imidazole + compound *6* ⟶ Bilirubin esters $\xrightarrow{\text{DDQ}}$ Biliverdin esters

$\xrightarrow{H^+}$ Biliverdin glucuronides $\xrightarrow{NaCNBH_3}$ Bilirubin glucuronides

At this stage, acid-catalyzed removal of acetal groups gave rise to disproportionation of bilirubins. Deprotection was carried out, therefore, on the corresponding biliverdin esters produced by oxidation with DDQ. Biliverdin mono- and diglucuronides were obtained as 1:1 anomeric mixtures with yields of 12% and 18%, respectively. Reduction of the biliverdin glucuronides to the corresponding bilirubin glucuronides was

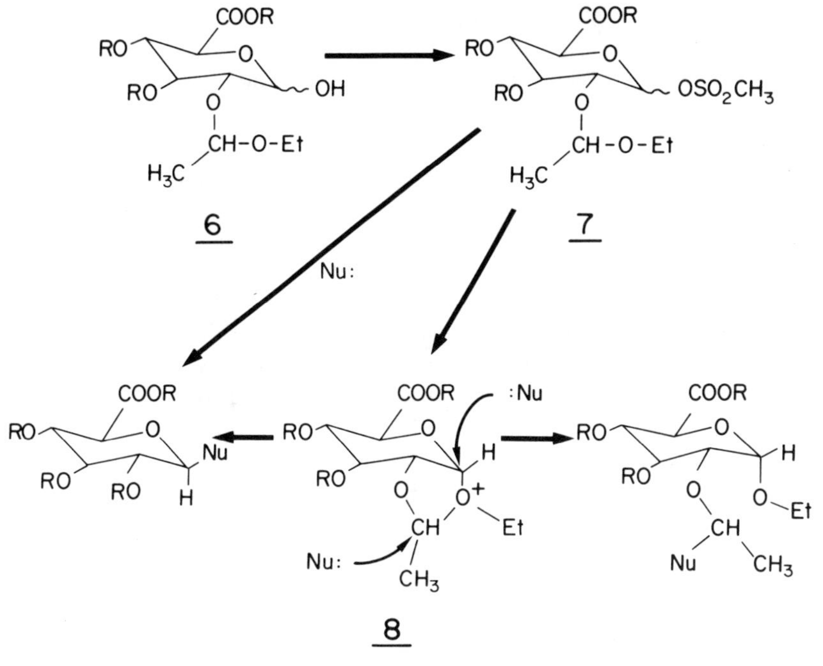

FIGURE 9. Suggested mechanism for formation of β-glucuronides. Compound *6* is converted to 1-*O*-mesylate 7. Displacement with various nucleophiles, i.e., OAc^-, MeOH and biliverdin di-anions proceeds either via S_N2 reaction or via intermediate *8*. β-Glycosides and α-ethyl glucoside are produced from intermediate *8*, whereas S_N2 reaction of the α-and β-anomers of mesylate *7* yields β- and α-glycosides respectively. R = CHMeOEt, Nu = nucleophile.

performed with $NaCNBH_3$ in propan-2-ol and acetic acid (9:1, v/v). Whereas TLC separation of anomers was possible for biliverdin and bilirubin monoglucuronides, the more complex mixture of diglucuronides (α,α; α,β; β,β) was not resolved.

In the proton NMR spectra of 1:1 anomeric mixtures of biliverdin mono- and diglucuronides signals for the anomeric protons were observed as doublets at δ 5.40 (β-form, $J_{1,2}$ = 7 Hz) and δ 5.98 (α-form, $J_{1,2}$ = 2.5 Hz).

Biliverdin mono-β-glucuronide was hydrolyzed completely with β-glucuronidase. The mono-α-glucuronide remained unchanged after treatment with enzyme at pH 5.2, but rearranged readily to biliverdin 2-*O*-acylglucuronide in unbuffered aqueous media (pH 6-7). Treatment of biliverdin di-αβ-glucuronides with β-glucuronidase gave a 1:2:1 mixture of, respectively, biliverdin and the mono- and di-α-glucuronides.

Reduction to the corresponding bilirubin glucuronides with $NaCNBH_3$ was shown to proceed without dipyrrole exchange, as no free bilirubin or diglucuronides were formed from bilirubin monoglucuronides. Solutions of bilirubin glucuronides were fairly stable when kept in propan-2-ol with small amounts of $NaCNBH_3$ and acetic acid. The reducing agent prevents oxidation to biliverdins and probably also inhibits radical-initiated disproportionation of bilirubins; acetic acid prevents formation of 2-*O*-acylglucuronides from the α-anomers.

Bilirubin mono- and diglucuronides were examined further as dipyrrolic azo pigments. The anomeric azodipyrrole glucuronides produced were separated by TLC as the methyl esters and analyzed by mass spectrometry of methyl ester trimethylsilyl ether derivatives. Molecular ions were observed at m/e 796 and 868, corresponding to introduction of two and three silyl groups.[34]

C. Specific Synthesis of β-Glucuronides of Bilirubin[44]

Production of 1:1 anomeric mixtures by direct esterification of compound 6 forms a major drawback of the former method, since the α- and β-anomers can be separated only for the monoglucuronides.

Transformation of compound *6* to a 1-*O*-mesylate *7* allows displacement of 1-OSO_2Me, a good leaving group, with carboxylate anions and other nucleophiles (Figure 9).[44] Enhanced formation of the β-anomers is expected for this displacement reaction, resulting from participation of the C-2 acetal oxygen at the C-1 carbonium ion site (structure *8*) in a way analogous to that observed for 2-*O*-acyl-1-bromosugars. Reaction of the mesylate with tetrabutylammonium acetate in dichloromethane yielded the β-1-*O*-acetate anomer only, as shown by subsequent removal of acetal groups, silylation, and GLC-mass spectral analysis. However, alternative attack of the nucleophile on the positive carbon atom of the C-2 acetal function (Figure 9) gave rise to formation of an acetal ester, which after deprotection yielded ethyl α-D-glucopyranuronoside as the major side product.

Thus, in dilute solution, formation of β-1-*O*-acylglucuronides involves either intermediate ion *8*, itself more readily produced from the β-mesylate, or direct S_N2 displacement of the α-mesylate. For higher concentrations and reactivities of the nucleophile, displacement of the β-mesylate also occurs, giving rise to formation of the α-1-*O*-acyl anomers. For example, use of a large excess of methanol as the nucleophile or working without solvent (see below) yielded 5 to 20% of the α-anomers.

Reaction of the tetrabutylammonium salt of biliverdin with the 1-*O*-mesylate was performed either in dichloromethane solution at 22°C or without solvent at 60°C. Esterification was nearly complete, as shown by TLC spots with polarities corresponding mainly to diesters and, to a lesser extent, monoesters. However, as for the model reactions, both 1-*O*-acyl and C-2 acetal esters were formed. Indeed, subsequent deprotection yielded mainly biliverdin and biliverdin monoglucuronide and a lesser amount of biliverdin diglucuronide.

TLC analysis and treatment with β-glucuronidase (see before) showed that exclusively the β-anomers were formed after reaction in dichloromethane. Yields of mono- and di-β-glucuronides were 6 and 1.5%, respectively. About 10 to 20% α-1-*O*-acyl anomers were detected when the esterification was performed without solvent. Yields of biliverdin mono- and diglucuronides were 15 and 6%.

Reduction to bilirubin glucuronides wth $NaCNBH_3$ was performed as described above. For isolation, acetic acid may be omitted from TLC solvents and during elution if no α-anomers are present.

V. CONCLUSION

Pure and well-characterized conjugates of bilirubin are needed for the study of hepatic transport and for elucidation of the enzymic mechanism of bilirubin conjugation, and further as reference materials for analysis of conjugated bilirubins. Whereas the present report shows that ester glycosides of bilirubin can be isolated, either from bile or by chemical synthesis, large-scale purification of the conjugates, preferably in the crystalline form, is a goal not yet achieved.

Synthesis of bilirubin glucuronides, radiolabeled in the sugar moieties, and also of bilirubin glucosides and xylosides and of conjugates involving other neutral sugars appears entirely feasible with the synthetic methods developed for bilirubin glucuronides.

REFERENCES

1. **Heirwegh, K. P. M., Fevery, J., Meuwissen, J. A. T. P., De Groote, J., Compernolle, F., Desmet, V., and Van Roy, F. P.,** Recent advances in the separation and analysis of diazopositive bile pigments, *Methods Biochem. Anal.,* 22, 205, 1974.
2. **Gordon, E. R.,** The conjugates of bilirubin, in *Jaundice,* Goresky, C. A. and Fisher, M. M., Eds., Plenum Press, New York, 1974, 19.
3. **Billing, B. H.,** Twenty-five years of progress in bilirubin metabolism (1952-77), *Gut,* 19, 481, 1978.
4. **Fevery, J., Blanckaert, N., De Groote, J., and Heirwegh, K. P. M.,** Bilirubin conjugates: formation and detection, *Progr. Liver Dis.,* 5, 183, 1976.
5. **Kuenzle, C. C.,** Bilirubin conjugates in bile, in *The Hepatobiliary System,* Taylor, W., Ed., Plenum Press, New York, 1976, 309.
6. **McDonagh, A. F.,** Bile pigments: bilatrienes and 5,15-biladienes, in *The Porphyrins,* Vol. 6, Dolphin, D., Ed., Academic Press, New York, 1978, 293.
7. **Schmid, R.,** Bilirubin metabolism: state of the art, *Gastroenterology,* 74, 70, 1978.
8. **Billing, B. H., Cole, P. G., and Lathe, G. H.,** The excretion of bilirubin as a diglucuronide giving the direct van den Bergh reaction, *Biochem. J.,* 65, 774, 1957.
9. **Schmid, R.,** The identification of direct-reacting bilirubin as bilirubin glucuronide, *J. Biol. Chem.,* 22, 881, 1957.
10. **Talafant, E.,** Properties and composition of the bile pigment giving a direct diazo reaction, *Nature (London),* 178, 312, 1956.
11. **Weber, A. P., Schalm, L., and Witmans, J.,** Bilirubin monoglucuronide (pigment I): a complex, *Acta Med. Scand.,* 173, 19, 1963.
12. **Jansen, F. H. and Billing, B. H.,** The identification of monoconjugates of bilirubin in bile as amide derivatives, *Biochem. J.,* 125, 917, 1971.
13. **Salmon, M., Fenselau, C., Cukier, J. O., and Odell, G. B.,** Rapid transesterification of bilirubin glucuronides in methanol, *Life Sci.,* 15, 2069, 1974.
14. **Blanckaert, N.,** Analysis of bilirubin and bilirubin mono- and diconjugates. Determinantion of their relative amounts in biological fluids, *Biochem. J.,* 185, 115, 1980.
15. **Fevery, J., Van Hees, G. P., Leroy, P., Compernolle, F., and Heirwegh, K. P. M.,** Excretion in dog bile of glucose and xylose conjugates of bilirubin, *Biochem. J.,* 125, 803, 197.
16. **Compernolle, F., Van Hees, G. P., Fevery, J., and Heiwegh, K. P. M.,** Mass spectrometric structure elucidation of dog bile azopigments as the acyl glucosides of glucopyranose and xylopyranose, *Biochem. J.,* 125, 811, 1971.
17. **Gordon, E. R., Dadoun, M., Goresky, C. A., Chan, T.-H., and Perlin, A. S.,** The isolation of an azobilirubin β-D-monoglucoside from dog gall-bladder bile, *Biochem. J.,* 143, 97, 1974.
18. **Gordon, E. R., Chan, T.-H., Samodai, K., and Goresky, C. A.,** The isolation and further characterization of the bilirubin tetrapyrroles in bile-containing human duodenal juice and dog gall-bladder bile, *Biochem. J.,* 167, 1, 1977.
19. **Compernolle, F., Jansen, F. H., and Heirwegh, K. P. M.,** Mass spectrometric study of the azopigments obtained from bile pigments with diazotized ethyl anthranilate, *Biochem. J.,* 120, 891, 1970.
20. **Compernolle, F., Van Hees, G. P., Blanckaert, N., and Heirwegh, K. P. M.,** Glucuronic acid conjugates of bilirubin-IXα in normal bile compared with post-obstructive bile. Transformation of the 1-*O*-acylglucuronide into 2-, 3- and 4-*O*-acylglucuronides, *Biochem. J.,* 171, 185, 1978.
21. **Gordon, E. R., Goresky, C. A., Chan, T.-H., and Perlin, A. S.,** The isolation and characterization of bilirubin diglucuronide, the major bilirubin conjugate in dog and human bile, *Biochem. J.,* 155, 477, 1976.
22. **Heirwegh, K. P. M., Fevery, J., Michiels, R., Van Hees, G. P. and Compernolle, F.,** Separation by thin-layer chromatography and structure elucidation of bilirubin conjugates isolated from dog bile, *Biochem. J.,* 145, 185, 1975.
23. **Noir, B. A.,** Bilirubin conjugates in bile of man, rat and dog. Semi-quantitative analysis of bile composition by thin-layer chromatography, *Biochem. J.,* 155, 365, 1976.
24. **Blumenthal, S. G., Taggart, D. B., Ikeda, R. M., Ruebner, B. H., and Bergstrom, D. E.,** Conjugated and unconjugated bilirubins in bile of humans and rhesus monkeys, *Biochem. J.,* 167, 535, 1977.
25. **Blumenthal, S. G., Taggart, D. B., Rasmussen, R. D., Ikeda, R. M., Ruebner, B. H., Bergstrom, D. E., and Hansen, F. W.,** Conjugated and unconjugated bilirubins in humans and rhesus monkeys. Structural identity of bilirubins from biles and meconiums of newborn humans and rhesus monkeys, *Biochem. J.,* 179, 537, 1979.
26. **Fevery, J., Van de Vijver, M., Michiels, R., and Heirwegh, K. P. M.,** Comparison in different species of biliary bilirubin-IXα conjugates with the activities of hepatic and renal bilirubin-IXα-uridine diphosphate glycosyl-transferases, *Biochem. J.,* 164, 737, 1977.

27. **Cornelius, C. E., Kelley, K. C., and Himes, J. A.,** Heterogeneity of bilirubin conjugates in several animal species, *Cornell Vet.*, 65, 90, 1975.
28. **Kuenzle, C. C.,** Bilirubin conjugates of human bile. Isolation of phenylazo derivatives of bile bilirubin, *Biochem. J.*, 119, 387, 1970.
29. **Kuenzle, C. C.,** Bilirubin conjugates of human bile. The excretion of bilirubin as the acyl glycosides of aldobiuronic acid, pseudoaldobiuronic acid and hexuronosylhexuronic acid, with a branched-chain hexuronic acid as one of the components of the hexuronosylhexuronide, *Biochem. J.*, 119, 411, 1970.
30. **Compernolle, F.,** Structure revision of disaccharidic conjugates of bilirubin-IXα in human bile and identification of phenylazo derivatives B_4, B_5 and B_6 as 2-, 3- and 4-*O*-acylglucuronides, *Biochem. J.*, 175, 1095, 1978.
31. **Heirwegh, K. P. M., Van Hees, G. P., Leroy, P., Van Roy, F. P., and Jansen, F. H.,** Heterogeneity of bile pigment conjugates as revealed by chromatography of their ethyl anthranilate azopigments, *Biochem. J.*, 120, 877, 1970.
32. **Fevery, J., Van Damme, B., Michiels, R., De Groote, J., and Heirwegh, K. P. M.,** Bilirubin conjugates in bile of man and rat in the normal state and in liver disease, *J. Clin. Invest.*, 51, 2482, 1972.
33. **Blanckaert, N., Compernolle, F., Leroy, P. M., Van Houtte, R., Fevery, J., and Heirwegh, K. P. M.,** The fate of bilirubin-IXα glucuronide in cholestasis and during storage *in vitro*. Intramolecular rearrangement to positional isomers of glucuronic acid, *Biochem. J.*, 171, 203, 1978.
34. **Compernolle, F., Van Hees, G. P., and Heirwegh, K. P. M.,** Rearranged glucuronic acid conjugates of bilirubin-IXα in post-obstructive bile. Structure elucidation of azopigments β and γ as ethyl anthranilate *N*-glycosides derived from 2-, 3- and 4-*O*-acyl glucuronides, *Biomed. Mass Spectrom.*, 5, 453, 1978.
35. **Isselbacher, K. J. and McCarthy, E. A.,** Studies on bilirubin sulfate and other nonglucuronide conjugates of bilirubin, *J. Clin. Invest.*, 38, 645, 1959.
36. **Noir, B. A., De Walz, A. T., and Rodriguez Garay, E. A.,** Studies on the bilirubin sulphate conjugate excreted in human bile, *Biochim. Biophys. Acta*, 222, 15, 1970.
37. **Noir, B. A. and Nanet, H.,** A study of the ethyl anthranilate azo derivatives of bilirubin sulphate. Confirmation of the existence of bilirubin sulfate conjugates in bile, *Biochim. Biophys. Acta*, 372, 230, 1974.
38. **Etter-Kjelsaas, H. and Kuenzle, C. C.,** A polypeptide conjugate of bilirubin from human bile, *Biochim. Biophys. Acta*, 400, 83, 1975.
39. **Weber, A. P. and Schalm, L.,** Evidence against "bilirubin sulphate", *Acta Med. Scand.*, 177, 519, 1965.
40. **Brodersen, R. and Jacobsen, J.,** Separation and determination of bile pigments, *Methods Biochem. Anal.*, 17, 3, 1969.
41. **Ostrow, J. D. and Murphy, N. H.,** Isolation and properties of conjugated bilirubin from bile, *Biochem. J.*, 120, 311, 1970.
42. **Fevery, J.,** unpublished data, 1980.
43. **Compernolle, F.,** Synthesis of biliverdin and bilirubin glucuronides, *FEBS Lett.*, 114, 17, 1980.
44. **Compernolle, F.,** Synthesis of biliverdin and bilirubin 1-*O*-acyl-β-D-glucopyranuronic acids, *Biochem. J.*, 187, 857, 1980.
45. **Lucassen, J.,** The Diazo-Reaction of Bilirubin and Bilirubin Diglucuronide, Ph.D. thesis, University of Utrecht, Keminck and Zoon, Utrecht, 1961.
46. **Talafant, E. and Appelt, J.,** Preparation of bilirubin-diglucuronide concentrates from dog bladder bile, *Clin. Chem.*, 14, 208, 1968.
47. **Jacobsen, J.,** A chromatographic separation of bilirubin glucuronides from human bile, *Acta. Chem. Scand.*, 23, 3023, 1969.
48. **Cole, P. G., Lathe, G. H., and Billing, B. H.,** Separation of the bile pigments of serum, bile and urine, *Biochem. J.*, 57, 514, 1954.
49. **Blanckaert, N., Gollan, J., and Schmid, R.,** Bilirubin diglucuronide synthesis by a UDP-glucuronic acid-dependent enzyme system in rat liver microsomes, *Proc. Natl. Acad. Sci. USA*, 76, 2037, 1979.
50. **Wolkoff, A. W., Scharschmidt, B. F., Plotz, P. H., and Berk, P. D.,** Purification of conjugated bilirubin: a new approach utilizing albumin-agarose gel affinity chromatography, *Proc. Soc. Exp. Biol. Med.*, 152, 20, 1976.
51. **Tenhunen, R.,** Studies on bilirubin and its metabolism, *Ann. Med. Exp. Biol. Fenn.*, 43 (Suppl. 6), 1, 1965.
52. **Thompson, R. P. H. and Hofmann, A. F.,** Separation of bilirubin and its conjugates by thin layer chromatography, *Clin. Chim. Acta*, 35, 517, 1971.
53. **Thompson, R. P. H. and Hofmann, A. F.,** Free and conjugated bile pigments of body fluids: qualitative analysis by thin-layer chromatography, *J. Lab. Clin. Med.*, 82, 483, 1973.
54. **Lim, C. K.,** The separation of conjugated and unconjugated bilirubin in bile by high-performance liquid chromatography, *J. Liq. Chromatog.*, 2, 37, 1979.

55. **Onishi, S., Itoh, S., Itoh, S., Kawade, N., Isobe, K., and Sugiyama, S.,** An accurate and sensitive analysis by high-pressure liquid chromatography of conjugated and unconjugated bilirubin-IXα in various biological fluids, *Biochem. J.,* 185, 281, 1980.
56. **Compernolle, F., Hutchinson, D. W., and Toppet, S.,** Tautomerism of azopigments derived from bilirubin, *Tetrahedron,* 36, 2237, 1980.
57. **Jirsa, M. and Jirsova, V.,** Spectrophotometric behavior of azobilirubin and azotaurobilirubin, *Clin. Chem.,* 5, 532, 1959.
58. **Jansen, F. H. and Stoll, M. S.,** Separation and structural analysis of vinyl- and isovinyl-azobilirubin derivatives, *Biochem. J.,* 125, 585, 1971.
59. **Blanckaert, N., Kabra, P. M., Farina, F. A., Stafford, B. E., Marton, L. J., and Schmid, R.,** Measurement of bilirubin and its mono- and diconjugates in human serum by alkaline methanolysis and high-performance liquid chromatography, *J. Lab. Clin. Med.,* 96, 198, 1980.
60. **Jirsa, M. and Vecerek, B.,** Neue Bilirubinderivate. I. Ihr Vergleich met Gallen- und Serum-Bilirubin, *Hoppe-Sevler's Z. Physiol. Chem.,* 311, 87, 1958.
61. **Thompson, R. P. H. and Hofmann, A. F.,** Chemical synthesis of bilirubin glucuronide conjugates, *Biochim. Biophys. Acta,* 451, 267, 1976.
62. **Hancock, F. E., Hutchinson, D. W., and Knell, A. J.,** Synthetic conjugates of bilirubin, *Biochem. Soc. Trans.,* 4, 303, 1976.
63. **Compernolle, F.,** Preparation of allyl 2,3,4-tri-*O*-allyl-D-glucopyranuronate and of 1-*O*-acyl-D-glucopyranuronic acids. Attempted synthesis of bilirubin glucuronides, *Carbohydr. Res.,* 86, 177, 1980.
64. **Compernolle, F.,** Preparation of α-ethoxyethyl-protected D-glucopyranuronic acid having HO-1 unsubstituted, *Carbohydr. Res.,* 83, 135, 1980.

Chapter 3

PHYSICAL CHEMISTRY OF BILIRUBIN: BINDING TO MACROMOLECULES AND MEMBRANES

Rolf Brodersen

TABLE OF CONTENTS

I. PROPERTIES OF BILIRUBIN ACID*

A. Solubility

1. Solubility in Water

Bilirubin isomers vary considerably with respect to solubility of the acids in water. The main isomer, bilirubin-IXα (Z,Z), is nearly insoluble in water at pH-values below 7 (Figure 1).[1,2] IIIα(Z,Z) and XIIIα(Z,Z) isomers are likewise insoluble while non-α isomers and the photobilirubins (E,Z and E,E) are more soluble. Only α-isomers with undissociated carboxyl groups, containing the (Z,Z) configuration, are capable of forming a complete pattern of intramolecular hydrogen bonds, saturating all affinities for water (Figure 5, bottom) and are insoluble. In non-α isomers, the carboxyl groups are located differently, relative to the lactam groups and pyrrole nitrogen atoms and this is also the case in photoisomers where the outer rings have been turned, forming E-configurations. All these have one or several hydrophilic moieties available for binding of water and are water soluble, even in acid solution.

The insolubility of bilirubin-IXα(Z,Z) acid is important for the toxic properties of bilirubin,[4] (This topic has been reviewed[5,6]). This chapter deals exclusively with the main component, bilirubin IXα(Z,Z) which is the toxic species, and this isomer is signified when no particular structure is mentioned.

The solubility of bilirubin acid as such in water is too low for direct measurement. Since, however, the disodium salt is soluble, and since a small amount of the acid must be present in equilibrium with the dianion, the acid must be soluble to some extent. The solubility can be calculated from measurements of bilirubin solubilities in alkaline buffers when the acid dissociation constants and the state of dispersion of the anion are known. The solubility of bilirubin acid in alkaline, aqueous media is described as a function of pH by Equation 6 (Section II.D) for n = 1. The measured solubility at pH 8.5, where the precision of the determination is best, is 0.60 μM.[2] The mean pK of the two carboxyl groups is 4.4. When these values are entered in Equation 6 we obtain the solubility of the bilirubin acid as 4×10^{-15} M at 37°C.

Colloid suspensions of bilirubin acid are readily formed by neutralization of alkaline solutions of the disodium salt. If the alkaline bilirubin solution is fairly concentrated, 0.1 mM or more, and is neutralized to pH 7, colloid aggregation of the acid can be observed by an immediate rise of light scattering to high values, indicating formation of large particles. The light absorption spectrum shows a slight, immediate loss of intensity, followed during several minutes or hours by a more marked decrease of the peak at 440 nm and an increase of absorption at 500 nm (Figure 2). Electron microscopy of the suspension reveals irregular granules, rods, and sheets.[7] The suspension is

* The term bilirubin acid is used to indicate the undissociated form.

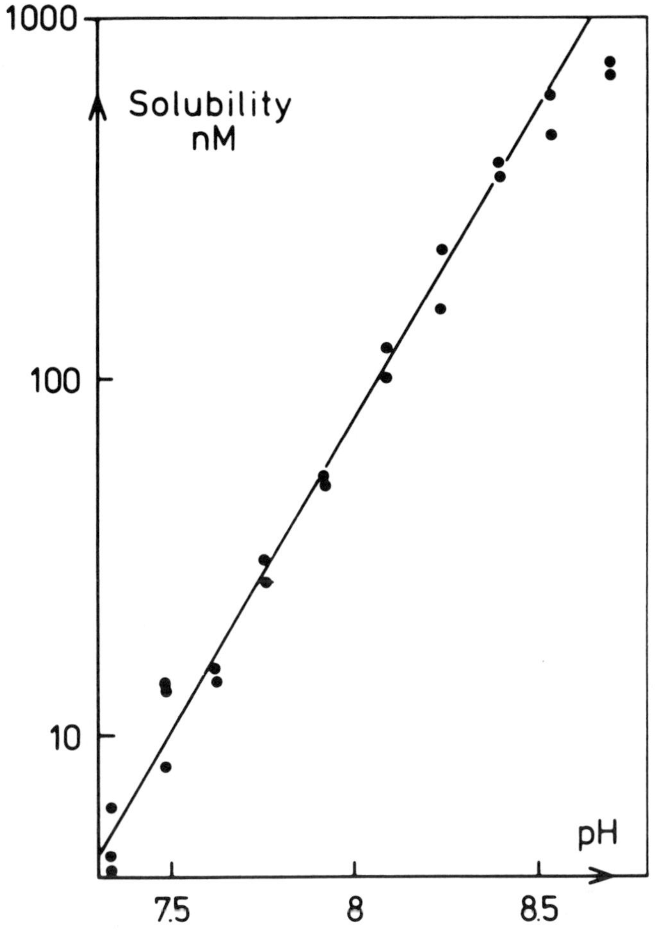

FIGURE 1. Solubility of crystalline bilirubin-IXα(Z,Z), purified according to McDonagh and Assisi,[3] in aqueous buffers (tris-NaCl, constant ionic strength, 0.15 *M*), as a function of pH. Temperature 37°C. (From Brodersen, R., *J. Biol. Chem.*, 254, 2364, 1979. With permission.)

unstable and solid bilirubin acid precipitates after several hours or days, leaving a colorless solution. Stable micelles of uniform size and shape are not formed.

2. Solubility in Organic Solvents

The solubility of bilirubin acid in several solvents has been measured (Figure 3).[2] The solubility in apolar media, such as *n*-hexane, is low, less than 1 μM, and generally increases with solvent polarity, to more than 10 m*M* in dimethylsulfoxide (DMSO). Aromatic hydrocarbons (benzene) are better solvents than the aliphatic, and an asymmetric structure seems to promote dissolution (toluene, xylene). Pyrrole and pyridine, which are asymmetric aromatic and polar, are good solvents. Dichloromethane and chloroform are asymmetric and are better solvents than carbon tetrachloride. Aliphatic alcohols do not dissolve bilirubin acid, indicating that ability to form hydrogen bonds is not sufficient. Acetone, on the other hand, dissolves some bilirubin, and here again the asymmetric ketones are better solvents. It is interesting to note that increasing chain length does not increase solubility, as illustrated by di-isobutyl ketone which dissolves less bilirubin than methyl isobutyl ketone or acetone. Also, ethyl acetate is a better

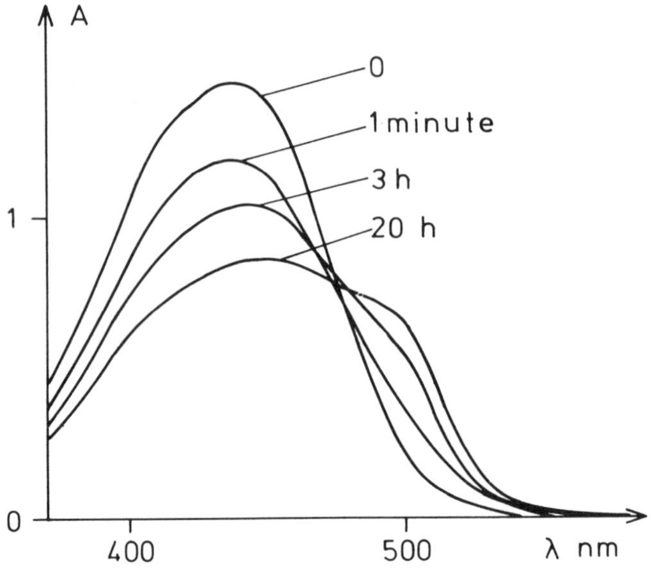

FIGURE 2. Light absorption spectra of a bilirubin solution during colloid aggregation of bilirubin acid. An alkaline solution of bilirubin was diluted with phosphate buffer to a final bilirubin concentration 0.8 m*M*, pH 7.4. After varying intervals of time, as indicated, aliquots of the reaction mixture were diluted with the same buffer to bilirubin concentration 26 μM, and spectra were recorded in 1-cm cells.

solvent than long-chain esters, olive oil and lard, which in fact dissolve very little bilirubin.

It is noteworthy that the pattern of solubility is essentially different from that observed with lipophilic substances which dissolve in hexane, ether, and olive oil but not in formamide and DMSO. The solubility profile is that of a polar aromatic substance. Numerous textbooks and review articles rate bilirubin as lipophilic and this character has been used to explain its neurotoxic properties. The misconception seems to have originated from the fact that bilirubin forms complexes with polar lipids. These complexes are soluble in ether. Formation of phospholipid-bilirubin complexes seems to be the basis for binding of bilirubin to lipid membranes in tissues. Also, adipose tissues are stained intensely yellow after administration of large doses of bilirubin to experimental animals. The pigment is, however, bound to membranes in the tissue and is not dissolved in the fat. Larger amounts of bilirubin are taken up by liver and skin. Deposition in fat has attracted the attention of observers, due to the translucent and colorless character of this tissue. Furthermore, a glance at the bilirubin formula shows a substance with two carboxyl groups, four pyrrole nitrogen atoms, and two C = O groups, capable of forming hydrogen bonds, compared with few and small hydrocarbon moieties, rather appearing like a polar and water soluble molecule. Formation of intramolecular hydrogen bonds in bilirubin-IXα(Z,Z) acid renders the molecule insoluble in water but does not make it lipophilic.

A final word should be added on inhomogeneity of solid bilirubin. Studies of the solubility in methyl isobutyl ketone, with varying ratios of bilirubin to solvent, have demonstrated that different forms of solid bilirubin exist with different solubilities.[2] It is also well known that freshly acid precipitated bilirubin dissolves readily in chloroform while preparations which have been kept for several years dissolve only after prolonged boiling.[8,9] Once dissolved, spectroscopic and other properties are identical.

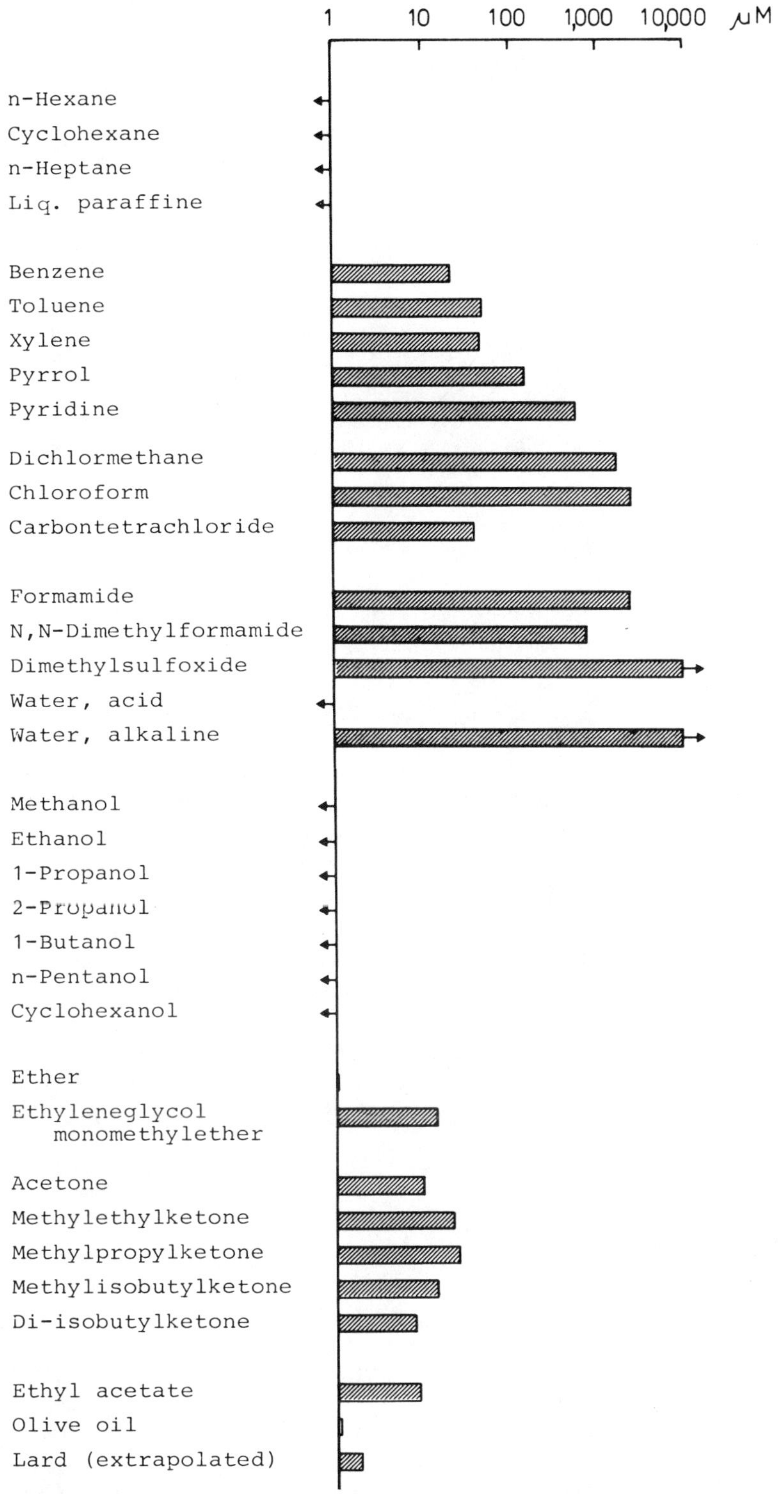

FIGURE 3. Approximate solubilities of bilirubin in organic solvents, temperature 25°C. Ten micromoles of crystalline bilirubin-IXα(Z,Z), purified according to McDonagh and Assisi,[3] was equilibrated with 1 mℓ of each solvent.

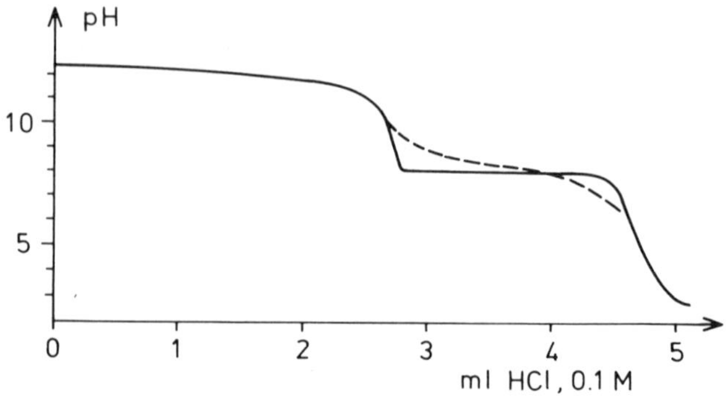

FIGURE 4. Acidimetric titration of bilirubin-IXα(Z,Z). Purified bilirubin was dissolved in an excess of sodium hydroxide and titrated with hydrochloric acid. The pH values obtained are shown by the full line. Colloid aggregation of bilirubin acid begins when pH = 8 is reached. This curve has been misinterpreted by some authors as indicating a pK value about 8. A calculated titration curve for a soluble acid, having pK = 8, is therefore shown in broken line.

All data on solubility should therefore be taken as provisional until knowledge can be obtained of different crystal modifications and solid states of bilirubin.

B. Acidity

1. Titration Curves

The pH titration of bilirubin dissolved in aqueous sodium hydroxide solution gives the curve shown in Figure 4. An apparent buffering effect is seen around pH 8 and a pK-value of 7-8 has accordingly been reported by some authors.[10,11] Other workers have adopted values around pH 5, more in agreement with the chemical structure of the carboxyl groups,[1] and this view has been confirmed by more detailed studies from several groups.[12-15] The originally published pK, about 8, has been maintained by many authors. An analysis of the titration curve, Figure 4, will accordingly be given here.

The shape of the curve is anomalous. Titration of a soluble acid with pK = 8 should give a curve as shown by the broken line. Measurement of light scattering shows furthermore an abrupt increase when pH 8 is reached, at the point of the sharp bend of the pH curve, indicating that insoluble aggregates of bilirubin acid are being formed. The process involved is therefore not only that of a simple pH titration,

$$\text{Bilirubin}^{2-} + 2H^{+} \rightleftharpoons \text{Bilirubin acid} \qquad (1)$$

but is followed by a second process,

$$\underset{\text{(dissolved)}}{\text{Bilirubin acid}} \rightleftharpoons \underset{\text{(solid)}}{\text{Bilirubin acid}} \qquad (2)$$

By definition, pK is the negative logarithm of the equilibrium constant of the process in Equation 1 (or rather of each of the two equilibrium constants involved, since two protons are taken up). The numerical value of pK cannot be read from the complex titration curve shown in Figure 4.[16] The use of an "apparent" or "practical" pK around 8 should be avoided, because variable figures are obtained, ranging from 7 to 8, depending upon bilirubin concentration in the titration and upon varying speed of acid addition. Furthermore, an entirely different value of "pK" is obtained if the titration is conducted in the opposite direction, with a suspension of bilirubin acid being titrated with sodium hydroxide solution, when "pK"-values as high as 10 may result.

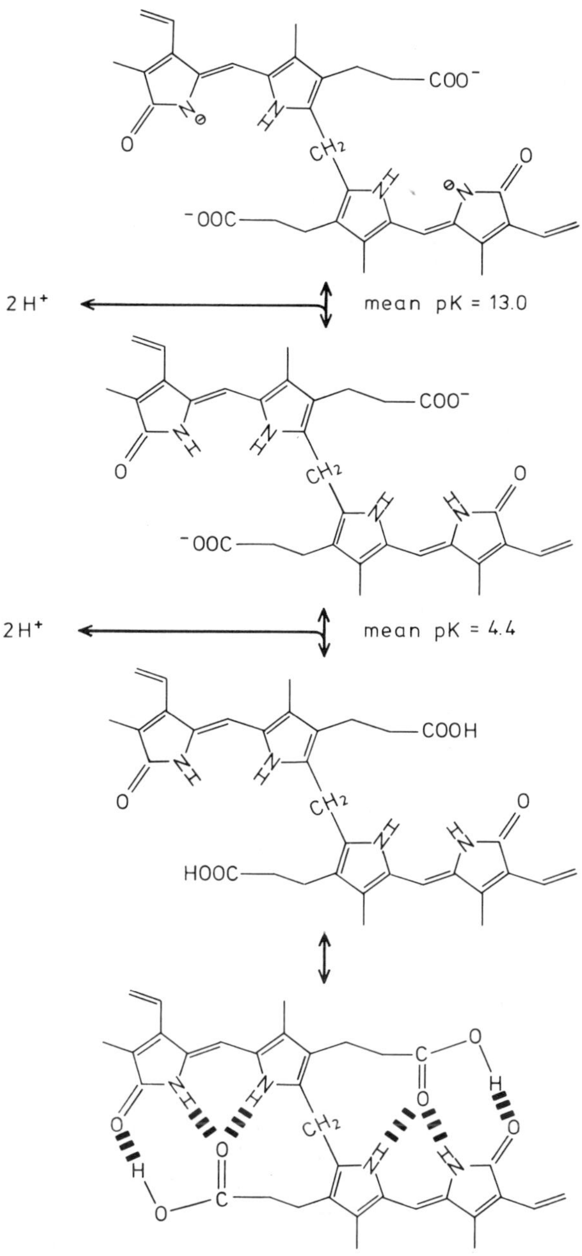

FIGURE 5. Acid dissociation of bilirubin-IXα(Z,Z). The acidic groups were identified by Hansen et al.,[15] using ^{13}C NMR spectrometry, and pK values were determined by electrometric titration in dimethylsulfoxide and transformed into values for aqueous media by means of the Born equation. The intramolecularly hydrogen bonded acid is shown at the bottom. Two carboxyl protons are dissociated, through formation of a hypothetical, open conformation of the molecule. The equilibrium of the hydrogen bonded species with the dianion has a mean pK = 4.4. The dianion is found in neutral and alkaline solutions of bilirubin in aqueous media. In strongly alkaline media, two further protons are dissociated with a mean pK = 13.0.

Bilirubin, besides being an acid, is a weak base, as seen from the fact that it forms a red cation with light absorption maximum at 512 to 517 nm.[12,16-19] The basicity is too weak to be evident from ordinary pH titration in aqueous medium and the corresponding pK-value has not been determined.

2. *Identity of Acidic Groups*

According to the chemical structure, bilirubin acid should have four acidic groups, two carboxylic and two lactam. Titration of bilirubin acid in DMSO with potassium hydroxide shows that four protons can indeed be titrated, two by two.[15] In water, the presence of two acidic protons with pK less than 7, and at least one additional proton with a high pK, about 12.9, could be demonstrated by electrometric and spectrophotometric titration.[15,20] Complete assignment of ^{13}C nuclear magnetic resonance (NMR) spectra at different steps of the titration in DMSO[15] showed that the two carboxyls dissociate first, and the two lactams at higher pH, as seen in Figure 5.

3. *Dissociation Constants*

Accurate determination of pK-values of bilirubin cannot be based on determinations in aqueous media, due to insolubility of the acid and instability of the tetraanion. Electrometric titration in DMSO[15] gives normally shaped curves and indicates that the two carboxyl groups have nearly identical pK's, and likewise the two lactams. This result at first seemed surprising since it was expected that the mono-anion would dissociate less readily than the uncharged acid and the trianion less readily than the dianion. On the other hand, the two carboxyl groups may be located with a fairly long distance between them, approximately as in an aliphatic dicarboxylic acid with eleven carbon atoms which, in fact, has nearly identical pK values of the two protons. Also the lactams are situated far apart in the molecule.

Numerical values of the four pK's were obtained in DMSO by cotitration with standard acids and values in water were calculated from the Born equation,[21] considering the ionic radii of the species involved, and the dielectric constants of the two media. This procedure involves an unknown degree of approximation but has in many cases given satisfactory values for soluble acids, when the pK's could be determined by titration in water. The mean pK for the two carboxyls is thus found to be 4.4, and for the two lactams 13.0, the latter value in agreement with that found by titration in water.

C. Spectroscopic Properties

Light absorption spectra of bilirubin-IXα(Z,Z) acid, dissolved in organic solvents, show two maxima, one weak band at about 290 nm and another, intense maximum at 450 to 460 nm. The former has not been studied in detail while the latter, discovered by Heilmeyer in 1931,[22] has attracted more attention due to its complex nature and variability. Spectra of non-α isomers of bilirubin, and of the dimethyl ester of bilirubin-IXα(Z,Z) in dimethylformamide solution (Figure 6), show similar maxima although the main peak is located at shorter wavelengths, 390 to 410 nm.[23] The different shape of the spectra of the isomers may partly be explained by the different extent and shape of the chromophores (see Figure 4 in Chapter 1). The particular location of the main peak of the α-pigment at a long wavelength may be related to formation of intramolecular hydrogen bonds between the carboxyl groups and lactam moieties in the nonneighboring terminal pyrrole rings.[23] This pattern of hydrogen bonds is disturbed by dimethyl esterification and the main peaks of the dimethyl ester spectra of the four isomers are accordingly more similar and are located at shorter wavelengths.

Each of the main peaks of the spectra shown in Figure 6 is composed of at least two symmetric Gaussian curves (when drawn with wave numbers as the abscissa). This splitting of the maximum cannot be explained solely by structural differences of the

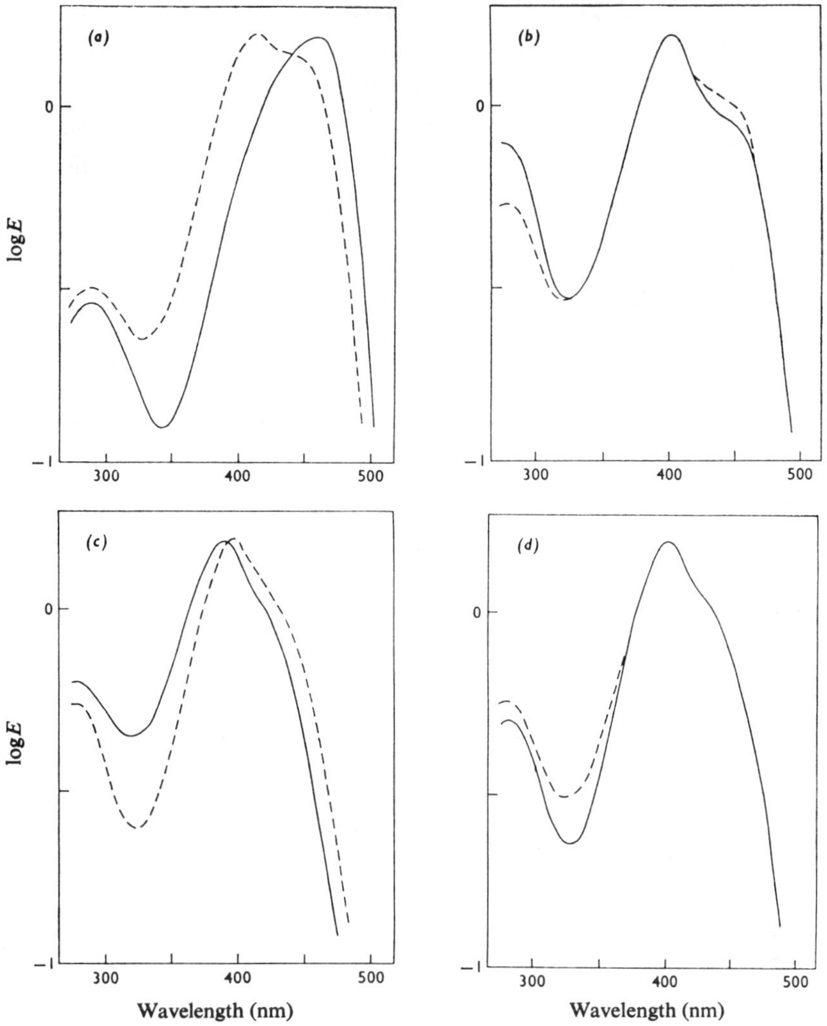

FIGURE 6. Light absorption spectra (logarithmic ordinates) of bilirubin-IX isomers, α, β, γ, and δ, in dimethylformamide, shown in (*a*), (*b*), (*c*), and (*d*), respectively. Spectra of the acids are drawn in full line, and spectra of their dimethyl esters are stippled. (From Blanckaert, N., Heirwegh, K. P. M., and Compernolle, F., *Biochem. J.*, 155, 405, 1976. With permission.)

two dipyrrolic chromophores present in each bilirubin molecule since a similar splitting is seen in the spectra of bilirubin-IIIα and -XIIIα in which the two chromophores are identical. Also the fact that the splitting is absent, or nearly so, in the spectrum of bilirubin-IXα disodium salt in alkaline, aqueous solution argues against this possibility. Blauer and coworkers,[24] after extensive studies of light absorption and circular dichroism (CD) spectra of bilirubin-albumin complexes explain the splitting of the main absorption band by intramolecular coupling between electric transition dipoles of the two chromophores leading to exciton splitting (Section III.A.6).

Bilirubin-1Xα(Z,Z) acid, dissolved in chloroform, has light absorption maximum at 460 nm and a molar absorption coefficient close to 60,000 M^{-1} cm^{-1}.

II. PROPERTIES OF BILIRUBIN SALTS

A. Metal Complexes

An insoluble complex salt with calcium, obtained by precipitation from an alkaline bilirubin solution, contains two molecules of bilirubin per atom of calcium.[25] This complex is a component of some gall stones.[26,27] A possible role of bilirubin in lowering the level of ionized calcium in blood plasma of highly icteric infants has recently been suggested by Chan et al.[28] The thermodynamic conditions for formation of the calcium-bilirubin complex have not been investigated further in spite of the possible biological importance of this process.

Other metal complexes have been described by several investigators.[9,13,14,29-32] This field has not received the attention it may deserve, considering the potential biological role of bilirubin-metal complexes.

The disodium salt of bilirubin is soluble in water, to more than 10 m*M* although the solubility is considerably less at high sodium ion concentrations, as expected. Properties of dissolved sodium salt are described below.

B. Stability of Bilirubin Disodium Salt Solutions

Bilirubin acid readily dissolves in diluted sodium hydroxide solutions. The resultant aqueous solution of bilirubin disodium salt undergoes chemical changes, due to oxidation, dipyrrole exchange, and photoisomerization. Light, as well as traces of transition and other metal ions, seems to promote oxidation. Addition of ascorbic acid[33] or EDTA[9] has been recommended to stabilize the solution. Also, a concentrated solution is said to undergo relatively less decomposition than one of low bilirubin concentration. Some investigators deaerate the aqueous medium.[34] On the other hand, a dilute solution of bilirubin, 25 μM, in 1 m*M* sodium hydroxide, kept at room temperature under orange light without any other precautions, showed a good stability with maximal light absorption declining 5% in 3 hr.[2] Similarly, bilirubin solutions, 170 μM in 2 m*M* NaOH, kept at 0 to 5°C, showed no significant change of light absorption during 6 hr.[24]

C. Light Absorption Spectra of Dilute Solutions

Dilute solutions of bilirubin disodium salt in alkaline, aqueous media have light absorption maximum around 430 to 440 nm, depending upon buffer composition and temperature.[34] The molar absorption coefficient at maximum has been reported from 4.7 to $5.2 \times 10^4 M^{-1}$ cm^{-1} by several investigators.[16,24,34]

The spectrum is constant with pH varying from 8 to 12 (apart from minor variations due to changes of buffer composition). At low concentrations of bilirubin, from about 20 n*M*, which is the practical lower limit for spectroscopic recording, to an upper limit between 1 and 10 μM, the spectrum remains constant when normalized to one concentration (Figure 7). This spectrum is probably that of the monomeric bilirubin dianion, as discussed in the following section.

According to Blauer et al.[24] the bilirubin anion spectrum may be represented as one, symmetric Gaussian curve or two curves showing a splitting of 10 nm, or less. A 10-nm exciton splitting would be achieved if the transition moments of the two chromophores are parallel and located within a distance of 9 to 10 Å. (The reader is referred to the original publication for details of the calculation). Although the actual position of the transition moments for bilirubin is so far unknown, they would probably be closer than 10 Å if the bilirubin molecule is in a flat, porphyrin-like conformation and a larger splitting of the light absorption maximum would thus be seen. The largest possible distance between the chromophores of bilirubin is achieved in the extended conformation, obtained by rotation of the dipyrromethene chromophores around the

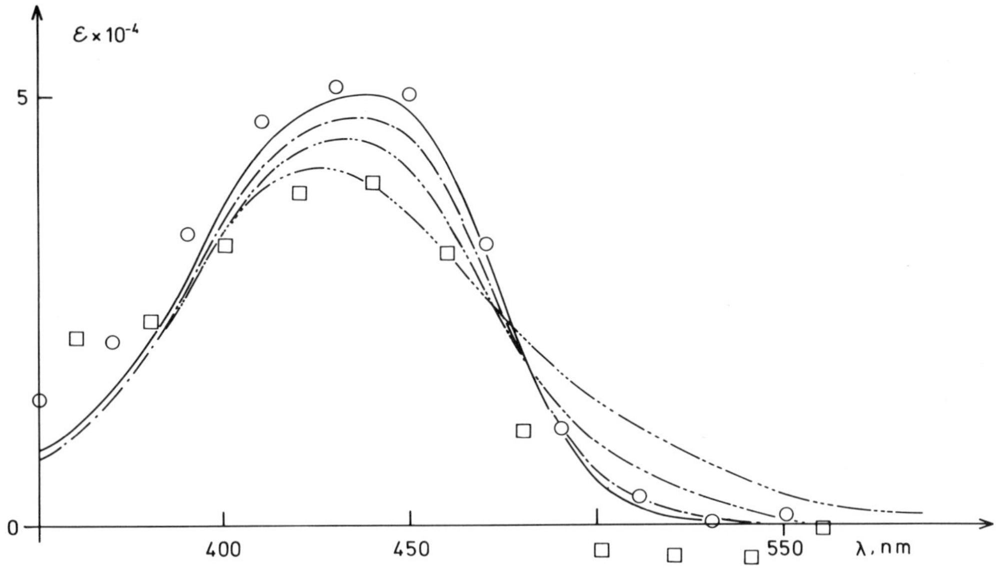

FIGURE 7. Light absorption spectra of bilirubin-IXα(Z,Z) disodium salt in aqueous solution, pH = 10.0, temperature 25°C, with *varying bilirubin concentration:* □, 20 n*M*; ○ 100 n*M*; ——— , 1 μ*M*;—·—, 10 μ*M*;—· ·—, 100 μ*M*; —· · ·—, 1 m*M* Optical cell length varied from 10 to 0.02 cm. Molar absorption coefficients are shown in the ordinate. The spectrum at 1 μ*M* concentration is that of the monomeric bilirubin dianion, as explained in the text. At 100 n*M*, a slight turbidity is seen, and at 20 n*M* the light absorption is decreased, due to oxidation of bilirubin. Higher concentrations of bilirubin, 10 μ*M* to 1 m*M*, show increasing degrees of dimerization of the dianion. Buffer, 0.7 m*M* tris hydrochloride, 50 m*M* tris base, 0.1 *M* NaCl.

central methylene group in either direction. This conformation may be stabilized by internal hydrogen bonding between carboxylate groups and pyrrole nitrogens. Definite knowledge of the internal hydrogen bonding in the bilirubin dianion is lacking, however.

D. Self-Association of the Bilirubin Anion

1. State of Bilirubin Dianion in Aqueous Solution

At higher concentrations, from 10 μ*M* to the practical upper limit around 5 m*M*, the bilirubin dianion spectrum undergoes changes which can be ascribed to dimerization or oligomerization.[34,35] Light absorption increases at wavelengths from 480 to 550. Changes at maximum seem to depend upon buffer composition. Little variation is seen in a tris buffer[35] while the molar absorption coefficient decreases markedly in a sodium bicarbonate-carbonate buffer when bilirubin concentration is increased (Figure 7). These changes are reversible and equilibrium is obtained within less than a minute. The spectra of concentrated bilirubin solutions in the range of pH from about 8 to 12 do not change with pH (apart from minor changes due to shift of buffer composition), demonstrating that this type of self-association does not involve hydrogen ions or bilirubin acid. The process is

$$n \text{ Bilirubin}^{2-} \rightleftharpoons (\text{Bilirubin})_n^{2n-} \qquad (3)$$

2. Determination of the Degree of Self-Association of Bilirubin Dianion in Dilute, Aqueous Solution

Determination of the degree of self-association, *n*, is difficult because direct methods such as ultracentrifugation, measurement of light scattering and of colligative properties, cannot be applied in dilute solutions with low values of *n*. The degree of self-association must be inferred from spectroscopy, solubility, or binding data. The best of these indirect methods is probably determination of the solubility of bilirubin at varying pH. The processes involved are

$$\underset{\text{solid}}{n\ \text{BilirubinH}_2} \rightleftharpoons \underset{\text{dissolved}}{n\ \text{BilirubinH}_2} \longleftrightarrow (\text{Bilirubin})_n^{2n-} + 2n\text{H}^+ \qquad (4)$$

Equilibrium of dissolution is obtained in 30 min when solid anhydrous bilirubin is agitated with tris buffers of varying pH and constant ionic strength at 37°C in the dark. Bilirubin concentrations in the aqueous phase can be measured by spectrophotometry with satisfactory reproducibility.[2] In a range of pH from 7.4 to 8.6 the solubility varies from 5 to 1000 n*M* (Figure 1). The solubility of the bilirubin acid is low. In the range of pH mentioned, the concentrations of bilirubin acid and of the monoanion may be considered negligible compared to that of the (possibly aggregated) dianion. At equilibrium, the concentration of dissolved bilirubin acid is constant since the solution is saturated. The equilibrium equation for the right half of the process in Equation 4 is accordingly

$$\frac{\left[(\text{B})_n^{2n-}\right] \times \left[\text{H}^+\right]^{2n}}{\left[\text{BH}_2\right]^n} = K_a^{2n} \qquad (5)$$

where $\left[(\text{B})_n^{2n-}\right]$ is the concentration at equilibrium of dissolved, aggregated bilirubin dianions, each containing *n* bilirubin molecules, $\left[\text{BH}_2\right]$ is the solubility of bilirubin acid as such, and K_9 is the mean acid dissociation constant of the carboxyl groups. Taking the logarithm and rearranging gives

$$\log \left[(\text{B})_n^{2n-}\right] = 2n\text{pH} + n\log \left[\text{BH}_2\right] - 2n\text{pK} \qquad (6)$$

The logarithm of the solubility of bilirubin should thus vary linearily with pH, the slope being 2*n*. Experimentally, a straight line is found[2] with a slope close to 2 (Figure 1) which means that *n* is equal to 1. Alkaline bilirubin solutions at concentrations less than about 1 μM thus consist mainly of the *monomer* dianion of bilirubin.

This result is further substantiated by examination of phase distribution of bilirubin among an alkaline, aqueous solution and an organic solvent (methyl isobutyl ketone).[35]

A third line of evidence in favour of the monomeric nature of dilute, aqueous bilirubin solutions stems from studies of bilirubin anion binding equilibria with human and bovine albumin. As detailed later (Section III.A.2) this equilibrium has been studied by several groups, using widely differing methods. In all these studies, the binding isotherms are in agreement with the assumption that the bilirubin-albumin complex is in equilibrium with monomeric bilirubin dianion. Entirely different binding isotherms would have resulted if the free bilirubin dianion were present in an aggregated state.

Finally, studies of fast reactions in binding of bilirubin to albumin indicate that the reactant is monomeric (see Section III.A.4).

A different conclusion has been arrived at by Carey and Koretsky in an extensive paper,[34] investigating spectra of bilirubin in aqueous solutions at pH 10, with ethanol or dioxan added in different proportions. With either of these solvents the bilirubin anion spectra gradually shift towards longer wavelength. This spectral shift is interpreted by Carey and Koretsky as being due to monomerization of bilirubin. An ethanol concentration of 20% (v/v) gives an intermediate spectrum, about half way between the spectra in water and in 90% ethanol, which by these authors are interpreted as the spectra of dimer and monomer bilirubin, respectively. In 20% ethanol, a mixture of monomer and dimer bilirubin should thus be present. It follows that the spectrum of this solution should shift towards the monomer spectrum on dilution with buffered 20% ethanol and should shift towards the dimer spectrum at higher bilirubin concentrations. This, however, is not so; the spectrum remains unchanged with variation of the bilirubin concentration within wide limits.[25] The solution in 20% ethanol cannot, therefore, contain a mixture of monomer and dimer bilirubin. Another explanation of the spectral shift with ethanol or dioxan concentration must be found and it seems reasonable to seek this in changes of solvation of the bilirubin anion, in shifts of intramolecular hydrogen bonding, and/or in changes of exciton splitting with varying polarity of the medium.

3. Dimerization of Bilirubin Dianion at Higher Concentrations

The spectral changes seen at higher concentrations of bilirubin in aqueous, alkaline solutions are thus due to reversible dimerization of the bilirubin dianion.

$$2\,B^{2-} \rightleftharpoons B_2^{4-} \qquad (7)$$

An equilibrium of dimerization is established in less than a minute. The spectral changes are independent of pH in the range from 8 to 12. The equilibrium equation is

$$\frac{\left[B^{2-}\right]^2}{\left[B_2^{4-}\right]} = K_{Dim} \qquad (8)$$

Experimental verification of this reaction scheme and determination of the dimerization constant, K_{Dim}, has been accomplished by measuring the ratio of light absorption at 520 and 430 nm in a wide range of bilirubin concentrations (Figure 8).[35] As may be seen from the figure, good agreement of observed points with theory is obtained. Since, however, the upper curvature cannot be observed with good precision, it is possible that further oligomerization takes place at high concentrations. On the other hand, this possibility seems remote since formation of aggregates with six or more negative charges on an aggregate of the limited size in question is improbable, except at high ionic strength. The dimerization constant has been determined as a function of temperature and salt concentration, and thermodynamic constants for the process have been calculated.[35] At 37°C and ionic strength 0.15 *M*, the dimerization constant is about 0.25 m*M*. Bilirubin dianion concentrations in body fluids are below 0.1 μM; the concentration of the dimer is thus extremely low and can usually be disregarded.

4. Acid Dependent Aggregation

While the above mentioned dimerization is independent of pH, a different type of aggregates, partially protonated and containing several bilirubin molecules, are formed at pH-values below 8. This type of self-association was first described by Jirsa and coworkers[36-38] and has since been studied by several investigators. Lee and Cowger[39] pointed to the possible biological importance of such aggregates, and Lee and Gartner[40] in 1976 proposed that "it is in the colloidal sol form (micropolymer), that bilirubin toxicity to brain, kidney, intestinal mucosa, erythrocyte, and other organs initially develops, by a process of colloid-to-surface interaction".

Formation of partially protonated aggregates of the bilirubin dianion is an interme-

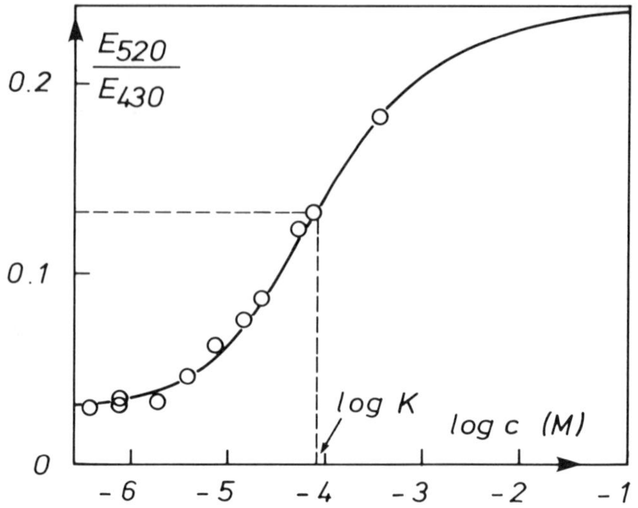

FIGURE 8. Equilibrium of dimerization of bilirubin-IXα(Z,Z) dianion. O, observed ratios of absorbances at 520/430 nm (ordinate) are pictured as a function of the bilirubin concentration on a logarithmic scale (abscissa). The curve is calculated from Equation 8 for $\log K_{dim} = -4.1$. The temperature was 25°C, pH = 8.25, ionic strength 0.1 *M*. (From Brodersen, R., *Acta Chem. Scand.*, 20, 2895, 1966. With permission.)

diate step in acid precipitation of bilirubin. The spectral changes and increase of light scattering involved have already been described in that context (Sections I.A.1 and I.B.1). At high concentrations of bilirubin, of the order of 0.1 m*M* or more, formation of such aggregates occurs promptly when an alkaline solution of bilirubin is neutralized. At lower concentrations, in the μ*M* or n*M* range, there is a pronounced tendency to supersaturation. Bilirubin solutions, 0.3 μ*M*, at pH 7, 8, and 9, show identical light absorption spectra (Figure 9) indicating that the dissolved sodium salt remains in true solution in spite of the fact that the concentration is a few times higher than the solubility at pH 8, and is 300 times the solubility at pH 7. Aggregation at the latter pH may take place at any time, after minutes or hours, and does take place if a small amount of an already aggregated suspension is added. The process thus has the character of micro-crystal formation when occurring at low bilirubin concentrations. In the presence of albumin, cocrystals of bilirubin-albumin are formed.[7] If the solution is in contact with a phospholipid membrane, formation of a bilirubin acid-phospholipid complex is a much faster process than aggregation of pure bilirubin in the free water phase.[2] It seems unlikely, therefore, that bilirubin aggregation could occur in blood plasma except on phospholipid structures. These complex aggregates will be dealt with later.

III. LIGAND BINDING OF THE BILIRUBIN DIANION TO MACROMOLECULES

A. Complexes with Albumin

1. Stoichiometry of Binding

Two bilirubin dianions may be reversibly bound to one molecule of human albumin, as shown by many investigators (see Kamisaka et al.[41] and references therein). It is possible that a third molecule may be bound at higher bilirubin concentrations; this can only be studied at high pH values, due to the low solubility of bilirubin acid, and

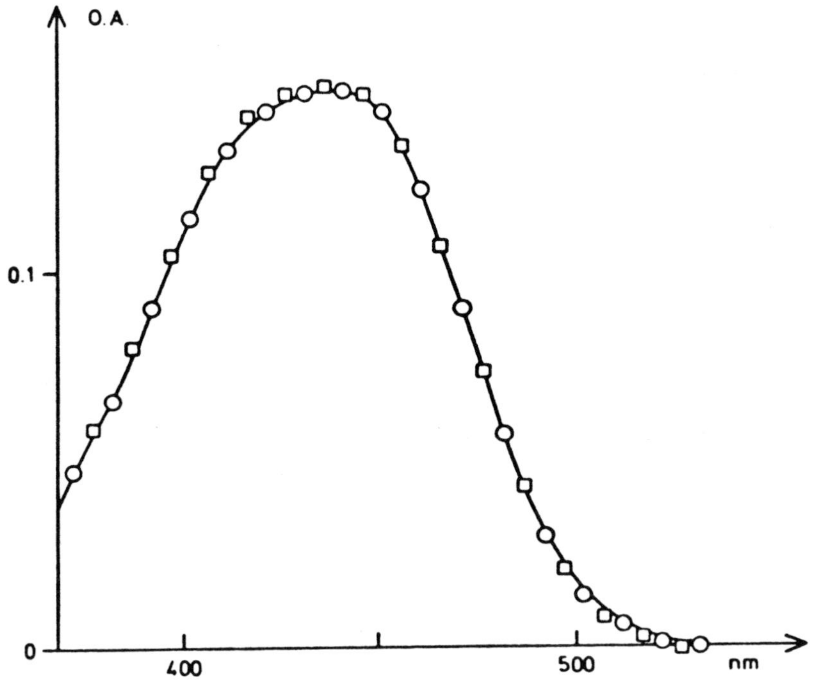

FIGURE 9. Light absorption spectra of bilirubin-IXα(Z,Z) in dilute, aqueous solution, bilirubin concentration 300 n*M*, and varying pH: □, pH = 7.0; ○, pH = 8.0; ———, pH = 9.0. Tris buffer, ionic strength 0.1 *M*, temperature 37°C. Optical path length, 10 cm. The spectra show no sign of self-aggregation of bilirubin, although the solutions at pH 8 and 7 are supersaturated by factors about 3 and 300, respectively.

has not been sufficiently investigated. Reports on binding of more than two molecules of bilirubin should be evaluated with care due to the possibility that coaggregation of bilirubin acid and albumin was involved, as detailed later.

The literature on the properties of bilirubin-albumin complexes contains conflicting results. Important sources of variation are found in the method of preparing the complexes. As stressed by Beaven et al.,[42] reproducible results are obtained when an alkaline solution of bilirubin is added to an alkaline solution of albumin. A complex of albumin with one or two molecules of the bilirubin dianion is then formed. Beaven et al. left the alkaline reaction mixture in darkness for 1 hr for attainment of equilibrium. (less than 5 min is probably sufficient, according to the results of Faerch and Jacobsen).[43,44] If the pH of the albumin solution on mixing with bilirubin is about 7 to 7.5, a variable amount of insoluble bilirubin acid is aggregated and final equilibrium of binding is then reached extremely slowly.

Other sources of variation are isomerization of bilirubin through dipyrrole exchange, or illumination, or use of albumin preparations with commercially added stabilizers which bind to the albumin, interfering with binding of bilirubin.

2. *Affinity of Binding*

Blauer et al.[45] have studied the circular dichroism of mixtures containing bilirubin and a mixture of albumins from two different animal species and have found that an equilibrium is established under these circumstances, with bilirubin bound to both proteins in a proportion which could be described by different binding affinities. These findings prove that bilirubin is bound reversibly to albumin.

Table 1
DETERMINATION OF BILIRUBIN-HUMAN ALBUMIN BINDING PARAMETERS

Author(s)	Year	Method	Fatty acids	pH	Ionic strength M	Temp.	n_1	K_1 M^{-1}	n_2	M^{-1}
Jacobsen[48]	1969	Peroxidase	Nat.	7.4	0.1	37°C	1	1.4×10^8	2	5×10^5
Krasner et al.[50]	1973	Equilib. dialysis[a]						2.4×10^7		
Beaven et al.[42]	1973	CD spectra	Nat.	8.5	0.5	24°C	1	6.7×10^6	1	3×10^5
Chen[51]	1973	Fluoresc. quench.	Nil	7.4	0.18	25°C	1	7.0×10^7	1	6×10^6
Nelson et al.[46]	1974	Peroxidase	Nat.	7.4	0.15	37°C	1	3.2×10^7		
Reed et al.[49]	1975	Peroxidase	Nat.	7.4	0.15	37°C	1	$(3.8 \pm 1.5) \times 10^7$		
Reed et al.[49]	1975	BSA-agarose	Nat.	7.4	0.15	37°C	1	$(4.2 \pm 0.3) \times 10^7$		
Yamaji[55]	1975	Sephadex[b]	Nat.				1	7×10^7	1	5×10^5
Jacobsen and Brodersen[47]	1976	Peroxidase	Nat.	7.4	0.18	37°C	1	3×10^7		
Levine[52]	1977	Fluoresc. quench.	Nil	7.3-7.5	0.35	Amb. room	1	1.0×10^8	1	3×10^6
Jacobsen[59]	1977	Peroxidase	Nil	7.4	0.18	37°C	1	5.6×10^7		
Brodersen and Funding[53]	1977	Peroxidase	Nil	7.4	0.1	37°C	1	7×10^7		
Brodersen and Funding[58]	1977	Spectrophotometry	Nil	7.4	0.1	37°C			2	5×10^5
Gray and Stroupe[56]	1978	Kinetics	Nil	7.4	0.1	4°C	1	$> 4 \times 10^9$		
Berde et al.[53]	1979	Fluoresc. quench.		7.45	0.07	37°C	1	6.4×10^7	1	2.5×10^6
Rubaltelli and Jori[54]	1979	Fluoresc. quench.	Nat.	7.4	0.1	18°C	1	2.07×10^8		
Lamola et al.[57]	1979	Fluoresc. of bilirb.	Nil	7.4	0.15	25°C	1	$(7 \pm 2) \times 10^6$		
			Nil	7.4	0.15	37°C	1	4×10^6		
		Fluoresc. quench.	Nil	7.4	0.15	25°C	1	$(5 \pm 2) \times 10^6$		
Brodersen[2]	1979	Peroxidase	Nil	7.4	0.18	37°C	1	5.5×10^7	1	4.4×10^6
Brodersen[5]	1980	Spectrophotometry[c]	Nil	8.9	0.10	37°C	1	abt 1×10^8		

[a] Equilibrium dialysis with varying concentration of DMSO, extrapolation to DMSO conc = 0.
[b] Sephadex® column of varying length, extrapolation to column length = 0.
[c] Spectrophotometry at extreme dilution.

The affinity of binding is independent of pH in a wide range from about 7 to 11.[2,46,47] This is in agreement with binding of the *dianion,* a mechanism confirmed by pH titration.[2]

Ten independent research teams have measured the binding constant for the first molecule, using seven different methods and have obtained fairly consistent results, as seen in Table 1. The seven methods are, (1) measurement of rate of oxidation of the free bilirubin anion with hydrogen peroxide (or ethyl hydroperoxide) and peroxidase,[2,46-49] (2) equilibrium dialysis with varying DMSO concentrations and exprapolation to zero concentration,[50] (3) CD spectrometry,[42] (4) fluorescence quenching,[51-54] (5) BSA-agarose exchange chromatography,[49] (6) Sephadex® chromatography,[55] and (7) spectrophotometry at extreme dilution.[5] Two groups using two other techniques have obtained deviating results, one giving a higher affinity,[56] the other a lower.[57] The most probable value for the first binding constant, at 37°C and 0.15 *M* ionic strength, is about $6.4 \times 10^7\ M^{-1}$.

Fewer investigators have determined the second binding constant,[2,42,48,51-53,55,58] and results are more variable. Recent determination by the peroxidase method has given $4.4 \times 10^6\ M^{-1}$ under the same conditions as above.[2]

Variation of binding affinity with temperature and salt concentration has been investigated by Jacobsen.[59] The numerical results of these measurements have been summarized in a diagram for easy calculation.[5] Jacobsen found that the binding affinity decreases with increasing temperature and calculated the *standard change of entropy on binding* of the first molecule of bilirubin, $\Delta S^\circ = -8.5$ cal mol^{-1} deg^{-1}. This finding is not compatible with predominantly hydrophobic binding of bilirubin to albumin, which would produce a positive change of entropy, but is consistent with binding through salt linkages, hydrogen bonds, and charge transfer (π-bonds), with minor contributions from hydrophobic interactions. This is in keeping with the polar character of the bilirubin molecule (Section I.A.2) but contradicts the notion of several earlier authors, that bilirubin binds in a hydrophobic pocket in the albumin molecule (see further Section III.A.8).

3. Binding Sites. Site-to-Site Interaction

The above figures are so-called *Scatchard's binding constants,* describing binding of bilirubin to two *independent* sites according to the equilibrium equation,

$$r = \frac{K_1 b}{1 + K_1 b} + \frac{K_2 b}{1 + K_2 b} \qquad (9)$$

when r is the average number of bilirubin molecules bound to each albumin molecule, b is the concentration of free bilirubin dianion in the solution, and K_1 and K_2 are the binding constants for the first and second site, respectively. This equation gives an excellent fit to the observed values, as seen in Figure 10.

This finding, however, does not prove that binding actually takes place to two independent sites. The above equation can be transformed into

$$r = \frac{(K_1 + K_2)b + 2K_1 K_2 b^2}{1 + (K_1 + K_2)b + K_1 K_2 b^2} \qquad (10)$$

This is identical with Adair's binding equation, applied to binding of two molecules,

$$r = \frac{k_1 b + 2k_1 k_2 b^2}{1 + k_1 b + k_1 k_2 b^2} \qquad (11)$$

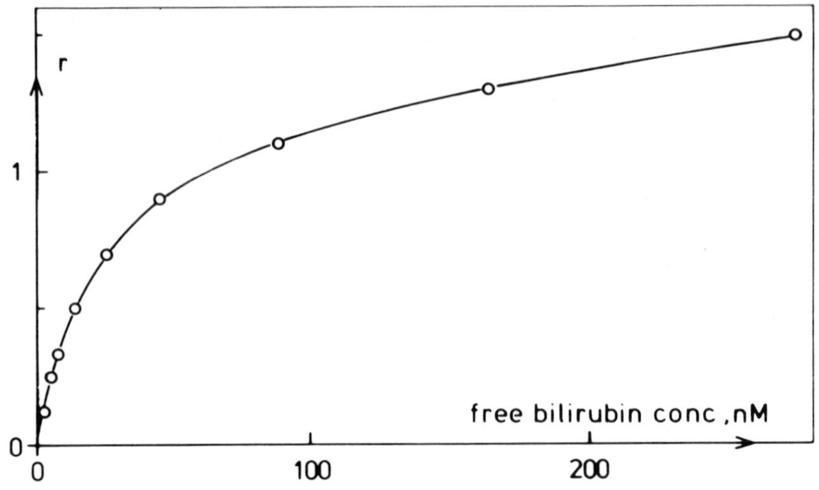

FIGURE 10. Binding isotherm of bilirubin-IXα(Z,Z) dianion to human albumin. The average number of bound bilirubin dianions per albumin molecule (ordinate) is plotted as a function of the free bilirubin dianion concentration (abscissa), as measured by the peroxidase method. Each point represents the average of eight determinations of the oxidation rate. The curve is calculated from the binding Equation 9, using the values of association constants for two independent sites, given in Table 2. Identical curves are obtained with any set of binding constants from the Table, together with the appropriate binding equations, (Equation 11 for stepwise and for stoichiometric binding to two sites, and Equation 13 for two equal, anticooperative sites).

Sodium phosphate buffer, 60 m*M*, pH = 7.4, temperature 37°C. (From Brodersen, R., *J. Biol. Chem.*, 254, 2364, 1979. With permission.)

when

$$k_1 = K_1 + K_2 \quad \text{and} \quad k_2 = \frac{K_1 K_2}{K_1 + K_2} \tag{12}$$

Equation 11 may be taken to describe stepwise binding, i.e., a mechanism in which only one site, with the binding constant k_1, is available in the absence of bilirubin. When one molecule of bilirubin is bound to this site, a second site becomes available with the binding constant k_2. As the experimental binding isotherm can equally well be described by Equation 11, it is concluded that knowledge of the binding isotherm does not allow establishment of any specific binding mechanism by sites.

Equation 11 may also be taken to express binding in general terms, *stoichiometric binding*, not inferring that specific sites are involved. One molecule of bilirubin, B, is bound to one molecule of albumin, A, forming a complex, AB, with a binding constant k_1. The complex AB is probably a mixture of different molecules with bilirubin attached to different sites. The complex, AB, binds a second molecule with the binding constant k_2. If a is the concentration of albumin without bilirubin, b that of free bilirubin dianion, c and d the concentrations of the complexes AB and AB_2, respectively, and A the total concentration of albumin, we have

$$k_1 = \frac{c}{a\,b} \qquad k_2 = \frac{d}{c\,b}$$

$$A = a + c + d \qquad r = \frac{c + 2d}{A}$$

Elimination of a, c, and d gives Equation 11.

The stoichiometric description of bilirubin binding is preferable to the conventional description by independent sites since the former does not imply knowledge of a specific binding mechanism to independent sites.

Our ignorance of the mechanism goes even further. Bilirubin may well bind to two *equal* sites on the albumin molecule, if these are anticooperative so that the first molecule of bilirubin, bound to either site, reduces the affinity for binding to the other. If the binding constant of each site is k in the absence of bound bilirubin, and qk when a bilirubin molecule is bound to the other site, we have

$$k = \frac{c}{a\,b} \qquad qk = \frac{d}{c\,b}$$

$$A = a + 2c + d \qquad r = \frac{2c + 2d}{A}$$

which gives the binding equation

$$r = \frac{2kb + 2qk^2b^2}{1 + 2kb + qk^2b^2} \tag{13}$$

where the constants, k and qk, are related to our original, independent binding constants as follows,

$$k = \frac{K_1 + K_2}{2} \qquad qk = \frac{2K_1K_2}{K_1 + K_2} \tag{14}$$

Equation 13 gives exactly the same binding isotherm as 9 and 11, when binding constants calculated according to 14 are entered. We thus have to conclude that two equal binding sites for bilirubin may be present in the albumin molecule. The often cited concept of one high-affinity and one or a few secondary sites with lower affinity may be incorrect.

Three mechanisms of binding to specific sites have been mentioned above, *independent, stepwise,* and *equal and anticooperative binding.* These, and the relevant sets of binding constants for each mechanism, are summarized in Table 2, where the constants for *stoichiometric* binding are given as well. Mechanisms with intermediate degrees of interaction between sites are equally possible.

The above considerations are in agreement with the general treatment of multiple binding, presented by Klotz and Hunston.[60,61] For a complete site description of binding of n ligand molecules to one protein it is necessary to measure $2^n - 1$ constants, which is *three* constants in the case of binding of *two* molecules. We have determined *two* constants only, two K-values, and seem to have no means of determining the third. Several *two*-site models are thus applicable. It may be added that mechanisms with *three* or more sites on the albumin molecule may equally well explain the experimental findings.

It should finally be mentioned that mechanisms involving binding of a bilirubin dimer to one site can be excluded. Such mechanisms would be *either*

$$2\,B^{2-} + A \rightleftharpoons (B^{2-})_2\,A \tag{15}$$

which gives the equilibrium equation

$$r = \frac{2Kb^2}{1 + Kb^2} \tag{16}$$

or, if the bilirubin dianion were dimeric in dilute solution,

$$B_2^{4-} + A \rightleftharpoons B_2^{4-}A \tag{17}$$

Table 2
POSSIBLE MECHANISMS OF BINDING OF TWO MOLECULES OF BILIRUBIN TO HUMAN ALBUMIN. BINDING CONSTANTS

Mechanism	Binding constants, M^{-1} 37°C, ionic strength 0.15 M
Two independent sites	$K_1 = 6.4 \times 10^7$
Equation 9	$K_2 = 4.4 \times 10^6$
Two stepwise sites	$k_1 = 6.8 \times 10^7$
Equation 11	$k_2 = 4.1 \times 10^6$
Two equal, anticooperative sites	$k = 3.4 \times 10^7$
Equation 13	$qk = 8.2 \times 10^6$
Stoichiometric binding of two	$k_1 = 6.8 \times 10^7$
molecules, mechanism unknown	$k_2 = 4.1 \times 10^6$
Equation 11	

which in equilibrium gives

$$r = \frac{2Kb}{2 + Kb} \qquad (18)$$

when b is twice the bilirubin dianion dimer concentration. Neither Equation 16 nor 18 can be fitted to the experimental binding isotherm. Since Equation 9, in which the ligand is presumed to be present as a monomer, gives an excellent fit to the experimental data, it is concluded that the bilirubin dianion in dilute, aqueous solution is present as the monomer in agreement with what was already concluded above (Section II.D.2).

4. *Kinetics of Binding*

By means of the stopped-flow technique and registration of fast changes of light absorption or fluorescence it is possible to resolve the binding of bilirubin to albumin into several steps. Chen[62] in 1974 found that the initial combination of bilirubin dianion and albumin proceeds very rapidly, so that its velocity could not be measured. The initial complex then undergoes several steps of relaxation until a final bilirubin-albumin compound is formed in the course of a few seconds.

Faerch and Jacobsen[43] and Reed[63] have studied kinetics of binding of bilirubin to bovine albumin, as well as the reverse process. These authors used a peroxidase technique for measuring the rate of bilirubin-albumin dissociation.

The multi-step mechanism of binding has been confirmed by Gray and Stroupe[56] and has been studied in detail by Faerch and Jacobsen.[44] The latter authors, working with human albumin at 5.5°C, were able to record the course of the primary combination step of bilirubin and albumin. They further reported the light absorption spectrum of the primary complex and followed its relaxation which could be described by a model of *four* consecutive steps. The rate constant of each step and the molar absorption coefficient of each intermediate species at 472 nm was determined. The results are seen in Figures 11 and 12 and in Table 3.

The reaction mechanism proposed by Faerch and Jacobsen is

$$B^{2-} + \text{Alb} \xrightarrow{k_1} \mathfrak{C}_1 \xrightarrow{k_2} \mathfrak{C}_2 \xrightarrow{k_3} \mathfrak{C}_3 \xrightarrow{k_4} \mathfrak{C}_4 \xrightarrow{k_5} \mathfrak{C}_5 \qquad (19)$$

Reverse reactions are neglected. This model has given excellent agreement with the observed data. When bilirubin (final concentration 8 μM) is mixed with an excess of

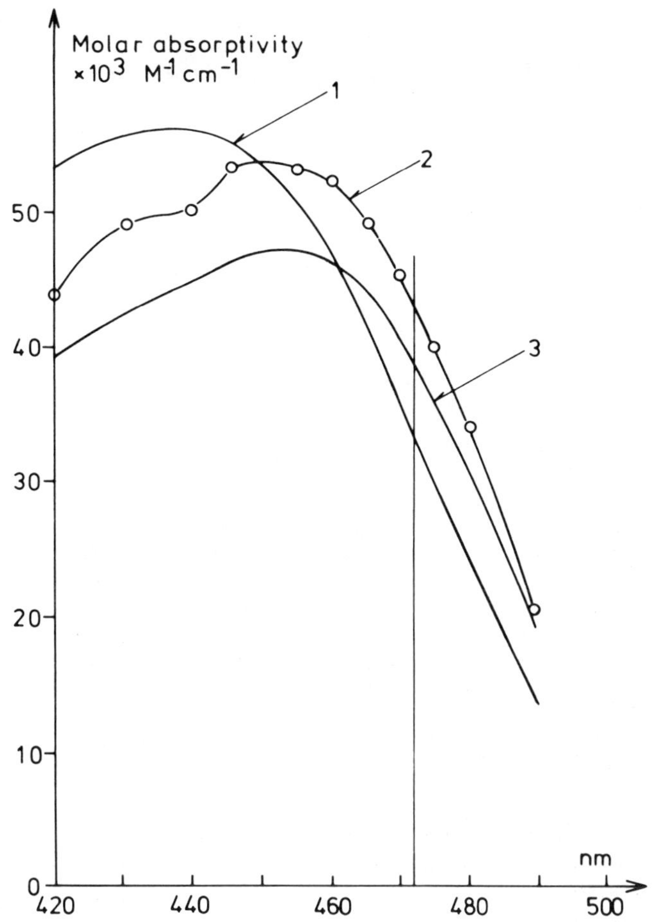

FIGURE 11. Light absorption spectrum (2) of the primary complex, $\mathfrak{C}_1$, of bilirubin-IXα(Z,Z) dianion and human albumin at pH 8.8. The spectra of bilirubin dianion (1), and of the final complex (3), $\mathfrak{C}_5$, are shown for comparison. The spectrum of the transient complex, $\mathfrak{C}_1$, was obtained in repeated experiments, each at a discrete wavelength, by mixing bilirubin, final concentration 2 μM, with albumin, final concentration 75 μM, in a stop-flow apparatus, recording the changes of light absorption, and retropolating to zero-time. (From Faerch, T., and Jacobsen, J., *Arch. Biochem. Biophys.*, 184, 282, 1977. With permission.)

human albumin at pH 8.8 and 5.5°C, the following changes in light absorption at 472 nm take place (Figure 12). An increase occurs within three milliseconds, due to a bimolecular combination of bilirubin and albumin to form the initial complex, $\mathfrak{C}_1$. This undergoes a 1st-order relaxation process whereby light absorption decreases, reaching a minimum at 45 ms when formation of the intermediate complex $\mathfrak{C}_2$ is largely completed. Further transformation into $\mathfrak{C}_3$ causes a renewed increase of light absorption, reaching a second maximum at 350 ms. The two final steps again cause a decline of light absorption under formation of $\mathfrak{C}_4$ which is transformed into the stable complex, $\mathfrak{C}_5$. The entire process is completed in about 10 sec.

The molecular mechanism of binding may be considered on the basis of Faerch and Jacobsen's findings. It might at first be tempting to suggest that the bilirubin dianion is initially attached to albumin at a single point, e.g., but binding one carboxylate

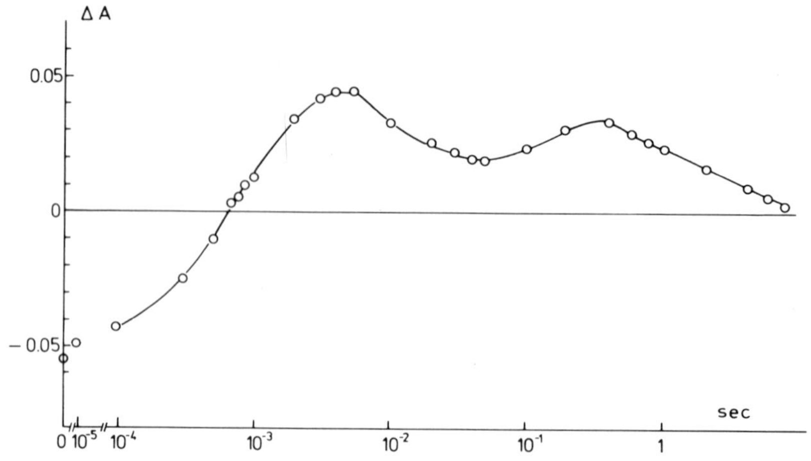

FIGURE 12. Calculated time course of the light absorption of bilirubin-IXα(Z,Z) dianion during binding to human albumin, at the wavelength 472 nm, pH = 8.8, temperature 5.5°C. Light absorption of the free bilirubin dianion is less than that of the final product and is pictured at zero-time. Formation of the primary complex, $\mathfrak{C}_1$, proceeds rapidly and is observed by an increase of light absorption to the first maximum. Conformational relaxation then results in a decrease to a transient minimum, when $\mathfrak{C}_2$ is the predominant species, followed again by an increase of light absorption to a second maximum, when an intermediate product $\mathfrak{C}_3$ predominates. The two final steps, formation of $\mathfrak{C}_4$ and the final product, $\mathfrak{C}_5$, causes a decrease of light absorption towards the final value which is reached in about 10 sec. (From Faerch and Jacobsen, *Arch. Biochem. Biophys.*, 184, 282, 1977. With permission.)

to a positively charged, anion binding site on albumin, thus forming the primary complex, $\mathfrak{C}_1$. The following steps would then involve binding of the second carboxylate, establishment of hydrophobic interactions with the hydrocarbon moieties, hydrogen bonding with pyrrole and lactam groups, etc., until the complex is finally stabilized by a maximal number of interactions. However, the light absorption spectrum of the primary complex, Figure 11, compared with the spectra of unbound bilirubin dianion and of the final product, shows that both chromophores of bilirubin have already undergone the shift to longer wavelength which characterizes the final complex. This means that bilirubin in $\mathfrak{C}_1$ is fully surrounded by the protein and indeed that the ligand molecule is located approximately in its final position, relative to the immediately surrounding albumin structures. The subsequent relaxation steps are conformational changes in the albumin-bilirubin complex. Interpretation of the kinetic results demands that the reacting bilirubin is in a monomeric state, as already shown.

If the mechanism proposed here is correct, it follows that conformational changes of the bilirubin-albumin complex influence its light absorption spectrum, in agreement with Blauer's exciton splitting theory (Section III.A.6). Several lines of evidence in favour of this are obtained from other sources, as we shall see later.

5. Competition and Cobinding with Other Ligands

When bilirubin dianion and a second ligand, such as a drug or a fatty acid anion, is added to a solution of albumin, both ligands will interact with the protein. The following types of mutual influence of binding may be observed; (1) binding of bilirubin may be enhanced by binding of the second ligand, and *vice versa* (heterotropic cooperativity), (2) the two ligands may bind independently without any mutual influence, (3) binding of bilirubin may be decreased by binding of the second ligand and *vice versa (negative heterotropic cooperativity,* or *anticooperativity).* At sufficiently

Table 3
KINETIC COURSE OF BINDING OF BILIRUBIN DIANION TO HUMAN ALBUMIN AT pH 8.8, 5.5°C[44]

Rate constants	Reactants	Millimolar absorption coefficient at 472 nm
		cm^{-1} mM^{-1}
	Human albumin + Bilirubin dianion	33.5
$\mathfrak{k}_1 = (1.6 \pm 0.4) \times 10^7\ M^{-1}\ s^{-1}$	↓	
	$\mathfrak{C}_1$	44.5
$\mathfrak{k}_2 = 47.9\ s^{-1}$	↓	
	$\mathfrak{C}_2$	40.8
$\mathfrak{k}_3 = 7.9 \pm 1.6\ s^{-1}$	↓	
	$\mathfrak{C}_3$	43.8
$\mathfrak{k}_4 = 2.3 \pm 0.5\ s^{-1}$	↓	
	$\mathfrak{C}_4$	42.1
$\mathfrak{k}_5 = 0.32 \pm 0.06\ s^{-1}$	↓	
	$\mathfrak{C}_5$	39.6

high ligand concentrations, both are bound in the same amount as in the absence of the other ligand. (4) Competitive binding, in which case binding of one ligand to an albumin molecule precludes binding of the other.

Intermediate or mixed types of cobinding exist. Binding of one molecule of bilirubin, and one of a second ligand, may occur independently while a negative cooperativity is observed when a second molecule of bilirubin is bound. Such mixed types of interaction are common, and closer investigation, when this has been carried out, has always disclosed a mixed mechanism. It is doubtful whether clear-cut cases of any of the four basic types exist.

The influence of binding of fatty acids on the binding of bilirubin, as studied by the peroxidase method (see Section III.A.9), is pictured in Figures 13 and 14.[5] A solution of human or bovine albumin, 30 μM, with 0.5 mole bilirubin per mole albumin, in a buffer, pH 7.4, is mixed with hydrogen peroxide and peroxidase. Oxidation of bilirubin takes place and is monitored by a decrease of light absorption at the maximum of bound bilirubin, 455 nm. The initial rate of oxidation is proportional to the concentration of free bilirubin dianion. Addition of fatty acids in varying concentrations causes variations of the oxidation rate, interpreted as variations of the bilirubin dianion concentration and hence of the bilirubin binding affinity. In the absence of albumin, fatty acids do not influence the rate of oxidation of bilirubin with hydrogen peroxide and peroxidase. It seems reasonable to conclude that the variations of oxidation rate indeed reflect variations of binding affinity of bilirubin to albumin, as effected by binding of fatty acid to the albumin. This is supported by the fact that similar findings have been made by Woolley and Hunter,[64] using an ultracentrifugation tech-

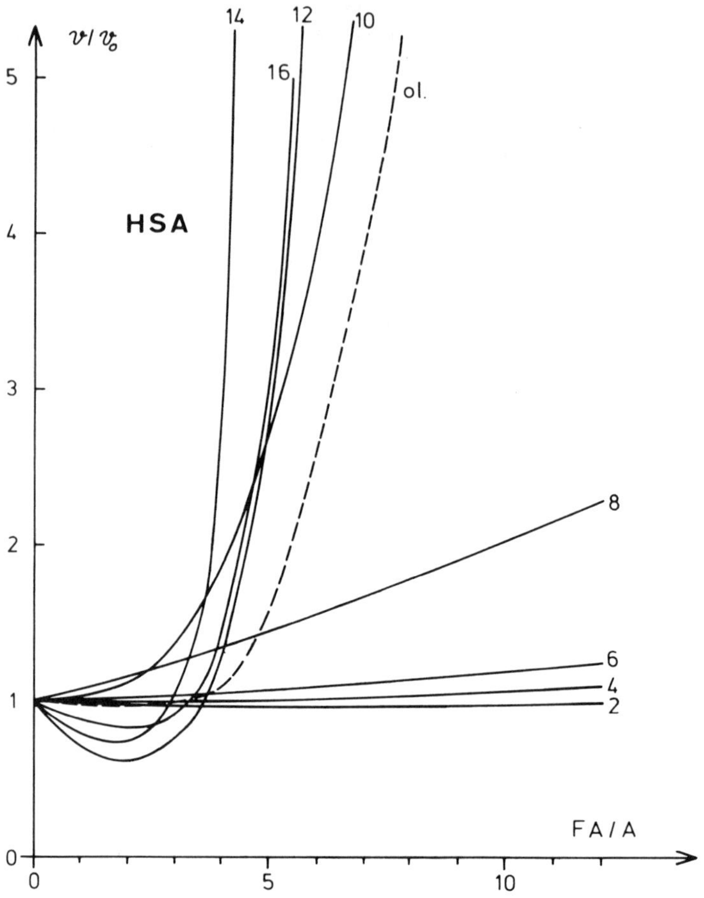

FIGURE 13.. Cobinding of bilirubin and fatty acids to human albumin at pH 7.4, ionic strength 0.15 *M*, temperature 37°C. The velocity of oxidation of bilirubin with hydrogen peroxide and perioxidase (ordinate) is taken as a measure of the equilibrium concentration of free bilirubin dianion and is pictured as a function of added concentration of fatty acids (abscissa). Numbers of carbon atoms in the fatty acids are given with each curve. The broken curve was obtained with oleic acid (Ol). Albumin concentration, 30 μM purified bilirubin-IXα(Z,Z)[3], 15 μM.

nique as well as light absorption and circular dichroism spectra, by Reed,[63] studying reaction rates of bilirubin binding and release from bovine albumin, and by others.[65-69] Fatty acids at pH 7.4, with even numbers of carbon atoms, produce various effects on bilirubin (one molecule), bound to human and bovine albumin: C_{2-6} acids show little effect. C_8 acid has a slight anticooperative effect at fatty acid/albumin ratios above 1. C_{10-18} acids are bound independently or cooperatively at ratios below 3-6, and anticooperatively at higher ratios of fatty acid to albumin. Definite variations of binding pattern are seen with varying chain length and also from human to bovine albumin.

Cobinding of bilirubin and drugs has also been studied by several groups, using a variety of techniques. The issue is clinically important because treatment of icteric newborns or experimental animals with sulfonamides has been found to cause a dis-

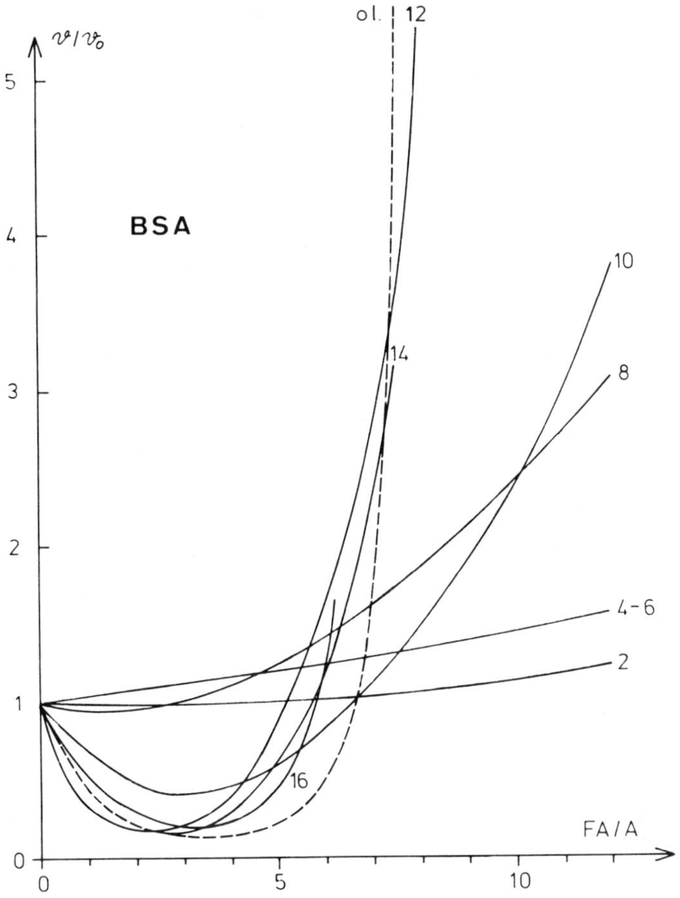

FIGURE 14. Cobinding of bilirubin and fatty acids to bovine albumin, see Figure 13.

placement of bilirubin from blood plasma, where it is bound to albumin, into the central nervous system, resulting in fatal kernicterus or lasting encephalopathy.[70-73] Studies by the peroxidase method have shown that the effect of many drugs can be described by a model of competitive binding of bilirubin and drug to one site on the albumin molecule.[74] This simple model has proved its practical value for screening of drugs, intended for use in newborns or in pregnant or lactating mothers.[75] It was found that, besides sulfonamides, roentgenographic contrast media for cholangiography and a few other drugs are bilirubin displacing to a considerable degree, when present in concentrations as seen in the clinic. Most drugs, on the other hand, are not given in sufficient amounts to cause significant displacement, or are not bound to albumin, or bound independently, of bilirubin.[76] Further studies in this field are needed, for the guidance of the prescribing physician. Techniques for this purpose are discussed later (Section III.A.9).

After surveying the competitive effect of 150 drugs,[75] it is possible to draw certain conclusions on the chemical nature of bilirubin displacing substances:

- Most displacing substances are anionic, and a few are molecules without a net electric charge. Cationic drugs do not displace bilirubin.
- Displacing substances contain a benzene ring or other aromatic structure.

- None of the displacers are lipophilic (discounting the fatty acids which do not seem to bind competitively with bilirubin, but rather show an allosteric, anti-cooperative effect through a conformational change of the albumin molecule, taking place with larger amounts of the fatty acid).

6. Spectroscopic Properties of Bilirubin Dianion-Albumin Complexes

The light absorption spectrum of bilirubin dianion, when bound to albumin, has a maximum at about 450 to 460 nm and a molar absorption coefficient approximately 5 $\times 10^4$ M^{-1} cm^{-1}. A shoulder is seen in the spectrum around 420 nm. Blauer et al.[24] have shown that the spectrum can be represented by two Gaussian peaks, usually separated by about 30 to 50 nm. Circular dichroism spectra are also complex. The main components are two close bands of opposite sign, located in the same positions as the components of the light absorption maxima. Blauer et al.[24] interpret the spectroscopic findings as a result of *exciton splitting*. When a dipyrrole chromophore of the bound bilirubin molecule absorbs a light quantum it is transformed into an excited state. This is characterized by an electronic shift which can be described by the transition dipole moment, $\vec{\mu}$, a vector of specific size and orientation. Energy can be transferred to the other dipyrrole chromophore of the bilirubin molecule (or to a neighbor bilirubin molecule or a suitable chromophore in the adjacent parts of the albumin). This causes a splitting of the light absorption maximum. The magnitude of the splitting is related to the two transition dipole moments, μ_1 and μ_2, the distance between their centers, r, and the angles between the moments and the distance, as follows,

$$\frac{\Delta\lambda}{2} \simeq \frac{\lambda_1 \lambda_2 \mu_1 \mu_2}{\mathfrak{r}^3 h\, \mathfrak{C}} \left[\cos(\vec{\mu}_1, \vec{\mu}_2) - 3 \cos(\vec{\mu}_1, \vec{\mathfrak{r}}) \cos(\vec{\mu}_2, \vec{\mathfrak{r}})\right] \qquad (20)$$

when λ_1 and λ_2 are the wavelengths at maxima of the two Gaussian components, $\Delta\lambda$ is the difference between them, h is Planck's constant, and $\mathfrak{C}$ is the velocity of light. It is seen that the splitting depends acutely upon proximity of the chromophores. The distance between the two maxima is small when the bilirubin molecule is stretched with the two dipyrrolic chromophores as far apart as possible. This occurs in alkaline solutions of bilirubin salts which show one light absorption maximum without a shoulder. Fixation of bilirubin in its binding site in the albumin molecule results in bending of the bilirubin molecule and proximity of the chromophores so that exciton splitting takes place with formation of a shoulder in the light absorption spectrum and a double band with opposite signs in the CD spectrum.

Fluorescence spectra of bilirubin-albumin have been studied especially by Chen[51] and by Beaven et al.[42] The bilirubin-albumin dianion in aqueous solution gives only a slight fluorescence which is considerably enhanced on binding of one molecule of bilirubin to one of albumin. A maximum in the fluorescence spectrum is seen at 530 nm (excitation about 450 nm). At the same time, the fluorescence of albumin, mainly originating from tryptophan in the peptide chain, is quenched, and further quenching occurs on binding of a second molecule of bilirubin. Chen has utilized the quenching, which can be measured in very dilute solutions, for studies of dissociation equilibria of the complex, as well as for fast reaction measurements, a method which later has been used by several authors.

It might be tempting to explain the enhancement of bilirubin fluorescence on binding to albumin as a result of embedding the bilirubin chromophores in a less polar surrounding. This would be consistent with the interpretation of the shift of light absorption maximum to longer wavelength, often considered in older literature, as resulting from binding of the "lipophilic" bilirubin molecule in an apolar pocket in the albumin molecule. As pointed out by Beaven et al.,[42] addition of dioxan to an aqueous solution of bilirubin sodium salt, to give a much reduced dielectric constant, has little effect

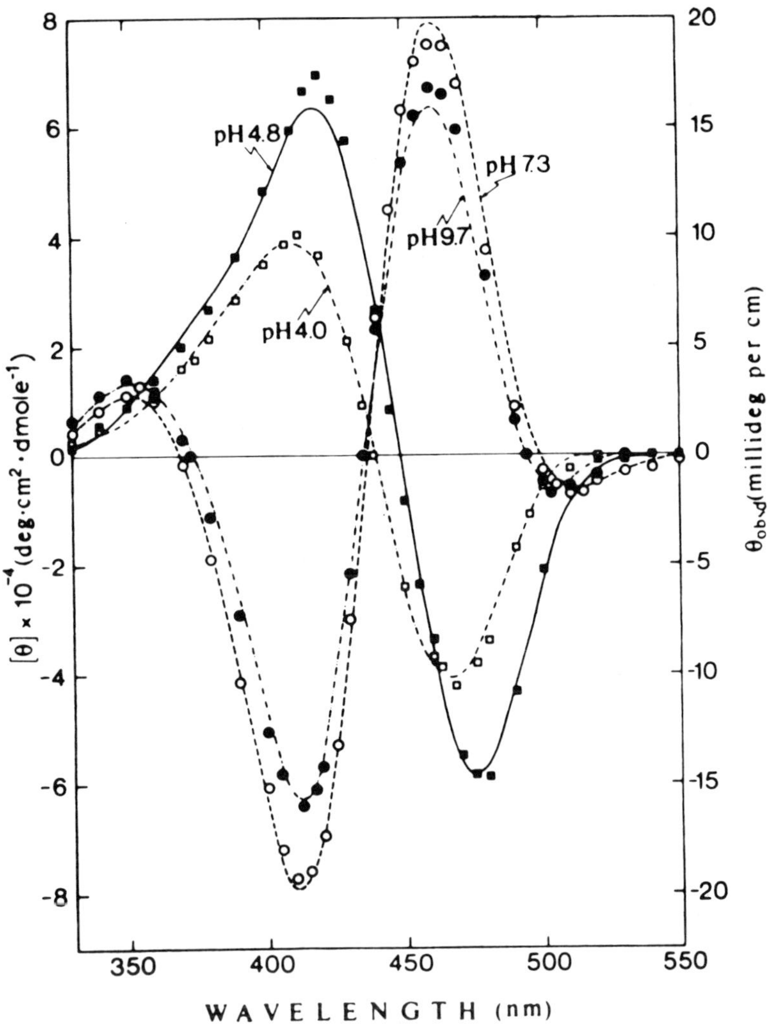

FIGURE 15. Circular dichroism spectra of bilirubin-human albumin in the region of bilirubin light absorption, at varying pH. The two proximate bands of opposite sign are reversed with increasing pH, as a result of conformational rotation of the two dipyrrole chromophores of bound bilirubin at the central methylene bridge, according to the theory of Blauer. (From Blauer, G., Harmatz, D., and Snir, J., *Biochim. Biophys. Acta,* 278, 68, 1972. With permission.)

on its fluorescence, which means that the strong fluorescence enhancement in the complex with albumin is rather a consequence of translational or vibrational immobilization. This latter explanation is in aggreement with Blauer's theory of the origin of the circular dichroism spectra.

The circular dichroism spectrum of bilirubin-albumin shows marked variation with pH (Figure 15). According to Blauer et al.[24] these changes can be explained by variation of the coupling between electric transition dipole moments, caused by rotation of the two dipyrrole chromophores around the bonds at the central methylene bridge, as understood from Equation 20. Also the light absorption spectrum varies with pH (Figure 16), as reported by Wennberg and Cowger,[77] and this must be related to the same molecular mechanism as the changes of CD-spectrum.

Changes of light absorption spectrum of bilirubin-human albumin in the range of

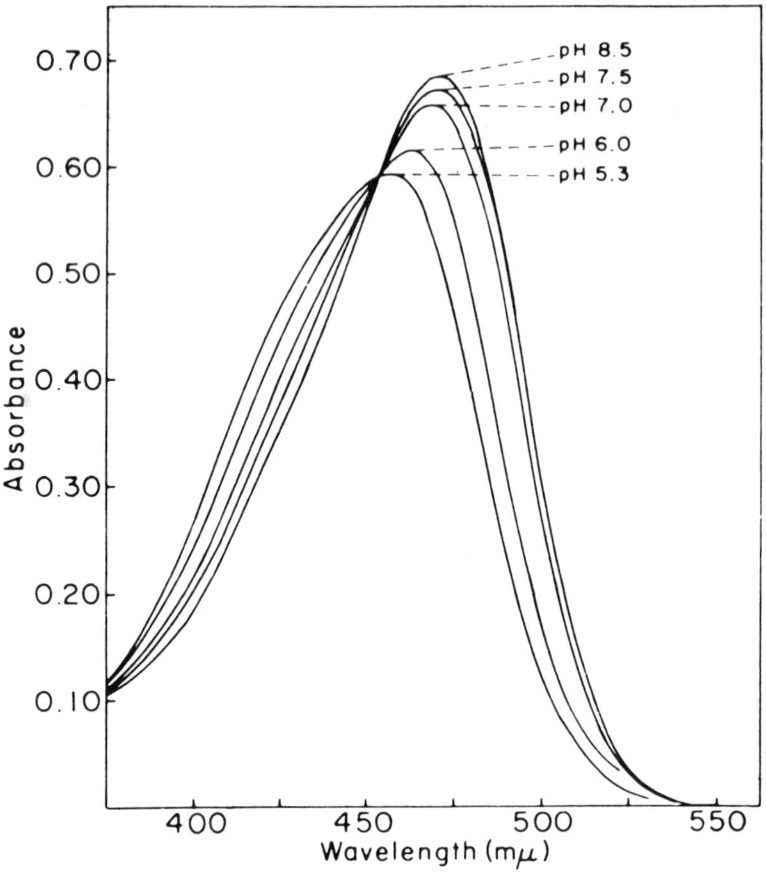

FIGURE 16. Light absorption spectra of bilirubin-bovine albumin with varying pH. Similar changes are observed with human albumin. (From Wennberg, R. P., and Cowger, M. L., *Clin. Chim. Acta,* 43, 55, 1973. With permission.)

pH 6-9 have been studied in detail by Jacobsen and Faerch[78] who have also examined the kinetic course of the changes, and the effects of calcium ions, fatty acids, and of varying temperature. All the changes observed are spectroscopically similar to the spectral shift seen in Figure 16. An increase of light absorption at the maximum with a shift towards longer wavelengths and a (relative or absolute) decrease of the shoulder is thus seen on increase of pH, on decrease of calcium ion concentration, on decrease of the temperature, and on addition of oleic acid. It is concluded that these changes are related to the N-B transformation of the albumin conformation.

Harmatz and Blauer[79] have studied circular dichroism and light absorption spectra of bilirubin complexes with albumin from several species and variation of the spectra with pH, and found that coupling between electric transition dipole moments within the dissymmetrically bound bilirubin molecule may contribute significantly to the optical activities and spectral variations in most cases.

The light absorption spectrum of the second molecule of bilirubin bound to human albumin is different from that of the first molecule.[5,58] The difference again is similar to that of bilirubin-albumin spectra at different pH.

7. *Spectra of Ternary Complexes*

Light absorption and circular dichroism spectra of complexes of albumin with bilirubin and a second ligand have been studied by several groups. Discrepancies have

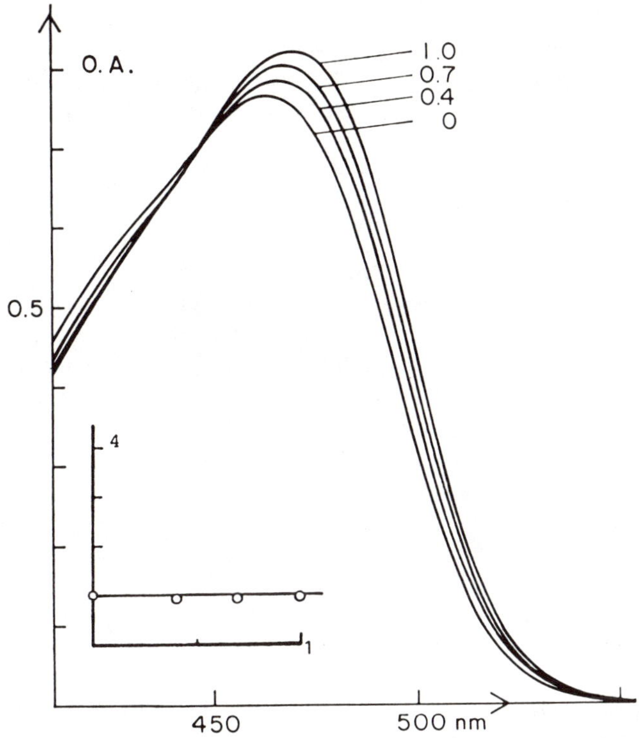

FIGURE 17. Cobinding of bilirubin and polymyxin B to human albumin. Light absorption spectra of bilirubin, 15 μM, with human albumin, 30 μM, are pictured with varying concentrations of added polymyxin B, concentration as given (mM). The insert shows the velocity of oxidation of bilirubin in the same solutions with hydrogen peroxide and peroxidase (ordinate) as a function of polymyxin B concentration (abscissa). The rate of oxidation, and thereby the equilibrium concentration of free bilirubin dianion, remains constant, indicating that bilirubin is not displaced from the complex with albumin. A ternary complex is formed. Note that the spectral change is similar to that produced by variation of pH (Figure 16). (From Brodersen, R., *J. Clin. Invest.*, 54, 1353, 1974. With permission.)

existed in the former literature, originating from two main causes. First, effects of the second ligand on the bilirubin spectrum have often been interpreted to indicate dissociation of bilirubin, disregarding a possible allosteric effect of the second ligand through a conformational change of albumin. The light absorption spectrum of bilirubin-human albumin is shifted by addition of sodium salicylate towards the spectrum of free bilirubin dianion, and this has been interpreted as a result of competitive displacement of bilirubin on binding of salicylate.[80] Similarly, decreases of ellipticity, or reversal of the CD-spectrum of bilirubin-albumin on addition of a second ligand has sometimes been interpreted as indicating dissociation of bilirubin from the complex.[41,42] It is clear from the work of Blauer et al, on exciton splitting, that dissociation of the complex is only one possible interpretation. Lavie and Blauer[81] could in fact demonstrate by electrophoretic and ultracentrifugation techniques, that dissociation of bilirubin took place in some cases and a ternary complex was formed in other cases.

Light absorption spectra of bilirubin-human albumin, with polymyxin B as the second ligand, are illustrative in this context (Figure 17).[74] A solution of bilirubin-human albumin in molar proportion 1:2 has a light absorption spectrum with maximum at 460 nm and a shoulder at about 420 nm, at pH 7.4. Addition of polymyxin B at constant pH causes a spectral shift, similar to that observed on increase of pH (Figure 16), with the maximum moving to longer wavelength and with increasing intensity, while the shoulder is decreased. In this case, the shift cannot be interpreted by dissociation of bilirubin, alone because free bilirubin dianion has a maximum at *shorter* wavelength. A change of conformation with altered exciton splitting (and hyperchromism) may explain the spectral shift, and this is substantiated by finding unchanged rates of oxidation with hydrogen peroxide and peroxidase (Figure 17), indicating that the equilibrium concentration of free bilirubin dianion remained constant with increasing concentration of polymyxin B. Misinterpretation of the spectral shift by dissociation of bilirubin was in this case excluded by the sign of the shift. With salicylate, however, the shift is in the opposite direction, and final interpretation on the basis of the spectrum alone was therefore not possible. Observation of oxidation kinetics in the case of salicylate shows that a dissociation of bilirubin does take place but that the concentration of free bilirubin dianion in equilibrium remains very low, compared with the bound bilirubin, so that the spectral shift must be explained solely by the allosteric effect of binding of salicylate anion on the conformation of the bilirubin-albumin complex.

A second source of discrepancies among results of several groups is interpretation in terms of site binding, when the spectroscopic methods allowed no more than stoichiometric descriptions. Spectral shifts of bilirubin-albumin on binding of a second ligand have thus been interpreted as suggesting a shift of the bilirubin molecule from one site in the albumin to another.[41,82] As seen from the above considerations, these results may equally well be due to conformational changes, while the bilirubin molecule remains in one site.

8. Molecular Models of Bilirubin Dianion-Albumin

In conclusion of all the studies of binding equilibrium and kinetics and spectra of the complex, it is seen that bilirubin dianion is bound reversibly to at least two sites in the albumin molecule where it is fixed in a definite position and conformation. Changes of the light absorption and CD spectra with pH, calcium ion concentration, cobinding of fatty acid and several other ligands, temperature, binding ratio, and zoological species of the albumin, can largely be explained by changes of albumin conformation resulting in changes of bilirubin conformation with internal rotation of the two dipyrrole chromophores at the central methylene group. This requires a model of the bilirubin-albumin complex in which each half of the bilirubin molecule is bound to either of two segments in the albumin. Alterations of any of the above factors causes the segments of albumin to rotate against each other.

The molecular structure of albumin is not known in detail since X-ray crystallographic studies have proved difficult with this protein. Mugnoli et al.[83] have reported the X-ray crystallographic structure of a di-isopropylamine salt of bilirubin, containing two molecules of chloroform, and have suggested that this could serve as a model of the structure of bilirubin in its complex with albumin. Acceptable models should be consistent with the following experimental observations and criteria:

- Albumin consists of three globular elements, linearly arranged.[84,85]
- Bilirubin should be bound in a highly specific way, as seen from the fact that photobilirubin, containing E-isomers, is not bound with high affinity.[86]
- Two molecules of the bilirubin dianion should be accommodated, at least one of these together with independently bound ligands, such as polymyxin B,[74] diazepam,[76] and tryptophan,[87] besides a few molecules of fatty acids.

- Each of the two dipyrrole chromophores of the bilirubin molecule should be bound to a motile part of the albumin so that the chromophores can be rotated relative to each other with conformational changes of the albumin molecule, effected by variations of temperature, pH, calcium ion concentration, and binding of fatty acids and independently bound ligands.
- The model should account for fast binding of the bilirubin dianion, followed by several relaxation steps of conformational changes.
- The bound bilirubin should be totally covered by the albumin molecule, excluding contact with the solvent, as seen from lack of solvent perturbation of the bilirubin light absorption spectrum on addition of organic solvents.[25]
- Binding should be abolished by extensive unfolding of the albumin molecule, as caused by comprehensive acetylation[88] or by increase of pH from 11 to 12.[5]
- Bilirubin should be bound mainly through salt linkages, to cationic groups in the albumin, and through hydrogen bonds and charge transfer (π-bonds), supplemented by minor contributions from hydrophobic interactions, as evidenced by the negative binding entropy,[59] by the anionic, polar, and aromatic character of bilirubin displacers, and by studies of infrared spectra.[5] This means that each binding site should contain two positively charged groups (lysine or arginin), besides aromatic amino acid side chains, and hydrogen bondforming elements.
- The N-terminal of the albumin molecule, which binds copper ions,[89] should not be involved since Cu^{++} ions are bound independently of bilirubin.[25] According to Reed et al.[49] amino acid residues in the sequence from 186 to 248 in bovine albumin are involved in bilirubin binding, in agreement with the findings of Geizow and Beaven[90] and of Kuenzle et al.[91-93] The latter authors have also found binding to a lesser extent in the region 446-547, close to the C-terminal. Lysine 240, which is analogous to lys 238 in the bovine protein, should be involved.[94-96] The following amino acid residues are not engaged in binding of bilirubin, cys 34, trp 216, lys 212, lys 199.[87,88,96] A few tyrosine side chains should be present in the binding sites.[96]
- Finally, distances between the trytophan residue and bound bilirubin and fatty acids should comply with those calculated by Chen[51] and by Berde et al.[53] on the basis of fluorescence quenching studies.

Human albumin contains 585 amino acid residues in *one* peptide chain with a known sequence (Figure 18).[97,98] More than half of this chain is present as α-helices which are held together by disulfide bridges (Figure 19).[99,100] The structure has three repeating units or *domains*. Several authors have used a model in which the three domains are linearily arranged as globular units, as pictured by Berde et al.[53] (Figure 20). Two molecules of bilirubin may be bound in the crevice between domains *1* and *2* (one bound bilirubin molecule is pictured) and two molecules of fatty acid in domain *3* (shown here as two molecules of parinaric acid anion, studied by Berde et al.[53]). The one tryptophan residue present in human albumin is also shown, and distances are given between this and the ligands, as calculated from fluorescence quenching studies. This model satisfies most of the above criteria. Conformational changes involving the relative position of domains *1* and *2* could influence the conformation of bilirubin and thus affect the spectral changes described in the preceding section. The model does not, however, account for the immediate surroundings of the bound bilirubin molecules and does not explain how binding of fatty acid in domain *3* could induce conformational changes between domains *1* and *2*.

A somewhat more detailed idea of the immediate binding structures can be obtained from Brown's model.[99] As shown in Figure 19, each domain may be divided in two subdomains, each containing at least three helical elements, interconnected through

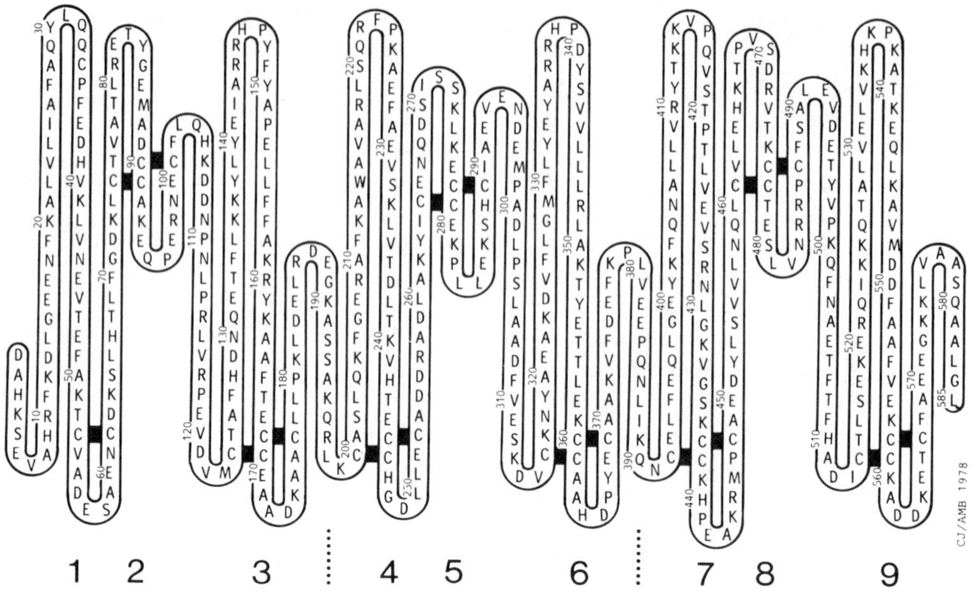

HSA

Ala - A - 62	Gln - Q - 21	Leu - L - 61	Ser - S - 24
Arg - R - 24	Glu - E - 61	Lys - K - 59	Thr - T - 28
Asn - N - 17	Gly - G - 12	Met - M - 6	Trp - W - 1
Asp - D - 36	His - H - 16	Phe - F - 31	Tyr - Y - 18
Cys - C - 35	Ile - I - 8	Pro - P - 24	Val - V - 41

Mol. wt. 66,438

FIGURE 18. Amino acid sequence and disulfide bridges of human albumin. Data compiled by C. Jacobsen from Behrens et al.[97] and Meloun et al.[98] Reproduced with kind permission from C. Jacobsen.

disulfide bridges. According to Brown, the three helices are positioned in parallel, out-of-plane, forming a trough, well suited as a binding element.[101] Examination of the composition of amino acid residues projecting into the interior of each of the six troughs reveals that two of these have peculiar patterns, especially suited for binding of bilirubin. As seen in Figure 21, the amino acids present in the inner aspects of the troughs of subdomains *1C* and *2C* have two permanent, positive charges, and several tyrosines and phenylalanines, providing an aromatic medium, besides carboxylate groups, aspartate and glutamate, capable of forming hydrogen bonds. Each of these two structures could accommodate one chromophore of the bilirubin molecule (Figure 22). A second trough, inverted on top of this could bind the second chromophore (Figure 23). Spectral changes can now be produced by rotation of the troughs so that the bilirubin molecule is twisted around the central methylene bridge. The two remaining subdomains could then form a fatty acid binding site, giving a total of three binding sites, each consisting of two subdomains and forming the three globular units of the albumin molecule. These units could be positioned in various ways, one example being shown in Figure 24. The two distal subdomains, containing the N- and C-terminals, are here placed together in the middle of the molecule with the other binding units on either side. Binding of fatty acids to the central unit would then cause a shift of its subdomains which would again shift the positions of the subdomains of the other binding units. This model seems to satisfy most of the criteria of bilirubin binding although the distances between bound molecules of bilirubin, fatty acids and the tryptophan of albumin are not in agreement with those calculated by Berde et al.[53] and by Chen.[51] Also some difficulties arise with the involvement of tryptophan and lysine 240, as previously discussed,[5] and with the most recent results of Jacobsen and Jacobsen,[87] on cobinding of tryptophan and bilirubin.

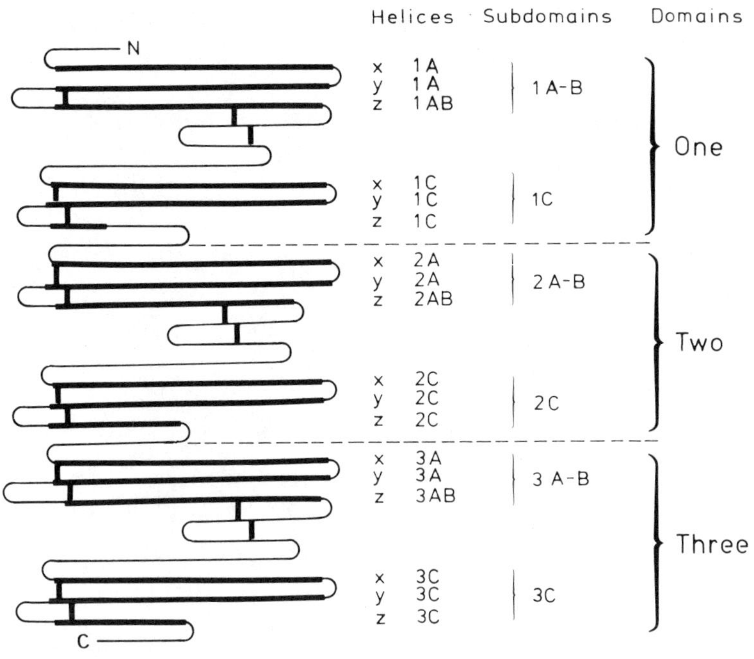

FIGURE 19. Helical structures in the molecule of human albumin, signified by solid lines. Data from Brown[99] and McLachlan and Walker.[100]

The model in Figure 24 underlines the flexibility of the albumin molecule. This feature which has not been found for any other protein, is essential for its biological role as a universal carrier. A model with six binding elements, each with specific liganding properties, depending upon the composition of amino acid side chains of the troughs, and interconnected through flexible hinged regions of the peptide chain so that they can combine in various ways according to actual binding tasks, seems to bear out the unique binding characters of the albumin molecule.

9. Practical Implications. Methods for the Study of Binding Equilibrium

Binding of bilirubin to albumin is of practical importance because of the toxicity of bilirubin to nervous and other tissues. Binding of bilirubin to albumin prevents transfer of the pigment from blood plasma to the brain while such transfer is enhanced by low pH and by the presence of competitively bound drugs. Numerous methods for clinical assessment of the state of binding of bilirubin have therefore been developed (see reviews[5,102]). Most of these methods aim at determination of the equilibrium concentration of free bilirubin or the vacant capacity for binding of bilirubin to albumin. Errors are introduced in most techniques, as follows: (1) by dilution, whereby an equilibrium with any loosely bound competitor is shifted, (2) by adding stoichiometric amounts of dyes, which also shift the equilibrium to be studied, (3) by using dyes which do not bind competitively with bilirubin, (4) by "titrating" the vacant albumin with bilirubin, whereby the equilibrium is again shifted, (5) by removing free bilirubin, by means of binding to Sephadex®, calcium carbonate etc., likewise shifting the equilibrium, or finally, (6) by working at room temperature rather than at 37°C. It should be added that measurement of bilirubin in ultrafiltrates or in supernatants from ultracentrifugation of the specimen gives values far in excess of the equilibrium concentration of bilirubin-IXα(Z,Z) dianion, due to the presence of bilirubin conjugates, non-α isomers, and photobilirubin, all of which are bound to albumin with lower affinity. On the other hand, though most of these methods do not measure a well defined chemical

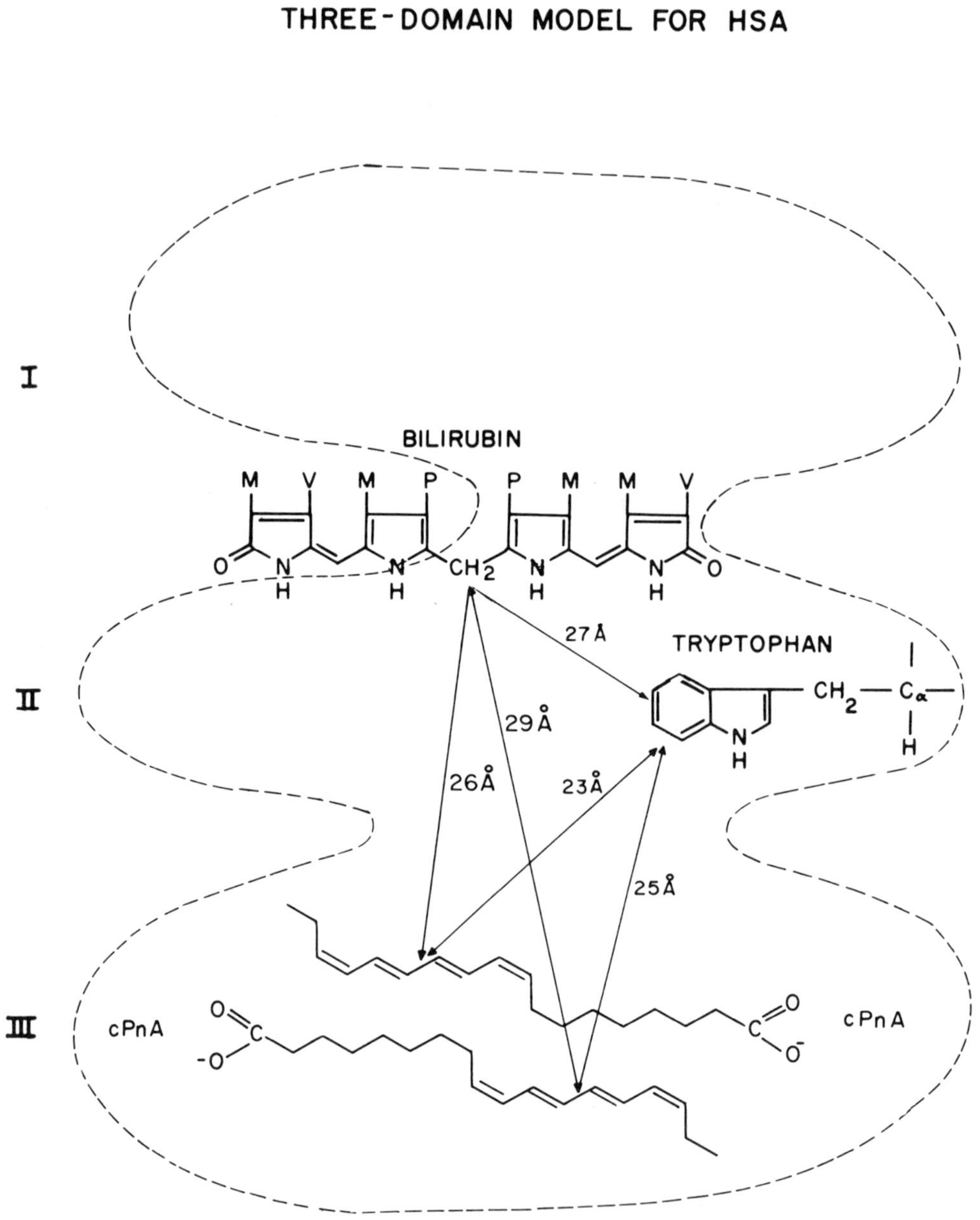

FIGURE 20. A model of the albumin molecule with bound bilirubin, positioned in the crevasse between domains I and II, and two molecules of bound fatty acid, located in domain III. The position of the lone tryptophan residue of the albumin peptide chain is also shown. (From Berde, C. B., Hudson, B. S., Simoni, R. D., and Sklar, L. A., *J. Biol. Chem.*, 254, 391, 1979. With permission.)

quantity, at least two techniques have an empirically proven value in prevention of brain damage in the newborn, as demonstrated by follow-up studies of 5 years or more.[80,103]

Several methods are available for determination of the equilibrium concentration of free bilirubin dianion in pure solutions of albumin and bilirubin, as used for determination of the binding affinity (see references in Section III.A.2) but none of these are applicable in serum or plasma.[5] It seems possible, however, to measure the vacant capacity for binding of bilirubin, the *reserve albumin concentration*, and this can be

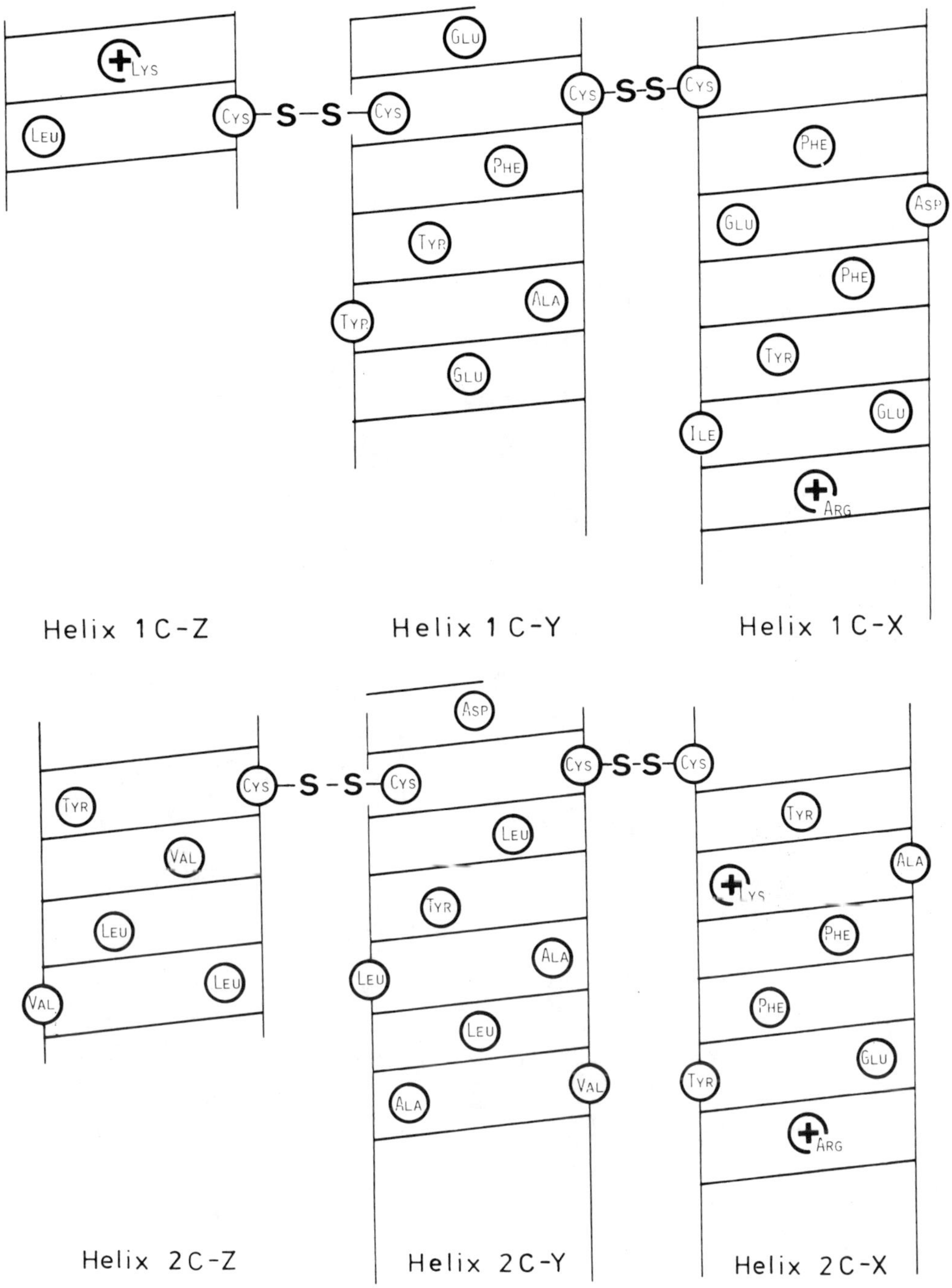

FIGURE 21. Amino acid side chain composition of proposed ligand binding structures in the albumin molecule. According to Brown,[99] three helices in each subdomain are positioned in parallel, forming a trough. The amino acid residue composition of the inner aspects of two of the six troughs is shown. These troughs seem particularly suited for binding of bilirubin.

done in serum and can be used for calculation of the affinity for transfer of bilirubin from blood plasma to tissues (see Section V). Methods for determination of the reserve albumin concentration for binding of bilirubin are based upon the principle of *selective*

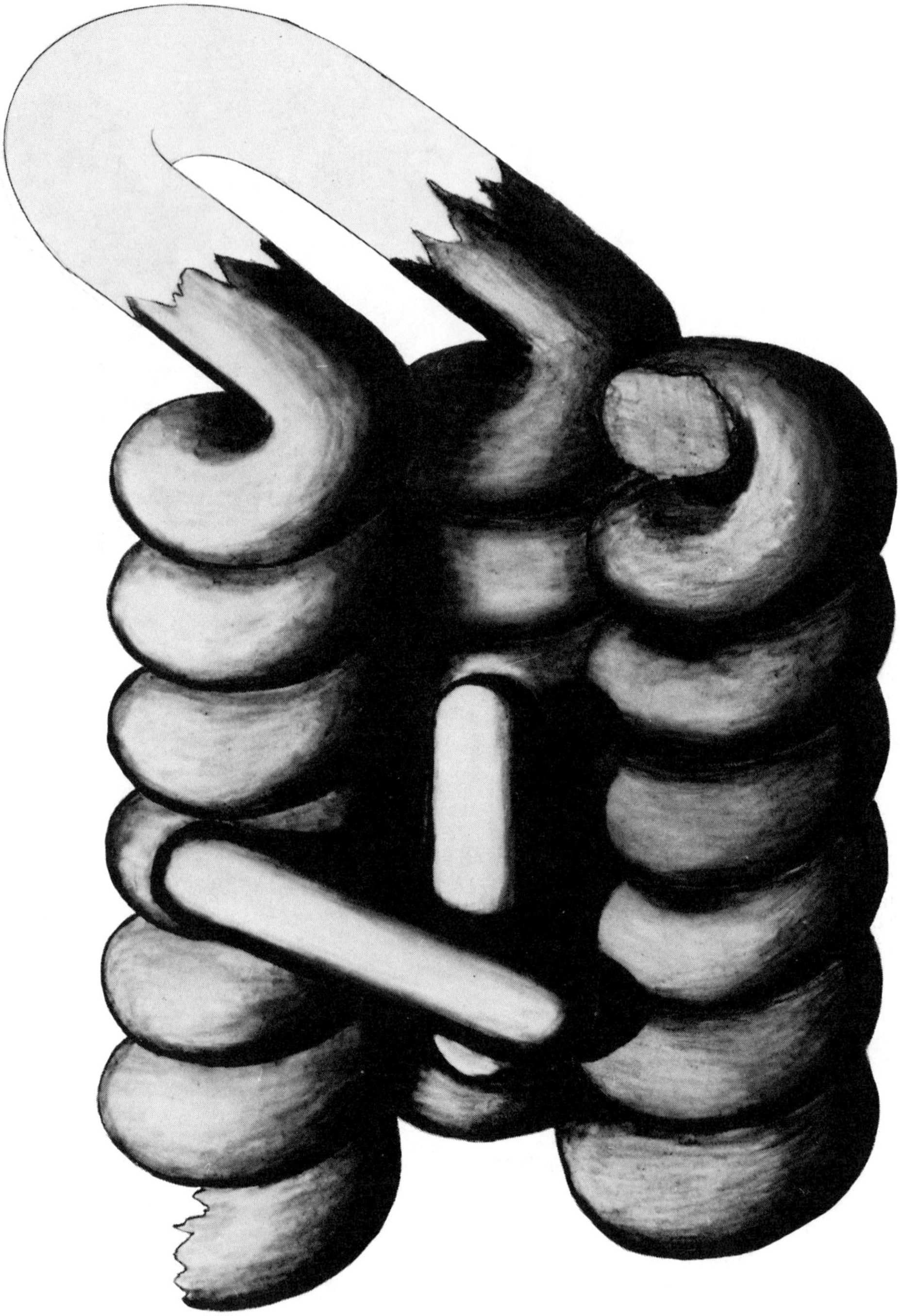

FIGURE 22. Proposed model for binding of one bilirubin molecule, shown as two light bars, in a triple-helical trough of albumin.

trace ligands (STL). A trace-amount of a ligand, not already present in the plasma, is added to the sample. Binding of the added ligand to albumin should be purely competitive with bilirubin. After establishment of equilibrium, the ratio of free to bound ligand is measured, and the reserve albumin concentration is obtained from a standard curve of ligand binding ratios obtained with pure albumin solutions. Due to the fact

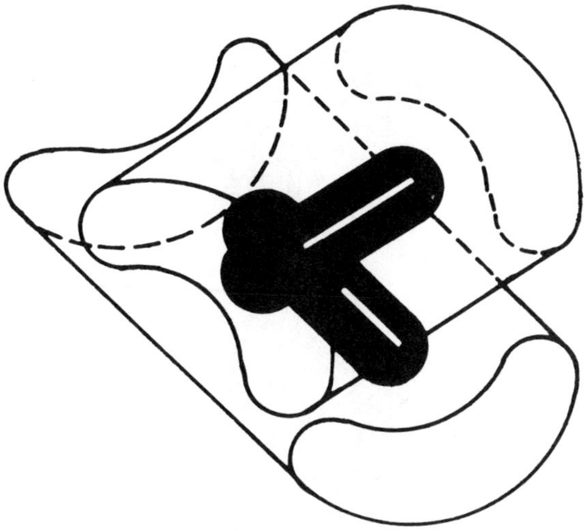

FIGURE 23. Proposed structure of a bilirubin binding site of albumin. One half of the bilirubin molecule is bound to a triple-helical trough, as shown in Figure 22, and the other half to a second trough, placed in an inverted position, facing the first. Rotation of one trough, relative to the other, around the central methylene bridge of the bilirubin molecule would produce the spectral changes seen on variation of pH (Figures 15 and 16) and on binding of a second ligand (Figure 17).

that the distribution of bound bilirubin on sites in the albumin molecule is unknown (Section III.A.3), as is the binding pattern of other ligands, difficulties arise with the definition of the reserve albumin concentration. These have been discussed[104] but do not seem to impede the practical utility of the determinations.

Two STL-methods for determination of reserve albumin for binding of bilirubin have been published, both applicable to small sample volumes of infant sera. One method, by Hsia et al.,[105] uses a spin-labeled trace-ligand and measures its binding to albumin by electron spin resonance spectroscopy. The other method utilizes monoacetyl-diaminodiphenyl sulfone, MADDS, as explained in Figure 25.[69,104] Clinical studies have proved the utility of the MADDS method,[107,112] also for estimating the bilirubin displacing effect of drugs in vivo.[112]

B. Complexes of the Bilirubin Dianion with Other Macromolecules, and with Polar Lipids

In recent years at least three other mammalian, bilirubin binding proteins have been found, ligandin, protein A (Z-protein), and α-fetoprotein. Although these have not yet been studied to the same extent as albumin, the binding of bilirubin has several features in common with binding to albumin and it may reasonably be presumed that these proteins also bind the bilirubin dianion. Further, phospholipids and gangliosides form complexes with bilirubin, with the bilirubin acid as well as with the dianion.

1. Ligandin

Bilirubin binding proteins in liver cytosol have been studied by several groups.[113-118] One component, termed *Y-protein,* and later *ligandin,* is especially well known. It is an enzyme, *glutathione S-transferase B,*[119] with enzymatic properties independent of the binding of bilirubin.[120] Ligandin is a basic protein, consisting of two subunits with a total molecular mass of 46,000 Da.[117] Binding of one molecule of bilirubin takes

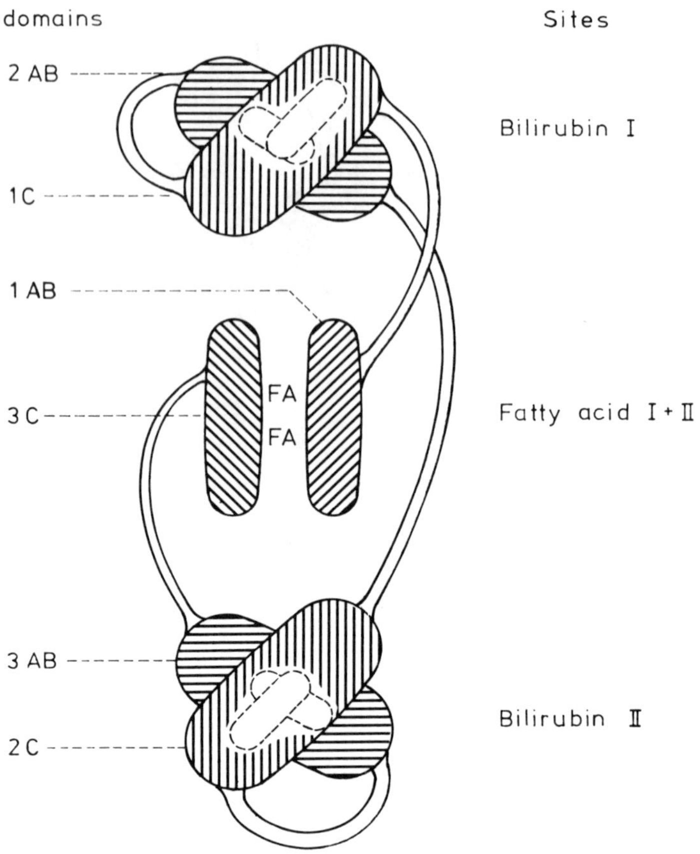

FIGURE 24. Proposed model of the albumin molecule, consisting of three binding units, as the one shown in Figure 23. One molecule of bilirubin is here bound to each of the distal units, and two molecules of fatty acid to the central unit. The six half-domains may combine in a different way for other binding purposes.

place with high affinity, followed by secondary binding of some additional bilirubin with lower affinity.[121] The primary binding constant has been somewhat differently reported but seems to be of the order of 10^6 to 10^8 M^{-1}, similar to that of bilirubin binding to albumin, or slightly lower.[121-123] Fluorescence and light absorption spectra of the bilirubin-ligandin complex are similar to those of bilirubin-albumin.[122] Also the circular dichroism spectrum resembles that of bilirubin-albumin in having two major adjacent peaks of opposite sign.[121,122] This seems to indicate that bilirubin is bound in a twisted configuration. The sign of optical activity at neutral pH-values is opposite to that of the complex with albumin, indicating that the bilirubin molecule is twisted in the opposite direction.

Ligandin binds a wide variety of anions, presumably in competition with bilirubin.[114,121] This property is important for hepatic excretion of anions. For a more detailed discussion, see Chapter 2, Volume II.

2. Aminoazo-Dye-Binding Protein A (Z-Protein)

Another anion binding protein in liver cytosol is amino-azo-dye-binding protein

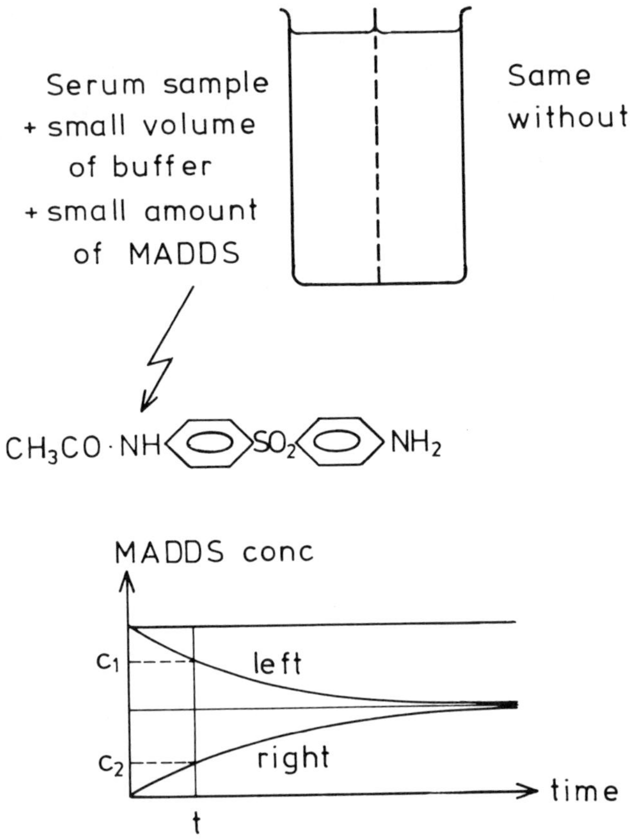

$$\text{Reserve albumin conc} = p = \frac{kt}{\log \frac{C_1 + C_2}{C_1 - C_2}}$$

FIGURE 25. Principle of the MADDS method for determination of the concentration of reserve albumin for binding of bilirubin (in infant sera). Undiluted samples of the serum, each 25 $\mu\ell$, are placed on either side of a dialysis membrane. A trace-amount of ^{14}C-labeled MADDS (monoacetyl-diaminodiphenylsulfone), which binds selectively and competively with bilirubin, is added to the serum on one side of the membrane. The rate is proportional to the free equilibrium concentration of MADDS and is thus inversely proportional to the available amount of MADDS (or bilirubin) binding site on albumin. Any competing ligand in the serum is present in equal concentration on either side of the membrane. A true value of the reserve albumin concentration is thus obtained, not influenced by errors from dilution of the sample, etc.

A[122,124,125] which is identical with Z-protein.[114,126,127] It has a low molecular mass, about 12,000 Da. The interaction with bilirubin has several similarities with that of albumin. The primary binding constant is probably between 2×10^7 and 10^8 M^{-1}.[122] Fluorescence, light absorption, and CD spectra are similar to those obtained with albumin and ligandin.[122] The sign of optical rotation is the same as with albumin.

3. α-Fetoprotein

α-Fetoprotein is present in the fetus where it functions as a universal carrier. It is also produced by some tumors. Its concentration in the plasma of the normal newborn is low, compared to that of albumin, and it is practically absent from the plasma of healthy adults. The amino acid sequence of α-fetoprotein shows homology with albumin.[128] Binding of bilirubin to human and bovine α-fetoprotein[129] and to the rat protein[130] has recently been studied. In all three species, one molecule of bilirubin is bound (or 0.6 mol to the human protein).[129] The complex can be equilibrated with albumin in different proportions, indicating that binding is reversible, proceeding to an equilibrium. The binding constant with human α-fetoprotein is about $3 \times 10^6\ M^{-1}$, when calculated from the finding that bilirubin is bound equally to human albumin and α-fetoprotein in a mixture of these two proteins, in the molar proportion 1:21, and using the known value of the binding constant to human albumin. Bovine α-fetoprotein binds bilirubin with a binding constant of $1.1 \times 10^6\ M^{-1}$, and the rat protein gives $2.9 \times 10^6\ M^{-1}$. In all three species the affinity is somewhat less than for binding to albumin.

Light absorption spectra, and the CD spectrum of bilirubin-rat α-fetoprotein, seem to be consistent with a binding mechanism similar to that observed with albumin.

4. Polar Lipids

French investigators half a century ago observed that some bilirubin could be extracted with ether from plasma of many icteric patients.[131] This "ether-soluble" bilirubin has also been investigated by German workers[132] and it has been shown that bilirubin is present in the ether phase as a complex of bilirubin and phospholipid.[133,134] This complex is probably not present as such in the plasma but is formed during the extraction procedure. The light absorption spectrum in organic solvents has a maximum at 420 nm.[2,134] The chemical composition and structure of the ether-soluble bilirubin has not been investigated and it is possible that it is a compound of bilirubin acid and phospholipid. It is biologically interesting because formation of such complexes possibly may explain how the polar bilirubin molecule is capable of penetrating phospholipid membranes.

Mustafa and King[135] have examined complexes of bilirubin with phospholipids in mitochondria and with other structural lipids. At pH 7.5, these complexes show light absorption spectra similar to the spectrum of aggregated bilirubin acid (Figure 1). Such complexes are dealt with in the following section. Nagaoka and Cowger,[136] have shown that the bilirubin dianion may combine with phospholipid vesicular membranes (liposomes), as seen from quenching of a fluorescent probe, 1,6-diphenyl-1,3,5-hexatriene (DPH), embedded in the membrane. At neutral pH, these complexes are unstable and within a few seconds or minutes form aggregates of bilirubin acid, attached to the membrane. The complex with bilirubin dianion is stable at higher pH, above 8.[137] Complexes of bilirubin with gangliosides, studied by Weil and Menkes,[138] and with phosphatidylcholine membranes, studied by Tipping et al.[139] are probably of a similar nature.

IV. COAGGREGATION OF BILIRUBIN ACID WITH MACROMOLECULES OR MEMBRANES, AND FORMATION OF MIXED MICELLES

A. Coaggregation with Albumin

When an alkaline solution of human albumin with a molar excess of bilirubin is neutralized to pH 7.5 or lower, a slow process is initiated, characterized as follows;[7] (1) light absorption spectrum decreases with formation of a shoulder around 500 nm,(2) light scattering increases markedly, and (3) optical rotation decreases and is, by bilirubin/albumin ratios higher than 5, inverted and may increase within a few hours to very high values of rotation, opposite to that observed with the bilirubin dianion-albumin complex. Electron microscopy of the reaction mixture shows formation of minute crystals. By ultracentrifugation in a sucrose gradient, two fractions are obtained, one containing large aggregates of bilirubin acid and albumin in molar proportion about 300:1, and a fraction of lower molecular size, consisting of bilirubin dianions and albumin, 1:1, i.e., the usual bilirubin-albumin complex.

A second type of bilirubin-albumin complex thus exists, containing several molecules of albumin and large numbers of bilirubin acid molecules, forming cocrystals. These aggregates are distinct from crystals of bilirubin acid with incidental admixture of albumin, as seen from the optical activity. A suspension of bilirubin crystals, formed in the absence of albumin, is optically inactive. Studies of the infrared spectrum likewise indicate involvement of the albumin in structuring of the aggregate, as seen from a considerable decrease of the albumin peak at 1550 cm^{-1}, corresponding to a conformational change of the albumin secondary structure.

Formation of these aggregates is unpredictable and may sometimes be difficult to achieve. If, on the other hand, crystallization has been successful once, it usually occurs promptly in subsequent experiments, as with formation of many other types of crystals.

The aggregates may be dissolved on addition of sodium hydroxide or dioxan, leaving a complex of albumin with two molecules of bilirubin dianion, and an excess of bilirubin dianion in solution.

B. Coaggregation of Bilirubin Acid with Polar Lipid Membranes

Mustafa and King[135] have shown that bilirubin combines with lipids in mitochondria and with many other structures containing polar lipids. Light absorption spectra obtained at pH 7.5 were identical with spectra of colloid suspensions of bilirubin acid and again with the above-mentioned aggregated suspensions of bilirubin acid with albumin. It seems likely that these complexes are of a similar nature to those obtained with albumin. When a suspension of phosphatidyl choline vesicles (liposomes) is added to a neutralized, supersaturated solution of bilirubin disodium salt, prompt formation of aggregates, containing bilirubin acid and phosphatidyl choline, is observed.[2] The process thus seems to differ from that observed with albumin in showing no tendency to supersaturation. Aggregation invariably takes place after mixing the components. A crystalline nature of the aggregates has not been observed with polar lipids. The reaction product is not optically active.[137]

The initial step in the formation of bilirubin acid-polar lipid aggregates is probably binding of a bilirubin dianion to the lipid structure, and this process can be studied at pH-values above 8. A convenient technique for the latter purpose is observation of quenching of fluorescence of an added probe, diphenylhexatriene.[136] In alkaline media, no further process is observed. In neutral solutions, the immediate quenching is followed by an increase of fluorescence, proceeding within minutes or hours. The final product, as revealed by infrared spectra, consists of aggregated bilirubin acid and lipid.[137] The first step in this process has been observed by Nagaoka and Cowger[136] with several phospholipids, phosphatidylserine, sphingomyelin, diphosphatidylcholine, phosphatidylethanolamine, diphosphatidylglycerol, and with mixed lipids prepared from bovine brain and from pig skin. An especially high affinity was found with sphingomyelin vesicles, although exact determination of binding constants under the conditions of the experiment seems to be difficult.[139] Formation of complexes with bilirubin, followed by aggregation of bilirubin acid, was observed with liposomes from phosphatidylcholine, phosphatidylethanolamine, phosphatidylserine, sphingomyelin, and a lipid preparation from cat brain, as well as with erythrocyte ghosts.[137] The course of the process was identical with phosphatidylcholine from eggs and with dipalmitoylphosphatidylcholine, and was unaffected by a cholesterol content of 5% in the liposomes. The affinity of formation of final aggregates containing bilirubin acid, was independent of the lipid used and was equal to the affinity of bilirubin acid aggregation in the absence of lipid. This is probably due to the presence of a large number of bilirubin acid molecules, connected to a few of the lipid molecules, so that the all-over affinity is dominated by bilirubin self-aggregation. The process of aggregation was slower with sphingomyelin than with the other lipids, in possible agreement with a higher affinity for binding of the dianion to sphingomyelin.[137]

These findings would be consistent with a special role of sphingomyelin in bilirubin neurotoxicity, as proposed by Nagaoka and Cowger.[136] Weil and Menkes have studied binding of bilirubin to gangliosides and have presumed that these are essential for the neurotoxic effect.[138]

C. Mixed Micelles with Bilirubin

Several detergents, which are capable of forming micelles, take up a limited amount of bilirubin in the micelles or on their polar surface.[34,57,140] Mixed micelles with bile salts may be biologically important for the transport of bilirubin in bile.[141]

V. MOLECULAR MECHANISM OF BILIRUBIN TOXICITY. FREE ENERGY OF TRANSFER FROM BLOOD PLASMA TO TISSUES

A. Mechanism of Binding of Bilirubin to Tissues

Binding of bilirubin to erythrocytes and to cellular elements in tissues increases at low pH.[46,65,142-144] Silberberg et al.[145] pointed out that this could be explained alternatively by decreased binding of bilirubin to albumin or by increased affinity of bilirubin for the tissues. Since bilirubin is bound as the dianion to albumin in plasma with an affinity which does not vary with pH,[46] and since bilirubin *acid* is bound to phospholipid structures in cellular membranes and other structures (Section IV.B), the latter alternative has to be adopted. This is also in good agreement with the theory of Lee and Cowger that toxicity of bilirubin depends upon aggregation of the insoluble bilirubin acid.[146] The all-over process of bilirubin transfer from plasma to tissues is thus

$$\underset{\text{in plasma}}{B^{2-}\text{-Albumin}} + \underset{\text{in plasma}}{2H^{+}} \rightleftharpoons \underset{\text{Aggregates in tissue}}{BH_2} + \underset{\text{in plasma}}{\text{Albumin}} \qquad (21)$$

The detailed mechanism of the transfer remains unknown.[147-149] Also, the ultimate (enzymatic?) mechanism of bilirubin toxicity in the cell has been the object of numerous investigations.[150,151] It has not been possible to establish any particular enzyme as the target of the toxic effect, and Cowger in 1971 formulated the hypothesis that "the primary lesion may be on multiple cell membrane systems, perhaps brought about by some alterations of membrane lipids".[152]

B. Free Energy of Bilirubin Transport from Plasma to Tissue

The process in Equation 21 is reversible,[135,137,153] although equilibrium may be obtained slowly. It is then possible to calculate the loss of free energy on transport of bilirubin from plasma to tissues, provided active transport is not involved in any step between the bilirubin-albumin complex in plasma and the bilirubin acid aggregate in the target organelle. A basic thermodynamic rule states that the loss of free energy is independent of the pathway of transport and depends only upon the chemical identity of the substances involved and their concentrations at the start and finish of the transport process. We may, therefore, imagine that the process takes place by precipitation of bilirubin acid on target membrane structures suspended in plasma. Under these circumstances the loss of free energy is

$$-\Delta G = RT\ln \frac{b}{b'} \qquad (22)$$

where b is the concentration of free bilirubin dianion in the plasma, and b' is the solubility of bilirubin at the pH of the plasma. The solubility of bilirubin varies with pH and is, according to Figure 1, obtained from

$$\log b' = 2\text{pH} - 23.24 \qquad (23)$$

The concentration of bilirubin dianion, b, cannot be measured by present means but can be calculated from the binding equation,

$$\frac{c}{a\,b} = K_B \qquad (24)$$

From Equations 22 to 24 we obtain the affinity of bilirubin transfer, using a known value of K_B (Table 2),

$$-\Delta G = 2.30RT(\log \frac{c}{a} - 2\text{pH} + 15.5) \qquad (25)$$

The concentration, cc of the bilirubin dianion-albumin complex is practically equal to the concentration of unconjugated bilirubin, B, as determined by conventional means. The concentration, a, of albumin unoccupied by bilirubin, can be determined by measuring the reserve albumin concentration, p, by the MADDS method. It is thus possible to determine the free energy of bilirubin transfer from plasma to tissue from measured values of the unconjugated plasma bilirubin concentration, the reserve albumin concentration, and the plasma pH.

The free energy is a measure of plasma bilirubin toxicity. If ΔG is positive, bilirubin cannot pass from plasma to tissues and any bilirubin already deposited will tend to dissolve. With negative values of ΔG, transport of bilirubin from plasma to tissue is thermodynamically possible. The rate of the transport processes, however, cannot be derived from thermodynamic considerations and probably depends upon local tissue factors, such as the integrity of the blood-brain barrier.[148] Also the final outcome may be modified by oxidation[154] of bilirubin which has already penetrated the cell. The free energy of transport is nevertheless a parameter of clinical interest for evaluation of the risk of brain damage in icteric newborns. For ease of calculation, *an index of plasma bilirubin toxicity* has been introduced,[4,5,155]

$$I = \log \frac{B}{p} - 2\text{pH} + 15.5 \qquad (26)$$

which is connected with the free energy of transfer,

$$-\Delta G = 2.30RTI$$

Due to the heterogeneity of solid bilirubin with respect to its solubility (see Section I.A.2), the absolute value of the constant 15.5 may have to be altered, should it become possible to measure the solubility of the actual aggregates of bilirubin acid in the tissues. This, however, will not limit the practical utility of the Index.

Clinical experience from a few hundred determinations of the Index in sera from newborns seems favorable.[106,110]

REFERENCES

1. **Overbeek, J. T. G., Vink, C. L., and Deenstra, H.,** The solubility of bilirubin, *Recl. Trav. Chim. Pays-Bas,* 74, 81, 1955.
2. **Brodersen, R.,** Bilirubin solubility and interaction with albumin and phospholipid, *J. Biol. Chem.,* 254, 2364, 1979.
3. **McDonagh, A. F. and Assisi, F.,** The ready isomerization of bilirubin IX-α in aqueous solution, *Biochem. J.,* 129, 797, 1972.
4. **Brodersen, R.,** Bilirubin interaction with albumin and tissues, in *Intensive Care in the Newborn III,* Stern, L., Salle, B., and Friis-Hansen, B., Eds., Masson Publ. U.S.A. Inc., New York, 1981, 105.
5. **Brodersen, R.,** Binding of bilirubin to albumin, *Crit. Rev. Clin. Lab. Sci.,* 11, 305, 1980.
6. **Brodersen, R.,** Bilirubin transport in the newborn, reviewed with relation to kernicterus, *J. Pediatr.,* 96, 349, 1980.
7. **Brodersen, R., Funding, L., Pedersen, A. O., and Røigaard-Petersen, H.,** Binding of bilirubin to low-affinity sites of human serum albumin in vitro followed by co-crystallization, *Scand. J. Clin. Lab. Invest.,* 29, 433, 1972.
8. **Küster, W.,** Beitrage zur Kenntnis der Gallenfarbstoffe. Über Bilirubin, Biliverdin und ihre Spaltungsprodukte, *Hoppe-Seyler's Z. Physiol. Chemie,* 59, 63, 1909.
9. **Fog, J. and Bugge-Asperheim, B.,** Stability of bilirubin, *Nature (London),* 203, 756, 1964.
10. **Gray, C. H., Kulczycka, A., and Nicholson, D. C.,** The chemistry of bile pigments. IV. Spectrophotometric titration of the bile pigments, *J. Chem. Soc.,* 442, 2276, 1961.
11. **Krasner, J. and Yaffe, S. J.,** The automatic titration of bilirubin, *Biochem. Med.,* 7, 128, 1973.
12. **Lee, J. J., Daly, L. H., and Cowger, M. L.,** Bilirubin ion equilibria; their effects on spectra and on conformation, *Res. Commun. Chem. Pathol. Pharmacol.,* 9, 763, 1974.
13. **Norman, J. D. v. and Szentirmay, R.,** Chemistry of bilirubin and biliverdin in N,N-dimethylformamide, *Anal. Chem.,* 46, 1456, 1974.
14. **Norman, J. D. v. and Szentirmay, R.,** Considerations concerning the formation of metal chelates of bilirubin: the zinc:bilirubin system, *Bioinorg. Chem.,* 4, 37, 1974.
15. **Hansen, P. E., Thiessen, H., and Brodersen, R.,** Bilirubin acidity. Titrimetric and ^{13}C NMR studies, *Acta Chem. Scand. B,* 33, 281, 1979.
16. **McDonagh, A. F.,** Bile pigments: bilatrienes and 5,15 biladienes, in *The Porphyrins,* Vol. 6, Dolphin, D., Ed., Academic Press, New York, 1979, chap. 6.
17. **Falk, H., Gergely, S., and Grubmayr, K.,** Das tautomere Gleichgewicht des Bilirubins, *Monatsh. Chem.,* 107, 827, 1976.
18. **Manitto, P. and Monti, D.,** Photoaddition of sulfhydryl groups to bilirubin in vitro, *Experientia,* 28, 379, 1972.
19. **Fischer, H. and Orth, H.,** *Die Chemie des Pyrrols,* Vol. 2/1, Die Pyrrolfarbstoffe Akad. Verlagsges., Leipzig, 1937, 619.
20. **Fog. J. and Bakken, A. F.,** Studies on the bilirubin-protein bond, in *Bilirubin Metabolism,* Bouchier, T. A. D. and Billing, B., Eds. Blackwell, Oxford, 1967, 85.
21. **Kolthoff, I. M. and Bruckensten, S.,** Acid-base equilibria in non-aqueous solutions, in *Treatise of Analytical Chemistry,* Vol. 1, Elving, P. J. and Sandell, E. B., Eds., Interscience, New York, 1959, 487.
22. **Heilmeyer, L.,** Das Absorptionsspektrum des Bilirubins in Chloroform, Alkohol und Alkalien, *Biochem. Z.,* 232, 229, 1931.
23. **Blanckaert, N., Heirwegh, K. P. M., and Compernolle, F.,** Synthesis and separation by thin-layer chromatography of bilirubin-IX isomers. Their identification as tetrapyrroles and dipyrrolic ethyl anthranilate azo derivatives, *Biochem. J.,* 155, 405, 1976.
24. **Blauer, G., Harmatz, D., and Snir, J.,** Optical properties of bilirubin-serum albumin complexes in aqueous solution. I. Dependence on pH, *Biochim. Biophys. Acta,* 278, 68, 1972.
25. **Brodersen, R.,** unpublished work.
26. **Sato, T.,** A study of bilirubin in pigmented calcium stones, *Tohoku J. Exper. Med.,* 77, 83, 1962.
27. **Maki, T., Sato, T., and Sato, T.,** A study on the activity of β-glucuronidase in bile in connection with precipitation of calcium bilirubinate, *Tohoku J. Exper. Med.,* 77, 179, 1962.
28. **Chan, G. M., Ash, K. O., Hentschel, W., and Wu, J.,** In vitro effects of bilirubin on ionized calcium, *Pediatr. Res.,* 13, 491, 1979.
29. **O'Carra, P.,** Zinc complex salt formation by bilirubin and mesobilirubin, *Nature (London),* 195, 899, 1962.
30. **Kuenzle, C. C., Pelloni, R. R., and Weibel, M. H.,** A proposed novel structure for the metal chelates of bilirubin, *Biochem. J.,* 130, 1147, 1972.
31. **v. Roy, F. and Heirwegh, K. P. M.,** Ability of bilirubin to form zinc complexes, *Arch. Internat. Physiol. Biochim.,* 73, 535, 1965.

32. **Velapoldi, R. A. and Menis, O.,** Formation and stabilities of free bilirubin and bilirubin complexes with transition and rare-earth elements, *Clin. Chem.*, 17, 1165, 1971.
33. **Ostrow, J. D., Hammaker, L., and Schmid, R.,** The preparation of crystalline bilirubin-C^{14}, *J. Clin. Invest.*, 40, 1442, 1961.
34. **Carey, M. C. and Koretsky, A. P.,** Self-association of unconjugated bilirubin-IXα in aqueous solution at pH 10.0 and physical-chemical interactions with bile salt monomers and micelles, *Biochem. J.*, 179, 675, 1979.
35. **Brodersen, R.,** Dimerisation of bilirubin anion in aqueous solution, *Acta Chem. Scand.*, 20, 2895, 1966.
36. **Jirsa, M. and Šponar, J.,** Zur Frage des direkt und indirekt reagierenden Gallenfarbstoffes, *Gesamte Inn. Med. Ihre Grenzgeb.*, 10, 967, 1955.
37. **Jirsa, M. and Sedláček, B.,** Aggregation von Bilirubin-teilchen im System Lösungsmittel - Fällungsmittel, *Collect. Czesh. Chem. Commun.*, 21, 1409, 1956.
38. **Jirsa, M. and Šponar, J.,** Das Absorptionsspektrum, der physikalische Zustand und die Geschwindigkeit der Diazoreaktion des Bilirubins, *Gesamte Inn. Med. Ihre Grenzgeb.*, 11, 519, 1956.
39. **Lee, J. J. and Cowger, M. L.,** Bilirubin-albumin binding and a possible mechanism of kernicterus, *Res. Commun. Chem. Pathol. Pharmacol.*, 8, 327, 1974.
40. **Lee, K. S. and Gartner, L. M.,** Spectrophotometric characteristics of bilirubin, *Pediatr. Res.*, 10, 782, 1976.
41. **Kamisaka, K., Listowsky, I., Betheil, J. J., and Arias, I. M.,** Competitive binding of bilirubin, sulfobromphthalein, indocyanine green and other organic anions to human and bovine serum albumin, *Biochim. Biophys. Acta*, 365, 169, 1974.
42. **Beaven, G. H., d'Albis, A., and Gratzer, W. B.,** The interaction of bilirubin with human serum albumin, *Eur. J. Biochem.*, 33, 500, 1973.
43. **Faerch, T. and Jacobsen, J.,** Determination of association and dissociation rate constants for bilirubin-bovine serum albumin, *Arch. Biochem. Biophys.*, 168, 351, 1975.
44. **Faerch, T. and Jacobsen, J.,** Kinetics of the binding of bilirubin to human serum albumin studied by stopped-flow technique, *Arch. Biochem. Biophys.*, 184, 282, 1977.
45. **Blauer, G., Lavie, E., and Silfen, J.,** Relative affinities of bilirubin for serum albumins from different species, *Biochim. Biophys. Acta*, 492, 64, 1977.
46. **Nelson, T., Jacobsen, J., and Wennberg, R. P.,** Effect of pH on the interaction of bilirubin with albumin and tissue culture cells, *Pediat. Res.*, 8, 963, 1974.
47. **Jacobsen, J. and Brodersen, R.,** The effect of pH on albumin-bilirubin affinity, *Birth Defects, Orig. Artic. Ser.*, 12, 175, 1976.
48. **Jacobsen, J.,** Binding of bilirubin to human serum albumin. Determination of the dissociation constants, *FEBS Lett.*, 5, 112, 1969.
49. **Reed, R. G., Feldhoff, R. C., Clute, O. L., and Peters, T.,** Fragments of bovine serum albumin produced by limited proteolysis. Conformation and ligand binding, *Biochemistry*, 14, 4578, 1975.
50. **Krasner, J., Giacoia, G. P., and Yaffe, S. J.,** Drug-protein binding in the newborn infant, *Ann. N.Y. Acad. Sci.*, 226, 101, 1973.
51. **Chen, R. F.,** The fluorescence of bilirubin-albumin complexes, in *Cell Biology*, Thaer, A. A. and Sernetz, M., Eds., Springer, Berlin, 1973, 239.
52. **Levine, R. L.,** Fluorescence quenching studies of the binding of bilirubin to albumin, *Clin. Chem.*, 23, 2292, 1977.
53. **Berde, C. B., Hudson, B. S., Simoni, R. D., and Sklar, L. A.,** Human serum albumin: spectroscopic studies of binding and proximity relationships for fatty acid and bilirubin, *J. Biol. Chem.*, 254, 391, 1979.
54. **Rubaltelli, F. F. and Jori, G.,** Visible light irradiation of human and bovine serum albumin-bilirubin complex, *Photochem. Photobiol.*, 29, 991, 1979.
55. **Yamaji, K.,** Interaction of bilirubin with albumin studied by gel filtration, peroxidase, and saturation index methods, *Nagoya Shiritsu Daigaku Igakkai Zasshi*, 25, 344, 1975 (Japan), cited from *Chem. Abstr.*, 83, 232, 1975.
56. **Gray, R. D. and Stroupe, S. D.,** Kinetics and mechanism of bilirubin binding to human serum albumin, *J. Biol. Chem.*, 253, 4370, 1978.
57. **Lamola, A. A., Eisinger, J., Blumberg, W. E., Pathel, S. C., and Flores, J.,** Fluorometric study of the partition of bilirubin among blood components: Basis for rapid microassays of bilirubin and bilirubin binding capacity in whole blood, *Anal. Biochem.*, 100, 25, 1979.
58. **Brodersen, R. and Funding, L.,** Binding of bilirubin and long-chain fatty acids to human serum albumin — with general remarks on displacement of firmly bound ligands, *Scand. J. Clin. Lab. Invest.*, 37, 257, 1977.
59. **Jacobsen, J.,** Studies of the affinity of human serum albumin for binding of bilirubin at different temperatures and ionic strength, *Int. J. Pept. Protein Res.*, 9, 235, 1977.

60. **Klotz, I. M. and Hunston, D. L.**, Protein interactions with small molecules. Relationships between stoichiometric binding constants, site binding constants, and empirical binding parameters, *J. Biol. Chem.*, 250, 3001, 1975.
61. **Klotz, I. M. and Hunston, D. L.**, Protein affinities for small molecules. Conceptions and misconceptions, *Arch. Biochem. Biophys.*, 193, 314, 1979.
62. **Chen, R. F.**, Fluorescence stopped-flow study of relaxation processes in the binding of bilirubin to serum albumin, *Arch. Biochem. Biophys.*, 162, 106, 1974.
63. **Reed, R.**, Kinetics of bilirubin binding to bovine serum albumin and the effects of palmitate, *J. Biol. Chem.*, 252, 7483, 1977.
64. **Woolley, P. W. and Hunter, M.**, Binding and circular dichroism data on bilirubin-albumin in the presence of oleate and salicylate, *Arch. Biochem. Biophys.*, 140, 197, 1970.
65. **Odell, G. B.**, The distribution of bilirubin between albumin and mitochondria, *J. Pediatr.*, 68, 164, 1966.
66. **Starinsky, R. and Shafrir, E.**, Displacement of albumin-bound bilirubin by fatty acids. Implications for neonatal hyperbilirubinemia, *Clin. Chim. Acta*, 29, 311, 1970.
67. **Chan, G., Schiff, D. and Stern, L.**, Competitive binding of free fatty acids and bilirubin to albumin: differences in HBABA dye versus Sephadex G-25 interpretation of results, *Clin. Biochem.*, 4, 208, 1971.
68. **Thiessen, H., Jacobsen, J., and Brodersen, R.**, Displacement of albumin-bound bilirubin by fatty acids, *Acta Paediatr. Scand.*, 61, 285, 1972.
69. **Brodersen, R.**, Determination of the vacant amount of high-affinity bilirubin binding site on serum albumin, *Acta Pharmacol. Toxicol.*, 42, 153, 1978.
70. **Silvermann, W. A., Andersen, D. H., Blanc, W. A., and Crozier, D. N.**, A difference in mortality rate and incidence of kernicterus among premature infants allotted to two prophylactic antibacterial regimens, *Pediatrics*, 18, 614, 1956.
71. **Harris, R. C., Lucey, J. F., and Maclean, J. R.**, Kernicterus in premature infants associated with low concentrations of bilirubin in plasma, *Pediatrics*, 21, 875, 1958.
72. **Johnson, L., Sarmiento, F., Blanc, W. A., and Day, R.**, Kernicterus in rats with an inherited deficiency of glucuronyl transferase, *Am. J. Dis. Child.*, 97, 591, 1959.
73. **Odell, G. B.**, The dissociation of bilirubin from albumin and its clinical implications, *J. Pediatr.*, 55, 268, 1959.
74. **Brodersen, R.**, Competitive binding of bilirubin and drugs to human serum albumin studied by enzymatic oxidation, *J. Clin. Invest.*, 54, 1353, 1974.
75. **Brodersen, R.**, Free bilirubin in blood plasma of the newborn. Effects of albumin, fatty acids, pH, displacing drugs and phototherapy. Appendix: a provisional survey of the bilirubin-displacing effect of 150 drugs, in *Intensive Care in the Newborn*, Vol. 2, Stern, L., Oh, W., and Friis-Hansen, B., Eds., Masson, New York, 1978.
76. **Brodersen, R., Sjödin, T., and Sjöholm, I.**, Independent binding of benzodiazepines and bilirubin to human serum albumin, *J. Biol. Chem.*, 252, 5067, 1977.
77. **Wennberg, R. P. and Cowger, M. L.**, Spectral characteristics of bilirubin-bovine albumin complexes, *Clin. Chim. Acta*, 43, 55, 1973.
78. **Jacobsen, J. and Faerch, T.**, Thermodynamics and kinetics of the neutral transition of human serum albumin, monitored by the spectral change of bound bilirubin, *Biochim. Biophys. Acta*, in press.
79. **Harmatz, D. and Blauer, G.**, Optical properties of bilirubin-serum albumin complexes in aqueous solution. A comparison among albumins from different species, *Arch. Biochem. Biophys.*, 170, 375, 1975.
80. **Odell, G. B.**, Studies in kernicterus. I. The protein binding of bilirubin, *J. Clin. Invest.*, 38, 823, 1959.
81. **Lavie, E. and Blauer, G.**, Circular dichroism and hydrodynamic measurements of ternary protein-two ligand systems: serum albumin-bilirubin — drug or alcohol, *Arch. Biochem. Biophys.*, 193, 191, 1979.
82. **Odell, G. B.**, Influence of binding on the toxicity of bilirubin, *Ann. N.Y. Acad. Sci.*, 226, 225, 1973.
83. **Mugnoli, A., Manitto, P., and Monti, D.**, Structure of di-isopropylammonium bilirubinate, *Nature (London)*, 273, 568, 1978.
84. **Bloomfield, V.**, The structure of bovine serum albumin at low pH, *Biochemistry*, 5, 684, 1966.
85. **Anderson, S. R. and Weber, G.**, Fluorescence polarization of the complex of 1-anilino-8-naphthalenesulfonate with bovine serum albumin. Evidence for preferential orientation of the ligand, *Biochemistry*, 8, 371, 1969.
86. **Pedersen, A. O., Schønheyder, F., and Brodersen, R.**, Photooxidation of human serum albumin and its complex with bilirubin, *Eur. J. Biochem.*, 72, 213, 1977.
87. **Jacobsen, C. and Jacobsen, J.**, Dansylation of human serum albumin in the study of the primary binding sites of bilirubin and L-tryptophan, *Biochem. J.*, 181, 251, 1979.

88. **Jacobsen, C.**, Chemical modification of the high-affinity bilirubin-binding site of human serum albumin, *Eur. J. Biochem.*, 27, 513, 1972.
89. **Bradshaw, R. A. and Peters, T.**, The amino acid sequence of peptide (1-24) of rat and human serum albumins, *J. Biol. Chem.*, 244, 55829, 1969.
90. **Geisow, M. J. and Beaven, G. H.**, Large fragments of human serum albumin, *Biochem. J.*, 161, 619, 1977.
91. **Kuenzle, C. C., Gitzelmann-Cumarasamy, N., and Wilson, K. J.**, Affinity labelling of the primary bilirubin binding site of human serum albumin, *J. Biol. Chem.*, 251, 801, 1976.
92. **Kuenzle, C. C., Gitzelmann-Cumarasamy, N., and Wilson, K. J.**, Mapping of the primary bilirubin binding site of human serum albumin, *11th FEBS Meeting, Copenhagen 1977*, B9-3, 412, 1/2/3.
93. **Gitzelmann-Cumarasamy, N., Kuenzle, C. C., and Wilson, K. J.** Mapping of the primary bilirubin binding site of human serum albumin, *Experientia*, 32, 768, 1976.
94. **Jacobsen, C.**, Covalent coupling of bilirubin to albumin, *Int. J. Pept. Protein Res.*, 8, 295, 1976.
95. **Jacobsen, C.**, Lysine residue 240 of human serum albumin is involved in high-affinity binding of bilirubin, *Biochem. J.*, 171, 453, 1978.
96. **Jacobsen, C.**, Trinitrofenylation of the bilirubin binding site of human serum albumin, *Int. J. Pept. Protein Res.*, 7, 159, 1975.
97. **Behrens, P. Q., Spiekerman, A. M., and Brown, J. R.**, Structure of human serum albumin, *Fed. Proc. Fed. Am. Soc. Exp. Biol.*, 34, 591, 1975.
98. **Meloun, B., Moravek, L., and Kostka, V.**, Complete amino acid sequence of human serum albumin, *FEBS Lett.*, 58, 134, 1975.
99. **Brown, J. R.**, Structure and evolution of serum albumin, in *Albumin, Structure, Biosynthesis, Function, FEBS 11th Meeting, Copenhagen 1977*, Peters, T., and Sjöholm, I. eds., Pergamon Press, Oxford, 1978, 1.
100. **McLachlan, A. D. and Walker, J. E.**, Serum albumin domain secondary structure prediction, *Biochim. Biophys. Acta*, 536, 106, 1978.
101. **Hsia, J. C.**, Serumalbumin structure and function — the allosteric domain model, *Fed. Proc. Fed. Am. Soc. Exp. Biol.*, 37, 852, 1978.
102. **Lee, K. S. and Gartner, L. M.**, Bilirubin binding by plasma proteins: a critical evaluation of methods and clinical implications, *Rev. Perinatal Med.*, 2, 319, 1978.
103. **Porter, E. G. and Waters, W. J.**, A rapid micromethod for measuring the reserve albumin binding capacity in serum from newborn infants with hyperbilirubinemia, *J. Lab. Clin. Med.*, 67, 660, 1966.
104. **Brodersen, R., Andersen, S., Jacobsen, C., Sønderskov, O., Ebbesen, F., Cashore, W. J., and Larsen, S.**, Determination of infant serum reserve albumin for bindng of bilirubin, using monoacetyldiaminodiphenylsulfone (MADDS) as a selective trace-ligand, *Anal. Biochem.*, in press.
105. **Hsia, J. C., Kwan, N. H., Er, S. S., Wood, D. J., and Chance, G. W.**, Development of a spin assay for reserve bilirubin loading capacity of human serum, *Proc. Natl. Acad. Sci. USA*, 75, 1542, 1978.
106. **Ebbesen, F.**, Bilirubin, reserve albumin for binding of bilirubin and pH in plasma during phototherapy (ordinary and double light) of term newborn infants, *Acta Paediatr. Scand.*, 70, 223, 1981.
107. **Ebbesen, F.**, The relationship between serum bilirubin and reserve albumin for binding of bilirubin during phototherapy of preterm infants, *Acta Paediatr. Scand.*, 70, 405, 1981.
108. **Ebbesen, F.**, Effect of exchange transfusion on serum reserve albumin for binding of bilirubin and index of serum bilirubin toxicity, *Acta Paediatr. Scand.*, 70, 643, 1981.
109. **Ebbesen, F. and Brodersen, R.**, Albumin administration combined with phototherapy in treatment of hyperbilirubinemia in low-birth-weight infants, *Acta Paediatr. Scand.*, 70, 649, 1981.
110. **Ebbesen, F. and Brodersen, R.**, Comparison between two preparations of human serum albumin in treatment of neonatal hyperbilirubinemia, *Acta Paediatr. Scand.*, 71, 85, 1982.
111. **Järnerot, G., Andersen, S., Esbjorner, E., Sandström, B., and Brodersen, R.**, Albumin reserve for binding of bilirubin in maternal and cord serum under treatment with sulfasalazine, *Scand. J. Gasroenterol.*, 16, 1049, 1981.
112. **Brodersen, R., and Ebbesen, F.**, Bilirubin displacing effect of ampicillin, indomethacin, chlorpromazine, gentamicin, and parabens *in vitro* and in newborn infants, submitted.
113. **Grodsky, G. M., Carbone, J. V., Fanska, R., and Peng, C. T.**, Tritiated bilirubin: Preparation and physiological studies, *Am. J. Physiol.*, 203, 532, 1962.
114. **Levi, A. J., Gatmaitan, Z., and Arias, I. M.**, Two hepatic cytoplasmatic protein fractions, Y and Z, and their possible role in the hepatic uptake of bilirubin, sulfobromophtalein, and other anions, *J. Clin. Invest.*, 48, 2156, 1969.
115. **Meuwissen, J. A. T. P. and Heirwegh, K. P. M.**, Transfer of adsorbed bilirubin to specific binding proteins, *Biochem. J.*, 120, 19P, 1970.
116. **Grodsky, G. M., Kolb, H. J., Fanska, R. E., and Nemechek, C.**, Effect of age of rat on development of hepatic carriers for bilirubin: a possible explanation for physiologic jaundice and hyperbilirubinemia in the newborn, *Metabolism*, 19, 246, 1970.

117. **Litwak, G., Ketterer, B., and Arias, I. M.,** Ligandin: a hepatic protein which binds steroids, bilirubin, carcinogens and a number of exogenous organic anions, *Nature (London),* 234, 466, 1971.
118. **Ketterer, B., Meuwissen, J., and Beale, B.,** Ligandin, *Biochem. Soc. Trans.,* 3, 626, 1975.
119. **Habig., W. H., Pabst, M. J., Fleischner, G., Gatmaitan, Z., Arias, I. M., and Jacobi, W. B.,** The identity of glutathione S-transferase B with ligandin, a major binding protein of liver, *Proc. Natl. Acad. Sci. USA,* 71, 3879, 1974.
120. **Bhargava, M. M., Listowsky, I., and Arias, I. M.,** Ligandin. Bilirubin binding and glutathione-S-transferase activity are independent processes, *J. Biol. Chem.,* 253, 4112, 1978.
121. **Kamisaka, K., Listowsky, I., Gatmaitan, Z., and Arias, I. M.,** Interaction of bilirubin and other ligands with bilirubin, *Biochemistry,* 14, 2175, 1975.
122. **Tipping, E., Ketterer, B., Christodoulides, L., and Enderby, G.,** Spectroscopic studies of the binding of bilirubin by ligandin and aminoazo-dye-binding protein A, *Biochem. J.,* 157, 211, 1976.
123. **Meuwissen, J. A. T. P., Ketterer, B., and Mertens, B. B. E.,** Hematin and bilirubin binding to ligandin, *Digestion,* 6, 293, 1972.
124. **Ketterer, B., Ross-Mansell, P., and Whitehead, J. K.,** The isolation of carcinogen-binding protein from livers of rats given 4-dimethylaminoazobenzene, *Biochem. J.,* 103, 316, 1967.
125. **Ketterer, B., Tipping, E., Hackney, J. F., and Beale, D.,** A low-molecular-weight protein from rat liver that resembles ligandin in its binding properties, *Biochem. J.,* 155, 511, 1976.
126. **Kamisaka, K., Listowsky, L., Gatmaitan, Z., and Arias, I. M.,** Circular dichroism analysis of the secondary structure of Z-protein and its complexes with bilirubin and other organic anions, *Biochim. Biophys. Acta,* 393, 24, 1975.
127. **Mishkin, S., Stein, L., Gatmaitan, Z., and Arias, I. M.,** Z-protein in hepatic uptake and esterification of long-chain fatty acids, *Biochem. Biophys. Res. Commun.,* 47, 997, 1972.
128. **Ruoslahti, E. and Terry, W. D.,** α-Foetoprotein and serum albumin show sequence homology, *Nature (London),* 260, 804, 1976.
129. **Ruoslati, E., Estes, Th., and Seppälä, M.,** Binding of bilirubin by bovine and human α-foetoprotein, *Biochim. Biophys. Acta,* 578, 544, 1970.
130. **Verseé, V. and Barel, A. O.,** Interaction of rat foetoprotein with bilirubin, *Biochem. J.,* 179, 705, 1979.
131. **Varela-Fuentes, B. and Viana, C.,** De la nature de la bilirubine ethero-extractible de quelque serum icteriques, *C. R. Soc. Biol. (Paris),* 114, 789, 1933.
132. **Beck, K. and Kühn, H. A.,** Über das ätherlösliche Bilirubin, *Klin. Wochenschr.,* 23/24, 630, 1956.
133. **Howe, R. B. and Pinto, S.de T.,** Ether-soluble bilirubin, *Medicine (Baltimore),* 45, 523, 1966.
134. **Talafant, E.,** Bile pigment-phospholipid interactions, *Biochim. Biophys. Acta,* 231, 394, 1971.
135. **Mustafa, G. and King, T. E.,** Binding of bilirubin with lipid. A possible mechanism of its toxic reaction in mitochondria, *J. Biol. Chem.,* 245, 1084, 1970.
136. **Nagaoka, S. and Cowger, M. L.,** Interaction of bilirubin with lipids studied by fluorescence quenching method, *J. Biol. Chem.,* 253, 2005, 1978.
137. **Eriksen, E. F., Danielsen, H., and Brodersen, R.,** Bilirubin-liposome interaction. Formation of a bilirubin dianion-phospholipid complex followed by bilirubin acid aggregation, *J. Biol. Chem.,* 256, 4269, 1981.
138. **Weil, M. C. and Menkes, J. H.,** Bilirubin interaction with ganglioside: possible mechanism in kernicterus, *Pediatr. Res.,* 9, 791, 1975.
139. **Tipping, E., Ketterer, B., and Christodoulides, L.,** Binding to egg phosphatidylcholine of some organic anions (bromosulphophthalein, oestrone sulphate, haem and bilirubin) that bind to ligandin and aminoazo-dye-binding protein A, *Biochem. J.,* 180, 327, 1979.
140. **Perrin, J. H. and Wilsey, M.,** The induced optical activity of bilirubin in the presence of sodium deoxycholate, *J. Chem. Soc. Chem. Commun.,* 769, 1971.
141. **Scharschmidt, B. F. and Schmid, R.,** The micellar sink. A quantitative assessment of the association of organic anions with mixed micelles and other macromolecular aggregates in rat bile, *J. Clin. Invest.,* 62, 1122, 1978.
142. **Diamond, I. and Schmid, R.,** Experimental bilirubin encephalopathy. The mode of entry of bilirubin-^{14}C into the central nervous system, *J. Clin. Invest.,* 45, 678, 1966.
143. **Stern, L. and Denton, R. L.,** Kernicterus in small premature infants, *Pediatrics,* 35, 483, 1965.
144. **Bratlid, D.,** The effect of pH on bilirubin binding by human erythrocytes, *Scand. J. Clin. Lab. Invest.,* 29, 453, 1972.
145. **Silberberg, D. H., Johnson, L., and Ritter, L.,** Factors influencing toxicity of bilirubin in cerebellum tissue culture, *J. Pediatr.,* 77, 386, 1970.
146. **Lee, J. J. and Cowger, M. L.,** Bilirubin-albumin binding and a possible mechanism of kernicterus, *Res. Commun. Chem. Pathol. Pharmacol.,* 8, 327, 1974.
147. **Wennberg, R. P., Ahlfors, Ch. E., and Rasmussen, L. F.,** The pathochemistry of kernicterus, *Early Human Dev.,* 3, 353, 1979.

148. **Levine, R. L.,** Bilirubin: worked out years ago? *Pediatrics,* 64, 380, 1979.
149. **Bloomer, J. R., Berk, P. D., Vergalla, J., and Berlin, N. I.,** Influence of albumin on the extravascular distribution of unconjugated bilirubin, *Clin. Sci. Mol. Med.,* 45, 517, 1973.
150. **Karp, W. B.,** Biochemical alterations in neonatal hyperbilirubinemia and bilirubin encephalopathy; a review, *Pediatrics,* 64, 361, 1979.
151. **Shepherd, R. E., Moreno, F. J., Cashore, W. J., and Fain, J. N.,** Effects of bilirubin on fat cell metabolism and lipolysis, *Am. J. Physiol.,* 237, E504, 1979.
152. **Cowger, M. L.,** Mechanism of bilirubin toxicity on tissue culture cells: factors that affect toxicity, reversibility by albumin, and comparison with other respiratory poisons and surfactants, *Biochem. Med.,* 5, 1, 1971.
153. **Oski, F. A. and Naiman, J. L.,** Red cell binding of bilirubin, *J. Pediatr.,* 63, 1034, 1963.
154. **Brodersen, R. and Bartels, P.,** Enzymatic oxidation of bilirubin, *Eur. J. Biochem.,* 10, 468, 1969.
155. **Brodersen, R.,** Binding of bilirubin to albumin and tissues, in *Physiol. Biochem. Basis Perinat. Med.,* Monset-Couchard, M. and Minkowski, A., Eds., S. Karger, Basel, 1981, 144.

Chapter 4

ANALYTICAL CHEMISTRY OF RUBINS

K.P.M. Heirwegh and N. Blanckaert

TABLE OF CONTENTS

I. NOMENCLATURE

The term *rubins* is used to denote diazo-positive tetrapyrroles that contain the 4,15-biladiene skeleton (Chapter 1). Commonly occurring rubins have eight side chains, attached at carbon positions 2, 3, 7, 8, 12, 13, 17, and 18 of the tetrapyrrole skeleton. In the rubins derived from heme these β-substituents comprise four methyl, two vinyl, and two propionic acid side chains. Depending on the sequence of the β-substituents, several positional isomers are possible which can be distinguished by type names such as bilirubin-IXα and IXβ (Chapter 1, Figure 4). The predominant rubin isomer in mammals is bilirubin-IXα. Several other positional bilirubin isomers are not derived from heme but are formed artificially by disproportionation of rubins (''dipyrrole exchange''). For example, bilirubin-IIIα and XIIIα are derived from bilirubin-IXα (see Chapter 1). The term *bilirubin conjugates* refers to bilirubin derivatives with a residue (e.g., a glycosyl residue) attached to the bilirubin aglycone, while the term *unconjugated bilirubin* is used to stress the absence of a conjugating group.

Reaction of rubins with diazo reagents leads to formation of two *dipyrrolic azo derivatives* from the parent tetrapyrrole (Chapter 1, Figure 11). For nomenclature used to denote these dipyrroles the reader is referred to Chapter 1. The name azobilirubin is misleading and has been replaced by azopyrromethene (Azpm). Alternatively, the equally acceptable trivial name, azodipyrrole, has also been used. Two isomeric azopyrromethenes, Azpm-12 and Azpm-8, are derived from bilirubin-IXα. They have been denoted previously as the ''isovinyl'', or exo-vinyl isomer (Azpm-12) and the ''vinyl'', or endo-vinyl isomer (Azpm-8) of azopyrromethene. From a bilirubin-IXα diglucuronide molecule one would obtain an exo- and endo-vinyl isomer of azopyrromethene glucuronide, corresponding with Azpm-12(GlcU) and Azpm-8(GlcU), respectively.

II. OVERVIEW

In the interest of conciseness the present chapter deals mostly with analytical developments reported since 1970. For additional information the reader is referred to other chapters of the book and to published reviews.[1-5]

The confusion about the significance and composition of rubins in biological sam-

Table 1
DIFFICULTIES IN ANALYTICAL WORK WITH RUBINS

1. Complexity of natural rubin mixtures:
   Unconjugated bilirubin; bilirubin mono- and diconjugates; bilirubin xylosides, glucosides, and glucuronides; diconjugates containing a single or two different sugar residues; positional and geometric isomers.
2. Unknown rubins
3. Lability of the rubin skeleton causes losses and numerous artifacts:
   Oxidation; disproportionation; photochemical alterations; formation of adducts (preferentially at exo-vinyl side chains)
4. Lability of the ester linkage of bilirubin sugar conjugates:
   Hydrolysis; transesterification; positional isomerization
5. Unavailability of primary standards of bilirubin glycosides
6. Lack of well-validated reference methods
7. Nonrubin components present in biological samples may affect the yield of azo color:
   Acceleration or inhibition of diazo cleavage; destruction of rubins, intermediates, and end-products; overestimation of rubins by contribution of nonrubin material

ples (Chapter 2) appears to be related largely to the lability of these pigments, the complexity of rubins present in biological samples, and to the use of ill-validated and inadequate methods (Table 1). In the present section the heterogeneity of rubins and major analytical principles will be outlined to set a background for discussion of the present status of analytical methodology.

A. Composition of Rubins in Biological Samples

A variety of conjugated and unconjugated rubins occur in mammals (Chapters 1 and 2), their amounts and distribution in biological samples depending in a multifactorial way on the nature of the specimen, species and strain,[6] sex,[7] developmental stage,[8] nutritional[9] and pathological state,[9-11] physical and medical treatment.

The rubin composition of bile from healthy mammals shows clear-cut species variation.[6] For instance, bilirubin mono- and diglucuronides are the predominant rubins in the bile of man, rhesus monkey, and rat whereas glucose and xylose conjugates are relatively more important in the bile of dog and cat.[12] Also, the ratios monoconjugates/diconjugates[6,8,12] and C-8 monoconjugates/C-12 monoconjugates[13] vary widely with species. Rubin patterns distinct from those in bile of healthy adult man have been observed during fetal development,[8] in the neonatal period,[14] and in acquired and inherited liver disorders (Chapter 6, Volume II). In patients with Gilbert's syndrome and Crigler-Najjar disease, the ratio of monoglucuronide to diglucuronide in bile is typically increased.[11,15,16] In cholestatic conditions, a more complex rubin pattern is observed in plasma and bile, which contain a mixture of positional isomers of bilirubin glucuronides (C-1, C-2, C-3, and C-4 sugar conjugates). This mixture is formed by nonenzymic sequential shifting of the bilirubin acyl group from position C-1 to positions 2, 3, and 4 of the sugar moiety.[17,18]

Unconjugated bilirubin is the predominant rubin in plasma of healthy adults and neonates. Various structural isomers may also occur in body fluids. Unconjugated bilirubin-IXβ (Figure 4, Chapter 1) has been demonstrated in the bile of healthy adult mammals and of newborn human and rhesus monkey babies.[19] However, this pigment represents only a small fraction (ca. 2%) of the biliary rubins. Formation of a mixture of geometric isomers of bilirubin-IXα (4Z-15Z; 4E-15Z; 4Z-15E; 4E-15E) has been postulated to occur during phototherapy (Chapter 1), and these isomers may be present in plasma of phototreated jaundiced Gunn rats and neonates.[20,21] In addition, unconjugated bilirubin-IXγ and IXδ, and several modified rubins and breakdown products have been found in bile of homozygous Gunn rats.[22,23] However, the total amount of rubins excreted in this species is small when compared to heme turnover.

Table 2
MAJOR RUBINS IN BIOLOGICAL SAMPLES FROM HUMANS

		Bilirubin-IXα C-1-glucuronides		Non-C-1-glucuronides	
	Unconjugated	mono[a]	di	mono	di
Bile					
Healthy adult		+[b]	+		
Gilbert's syndrome		+	+		
Criggler-Najjar disease, Type I	+				
Hemolytic disease		+	+		
Cholestatic disease		+	+	+	+
Serum					
Healthy adult	+				
Gilbert's syndrome	+				
Criggler-Najjar disease, Type I	+				
Hemolytic disease	+				
Cholestatic disease	+ (?)	+	+	+	+
Urine					
Cholestatic disease		+	+	+	+

[a] In general, monoglucuronides consist of a mixture of the bilirubin-*8*-12(GlcU) and bilirubin-8-*12*(GlcU) positional isomers.
[b] +, major rubin.

The possible natural occurrence of alkali-stable bilirubin conjugates is briefly discussed in Chapter 2. Indirect evidence for the presence in plasma of patients with conjugated hyperbilirubinemia of as yet unidentified diazo-positive compounds has recently been obtained.[24]

B. Analysis of Rubin Multicomponent Systems

None of the presently available methods permits individual measurement of each of the rubins present in mixtures that are as complex as most biological fluids. To extract the maximum of useful information one must rely, therefore, on combined results derived from more than one procedure. For instance, for normal human or rat bile the total amount of mono- and diester conjugates, and the proportion between C-8-monoester, C-12-monoester, and diester conjugates can be determined by the alkaline methanolysis HPLC procedure (Section VI.B.3.b). In addition, the proportion of the various sugar residues can be obtained by TLC of ethyl anthranilate azo derivatives (Section VI.A.3).

It may be useful to distinguish major and minor rubin components (Table 2) since determination of the latter places higher demands on sensitivity and, in particular, specificity of the methods used. For example, accurate determination of unconjugated bilirubin in the presence of conjugated bilirubin in bile proves very difficult since a minor degree of nonspecificity of the assay or occurrence of hydrolysis or disproportionation of bilirubin conjugates may produce large errors. Similarly, great technical difficulties are encountered in the measurement of conjugated bilirubins in serum of healthy adults. Also, it must be emphasized that assay procedures should be tested not only with unconjugated bilirubin but also with preparations of purified mono- and diglucuronides (Section IV.B).

Most assays currently employed in clinical chemistry proceed in homogeneous liquid medium rendering them relatively simple and amenable to automation. These so-called single-phase procedures are based on *measurement of an equilibrium property* (such as circular dichroism, light absorption (Section VI.B.1), or fluorescence),[26] on *analysis*

Table 3
DIRECT-REACTING (DB) AND INDIRECT-REACTING (IB) RUBINS

	Diazo reactivity	Sources and references
Unconjugated bilirubins		
IXα	IB	Body fluids of mammals[5]
IIIα and XIIIα	IB	Synthetic, by disproportionation of bilirubin-IXα[123]
IXβ, IXγ and IXδ	DB	Body fluids of mammals[19,23,34]
Geometric isomers of bilirubin-IXα	DB(?)	Skin and serum of neonates during phototherapy (?); illuminated solutions of bilirubin-IXα (?)
Conjugated bilirubins		
Mono- and diglucuronides	DB	Body fluids of mammals[6]
Other ester glycosides	DB	Bile of dog and cat[6]
Taurine conjugates	DB	Synthetic[66]

of the time course of diazo cleavage,[27,28] or on *end-point determination* (e.g., by monitoring formation of dipyrrolic azo derivatives (Section VI.A.1) or fluorescent[29] or oxidative reaction products).[5] Methods based on direct spectrophotometry or analysis of the time course of diazo cleavage, in principle, permit multicomponent analysis on individual samples, but it has been impossible so far to evaluate the applicability of this approach because, with the exception of unconjugated bilirubin, natural bilirubins are unavailable in pure form. The other single-phase methods yield chemically ill-defined analytical results and their specificity is either low or has not been assessed in sufficient detail.

The discussion of single-phase procedures will be limited largely to methods based on diazo cleavage since these have been investigated in greatest detail, are in common use, and can potentially provide much information (Section VI.A). Specific determination of rubins can be improved by introducing a purification stage, e.g., extraction (Section VI.B.2). Chromatographic procedures are required for determination of compositional parameters, e.g., the proportion of the various carbohydrate residues (Sections VI.A.3 and B.3).

C. Basic Analytical Procedures — Diazo Reaction and Tetrapyrrole Analysis

Most procedures for separation and measurement of rubins rely on diazo cleavage producing dipyrrolic red-violet azo derivatives which are more stable than the parent tetrapyrroles. Ehrlich discovered that bilirubin reacts with *p*-diazobenzene sulfonic acid in the presence of alcohol.[30] After the fortuitous discovery that bilirubins in bile react rapidly in absence of alcohol, and after screening various types of biological samples, Hijmans van den Bergh, and Müller[31] introduced the distinction between *direct-reacting* and *total bilirubin* (Table 3). The direct-reacting fraction corresponds with compounds that react with diazo reagent in the absence of an added accelerator in aqueous acidic medium. Total bilirubin is calculated from the total azo color obtained when the diazo reaction is carried out in the presence of an added accelerator[32] such as methanol. It should be realized that "direct-reacting" and "indirect-reacting bilirubin" are operationally defined, are dependent therefore on the diazo reaction conditions and sample (pigment and matrix) composition, and do not accurately reflect conjugated and unconjugated bilirubins, respectively.

Aromatic amines yielding *water-soluble* (e.g., sulfanilic acid) or *organic soluble azo derivatives* (e.g., ethyl anthranilate) have been used.[4] The former amines have found widespread application in clinical chemistry. Compared to single-phase assays, extraction of azo color improves sensitivity and lowers the blank values. Perhaps more importantly, by separation of the extracted azo pigment, information can be obtained about the composition of rubins in the sample (Section VI.A.3). For isolated rubins the diazo reaction offers a simple and convenient approach for elucidation or confirmation of the structure of the isolated pigment since characteristic pairs of dipyrrolic azo derivatives are formed.[33-36] Organic soluble azo pigments, in particular those derived from ethyl anthranilate, have been used successfully for this purpose (Chapters 1 and 2).

Analysis of rubin mixtures would be more straightforward if direct measurement of each individual tetrapyrrolic rubin would be possible. Recent development of TLC procedures for separation of rubins has been instrumental in broadening our knowledge of naturally occurring conjugated and unconjugates rubins. However, major analytical problems in this approach include destruction and alteration of the pigments in the course of their application and separation. Better insight into the factors causing lability of rubins will be necessary for development of quantitative techniques for direct analysis of rubins. It is likely that, for most applications, TLC will soon be superceded by HPLC. The latter technique not only is more powerful, but also shows several features that are favorable for separating rubins, such as easy exclusion of oxygen and light.

III. LABILITY OF RUBINS

In this section precautions that may improve storage, separation, and measurement of rubins will be considered. *Metastability of supersaturated solutions* (Chapters 3 and 2, Volume II) is of great concern in preparation of standard solutions of bilirubin and model assay systems. Chemical changes in rubins comprise *decomposition, disproportionation,* and geometric isomerization of the tetrapyrrole skeleton (Chapter 1), and *hydrolysis, transesterification* (alcoholysis), *positional isomerization* (shifting of the bilirubin acyl group on the conjugating sugar), and possibly *aminolysis* (Chapter 2). Studies regarding supersaturated solutions and transformation of the tetrapyrrole skeleton have been done almost exclusively with bilirubin-IXα. It is likely, however, that such changes will also occur with more water-soluble tetrapyrroles such as conjugated bilirubins[37] and structural and geometric isomers of bilirubin. All concentrations indicated below have been taken from the publications referred to and are given only to indicate orders of magnitude of the concentrations studied.

A. Metastability of Supersaturated Solutions

Although the solubility of bilirubin at physiological pH values is very low (about 7 nM at pH 7.4 and 37°C),[38] oversaturated aqueous solutions of bilirubin (3.2 μM at pH 7.4 or 15 μM at pH 8.5) can be prepared which may show pronounced delays in colloid formation and precipitation.[38,39] Aggregation rates are increased by mechanical agitation or bubbling of gases.[39] Onset of aggregation can easily be detected by monitoring absorption[38,40,41] and scattering of light.[42] Colloid formation is inhibited by detergents, by water-miscible solvents such as ethanol, acetone, and pyridine and by a molar excess of albumin.[40]

B. Decomposition, Disproportionation and Geometric Isomerization of the Tetrapyrrole Skeleton

Chemical alterations of unconjugated bilirubin have been critically reviewed by McDonagh[5,44] and Lightner[45] (Chapter 1). In darkness, molecular oxygen proved instrumental for modification of rubins.[39] Even when molecular oxygen is present only in trace amounts, bilirubin in aqueous solution at alkaline pH decomposes by autoxidation (pH 7.4-13.2) and disproportionates to form equilibrium mixtures of IIIα, IXα, and XIIIα isomers (pH 7.4.-12). Autoxidation, but not disproportionation, is catalyzed by trace amounts of bivalent metal ions and inhibited, but not stopped, by EDTA. Disproportionation does not occur in strongly alkaline medium (e.g., 0.1 *M* NaOH). Autoxidation and disproportionation of bilirubin are inhibited by autoxidants such as ascorbate (6 m*M*), cysteine and glutathione (3 m*M*), and by a molar excess of albumin. The reactions are slow in chloroform and benzene. Application of bilirubin[5] and its monoglucuronide,[46] in organic solution to thin-layer plates and rechromatography are often accompanied by a certain extent of disproportionation. Disproportionation of bilirubin monoglucuronides in protein-free aqueous solution (pH 7.4) can effectively be inhibited by addition of ascorbic acid (1 mM).[47]

Illumination of aqueous solutions of bilirubin, even in absence of molecular oxygen, causes decomposition, disproportionation to IIIα and XIIIα isomers, and geometric isomerization to 4Z-15E, 4E-15Z, and 4E-15E isomers.[44,45] A molar excess of albumin or dissolution of bilirubin in strongly alkaline medium (e.g., 0.1 *M* NaOH) inhibits formation of the IIIα and XIIIα isomers.[44] In aqueous solution, at pH 6.5, cationic, but not neutral or anionic detergents may accelerate photo-induced disproportionation of bilirubin.[48]

Under aerobic conditions either dark reactions (e.g., disproportionation) or light-induced reactions (e.g., photoxidations) can occur.

C. Hydrolysis, Transesterification, Positional Isomerization, and Aminolysis

Replacement of sugar residues of bilirubin ester conjugates by a variety of groups may occur in alkaline medium and lead to artificial formation of bilirubin derivatives. Bilirubin esters are rapidly hydrolyzed in aqueous solutions at pH 11-11.5 at room temperature.[49] Methyl ester derivatives may be formed in methanol solutions of bilirubin ester conjugates.[50] It has also been suggested that bilirubin polypeptide conjugates, detected in bile,[51] may have been formed artificially, by aminolysis of ester conjugates in the presence of protein (Chapter 2). In aqueous medium at pH 7 to 9, the bilirubin acyl group shifts sequentially from position C-1 to positions 2, 3, and 4 of the conjugating sugar moieties[17,18] (Chapter 2). Acyl-shifting was not observed during prolonged storage of bilirubin glycosides at pH 2.6 to 7,[18] and hydrolysis was absent during storage of conjugated pigments at pH 2.7 at 0 to 25°C for 3 hr.[47]

D. Recommendations

In the light of our present, though limited, knowledge of artificial alterations of rubins during storage and manipulation, the following precautions must be considered in analytical work with rubins. The samples should be shielded from light, manipulations being done in dim, preferably red light. It is recommended to deoxygenate the solvents and, whenever possible, to keep the pigments under an inert atmosphere (nitrogen, argon). Deoxygenation by bubbling of inert gases is likely to facilitate aggregation of supersaturated solutions of bilirubin (IIIα, IXα, and XIIIα) but may affect less, or not at all, aqueous solutions of conjugated bilirubins and polar bilirubin isomers. Autoxidation can be minimized by using ultrapure solvents and reagents. Addition of disodium EDTA (1 to 5 mM) and/or ascorbate (1-5 mM) can be advantageous and frequently permissible. Hydrolysis and acyl-shifting can be avoided by buffering aqueous solutions to pH values below 6. Also, enzymic hydrolysis catalyzed by β-glycosidases present in many biological samples (serum, bile, tissue homogenates, microsomal preparations) can be inhibited by addition of aldonolactones.[52,53]

Conditions for storage of conjugated bilirubin have been evaluated incompletely. According to Lucassen[54] bilirubin conjugates can be stored *in vacuo* at room temperature over concentrated sulfuric acid for 1 year without loss in diazo reactivity. However, a mixture of mono- and diglucuronides of bilirubin in 50 mM-sodium phosphate buffer, pH 6.5 stored at −15°C showed a loss of ca. 1% in diazo reactivity per day.[55]

For a lyophilized preparation of conjugated pigments (largely bilirubin diglucuronide) stored at −15°C, diazo reactivity decreased by less than 10% over a period of 2 weeks, but about 40% of diglucuronide was converted into monoglucuronide.[56]

IV. PRIMARY STANDARDS

Major problems are related to the unavailability of pure, well-characterized bilirubin conjugates.

A. Bilirubin-IXα

Bilirubin is commercially available but its purity must be evaluated before the pigment is used for calibration purposes. Tests for purity discussed by McDonagh,[5] include the following: (1) the pigment must be completely dissolvable in chloroform (containing 1% ethanol stabilizer) and show a molar absorption coefficient at 25°C equal to at least 60,000 at λ_{max} (453 to 455 nm), (2) treatment of dilute solutions in chloroform with 0.1 *M* $NaHCO_3$ should not extract any color, and (3) TLC on silica gel (with 1% acetic acid in chloroform) and on polyamide (with 1% NH_4OH in methanol) should yield a single yellow spot with no baseline residue or fluorescent impurities. Traces of IIIα and XIIIα isomers can be ignored for clinical assays. If the preparation is impure, bilirubin can be purified by crystallization.[5,57,58]

Usually, solutions of bilirubin containing serum or serum albumin are needed for calibration purposes. Procedures for preparation of such aqueous standard solutions have been discussed by McDonagh.[5] They include preparation of a concentrated solution of bilirubin in a co-solvent such as 0.1 *M* NaOH, or formamide containing 0.1 *M* KCN,[59] and quantitative transfer to a protein-containing diluent. Purified serum albumin (fraction V) has been claimed to be unsuitable for calibration of diazo assays because the azo color yields obtained were low when compared to serum-containing systems[60,61] and decreased at increasing concentrations of albumin.[62,63] With only two out of five diazo methods this discrepancy was indeed observed for albumin preparations from Armour and Sigma,[63] but not from Miles and Fluka.[63,64] It thus would appear that both the purified albumin preparation and the particular diazo procedure that is used play a role in the yield of azo color from bilirubin. It is worthwhile to further study selection of appropriate albumin preparations as this would facilitate studies of storage and assay conditions in the presence of a protein matrix. At present, it seems advisable to use serum of healthy human adults as the protein matrix for preparation of bilirubin standard solutions, as recommended by Billing et al.[3] For calibration of diazo assays in aqueous media that contain little or no binding protein such as bile, Boonyapisit et al.[65] advocated the use of bilirubin-disodium EDTA complex.

B. Mono- and Diglucuronides of Bilirubin

Fully characterized *primary standards* are not available as yet. For the present, it might be useful to develop suitable preparations of the probably more stable mono- and ditaurine conjugates of bilirubin,[66] for inter-laboratory comparison of results and for checking consistency of calibration over long periods of time.

Purified mono- and diglucuronides isolated from biological sources[54-56,67-69] or prepared by chemical synthesis (Chapter 2) are useful in developing and evaluating assay procedures, provided the composition of each pigment preparation is properly described. Whenever possible, the content of any impurity should be stated as the molar ratio, contaminant/named compound.

One can define the following *practical criteria of purity.* (1) Homogeneity by TLC or HPLC can be tested (Section VI.B.3). At the final stage no bands other than the mono- or diglucuronides of bilirubin should be detectable. The ratio, monoglucuronide/diglucuronide should be reported (Sections VI.A.3 and VI.B.3.b). (2) Chromatography of rubins formed by saponification allows quantification of the content of IIIα and XIIIα chromophores (Section VI.B.3.c). Alternatively, for monoglucuronides, one can separate the methyl esters obtained by alkaline methanolysis (Section VI.B.3.b). The alkali-stable fraction should be negligible. (3) Nonhexuronide residues and non-C-1 isomers can be detected by chromatography of the methyl esters of azopyrromethene glucuronide (Section VI.A.3). (4) For preparations obtained from bile, specific assays for bile acid, phospholipid, and cholesterol are of value. As yet, no single published procedure for preparation of bilirubin glucuronides from bile has been evaluated completely, in particular with regard to the extents of disproportionation of the aglycone and acyl-shifting at the ester linkages.

V. REFERENCE PROCEDURES

Such procedures should permit assay of rubins in solutions used for calibration and evaluation of routine methods for a variety of biological samples. The number and scope of presently available reference methods is limited. As yet, only unconjugated bilirubins (free acids and alkyl esters) can be obtained commercially or prepared in pure forms in amounts suitable for weighing but physical data relate mostly to organic solvents.[5] For assays of aqueous protein-free solutions of bilirubin and ester glycosides of bilirubin, Lucassen's diazo procedure[54] has a reasonably sound experimental basis, although independent confirmation with pure ester conjugates of bilirubin is still required.

For evaluation of methods applicable to model mixtures or patient samples, one often has used the procedure of Jendrassik and Grof[70] for assay of "total bilirubin". Although this method seems to be one of the best diazo procedures available for routine assays on serum, it is unsatisfactory for reference purposes. The notion "total bilirubin" only has an operational significance as the photometric response reflects diazo reaction of ill-defined fractions of rubins and nonrubin compounds and may be modulated by matrix effects. A more selective procedure for assay of unconjugated bilirubin and bilirubin mono- and diester conjugates is based on alkaline methanolysis. It has been worked out for serum only but applicability to other types of biological samples is likely and deserves evaluation.

A. Direct Spectrophotometric Assay of Pure Compounds[5]

For well-characterized rubins that are available in pure form, the pigment concentration can be determined spectrophotometrically, using calibration curves or known molar absorption coefficients. Thus bilirubin-IXα, -IIIα, and -XIIIα, mesobilirubin, and a number of alkyl ester derivatives of bilirubin have been obtained in pure form, and generally can be measured in chloroform solution (Table 4).

B. Diazo Assay of Unconjugated Bilirubin and Purified Bilirubin Conjugates in Protein-Free Aqueous Solutions

Lucassen[54] showed that in protein-free media the concentrations of unconjugated bilirubin and of purified conjugated bilirubin (enriched in diglucuronide) can be determined reliably by a modification of the diazo procedure of Jendrassik and Grof.[70] In this method diazo cleavage is performed with *p*-diazobenzene sulfonic acid in presence of a mixture of caffeine, sodium benzoate, and sodium acetate as the reaction accelerator for bilirubin. Because Lucassen's thesis is not readily available his procedures for assaying bilirubins and for standardization are given below.

Reagents. Sulfanilic acid solution: 5.0 g sulfanilic acid, about 500 mℓ distilled water

Table 4
MOLAR ABSORPTION COEFFICIENTS OF SOME WELL-CHARACTERIZED RUBINS DISSOLVED IN CHLOROFORM

	λ_{max}(nm)	ε_{mM}	Ref.
Bilirubin-IXα	453-455	62.6	33
	454	60.7	57
Bilirubin-IXα C-8 monomethylester	438	59.3	121
Bilirubin-IXα C-12 monomethylester	442	55.2	121
Bilirubin-IXα dimethylester	398	59.8(10 μM)[a]	124
	397	60.5(14 μM)	121
		71.7(104 μM)	121
Bilirubin-IIIα	445-458	65.2	33
Bilirubin-XIIIα	449-453	52.5	33
Mesobilirubin-IXα	433	54.6	125

[a] Bilirubin-IXα dimethylester does not follow beer's law.[121,124] The same probably applies to other dialkylesters of bilirubin. However, the spectrum of bilirubin-IXα dimethylester seems concentration independent in chloroform/ethanol (1:1, v/v).[121]

and 15 mℓ 12*M* HCl were mixed in a 1 ℓ volumetric flask. The sulfanilic acid was dissolved by gentle heating and the solution brought to the mark with distilled water. *Sodium nitrite solution:* 500 mg $NaNO_2$ was dissolved in 100 mℓ distilled water. *Diazo reagent:* 0.3 mℓ sodium nitrite solution was mixed with 10 mℓ sulfanilic acid solution (concentration of diazonium salt, ca. 2 m*M*). The diazo reagent was prepared shortly before use. *Caffeine reagent:* 24.3 g caffeine and 36.0 g sodium benzoate were dissolved in 300 mℓ distilled water in a 500 mℓ volumetric flask. After addition of 68.0 g sodium acetate. $3H_2O$ the solution was brought to volume with distilled water.

Diazo procedure. Caffeine reagent (7 mℓ) was mixed with 2 mℓ sample (bilirubin dissolved in 0.1 *M* NaOH, or an aqueous solution of conjugated bilirubin), 1 mℓ freshly prepared diazo reagent was added to the mixture, and after reaction for 10 min at 20°C the azo color was determined at 530 nm.

Standardization of the procedure. The assays were calibrated with pure β-naphthol as a standard. In a 250 mℓ-volumetric flask 1.7 g of sodium acetate.$3H_2O$ was dissolved in 15 mℓ of distilled water. Then 90 mg accurately weighed β-naphthol was added and dissolved, and the volume brought to the mark with 96% ethanol (2.5 m*M* β-naphthol). A 50 μ*M* solution of β-naphthol was prepared by dilution with 0.68% sodium acetate.$3H_2O$ in 90% ethanol.

Diluted β-naphthol solution (9 mℓ) was mixed with 1 mℓ of diazo reagent (ca. 5 m*M*). After complete reaction (5 min) the absorption was read at 486 nm (ε_{468}(21.9 ± 0.1 S.D.) × $10^3 M^{-1}.cm^{-1}$; n = 5). For determination of the concentration of diazonium salt, 9 mℓ of the stock β-naphthol solution (2.5 m*M*) was mixed with 1 mℓ of diazo reagent (final concn. 5 to 100 μ*M*). After completion of diazo-coupling the absorption was read at 486 nm and the concentration of diazonium salt calculated using the molar absorption coefficient of the β-naphthol azo pigment.

After purification of bilirubin (twice recrystallized) samples of bilirubinate solution (final concn. ca. 18 μm) were submitted to diazo cleavage (see above) with various dilutions of diazo reagent (final concn. 6 to 100 μ*M*) and the A_{530}-values (0.5 cm light-path) were determined. A plot of A_{530} against the concentration of diazo reagent showed complete and stoichiometric reaction of bilirubin with diazo reagent. The abscissa of the point of intersection thus yielded the concentration of diazo reagent, equivalent to the bilirubin present and the ordinate of this point gave the absorption of azopyrromethene formed. From these values Lucassen derived the molar absorption coefficient, ε_{530} (25.7 ± 0.5 S.D.) × 10^3 $M^{-1}.cm^{-1}$ (n = 5). Within experimental error the same value was found when the preparation of purified conjugated bilirubin was reacted with diazo reagent.

Comment. It is important to use ultrapure reagents and carefully purified water. Heavy-metal ions can form complexes with dipyrrolic azo pigments at near-neutral pH.[71,72] The presence of caffeine in the reaction medium protects the azo pigments against destruction by the excess of diazonium salt.[54] It is likely that the reaction conditions are suitable for all known ester conjugates of bilirubin. Obviously, the method does not permit differential determination of an individual rubin in samples containing more than one rubin species.

C. Differential Determination of Unconjugated Bilirubin and Bilirubin Mono- and Diester Conjugates in Serum

Blanckaert[24] recently developed a procedure which permits virtually quantitative conversion (ca. 97%) of bilirubin sugar conjugates in serum to methyl esters by alkaline methanolysis. Using an internal standard and pure, well-characterized bilirubin and bilirubin mono- and dimethyl esters for calibration and HPLC for separation of the various pigment fractions, this so-called alkaline methanolysis-HPLC technique seems to permit accurate differential determination of bilirubin and its mono- and diester conjugates in serum (Section VI.B.3.b). Definitive confirmation of the validity of this approach has to await the availability of pure bilirubin mono- and diglucuronides. Also, it should be emphasized that the sum of unconjugated bilirubin and bilirubin sugar conjugates, measured by this method, does not necessarily correspond with total rubins in the sample, since pigments distinct from unconjugated bilirubin-IXα, -IIIα and -XIIIα and their sugar esters are not assayed by this technique. For example, non-α isomers of bilirubin-IX and alkali-stable bilirubin derivatives cannot be determined by the alkaline methanolysis method. A limitation of the method is that it is impossible to accurately measure unconjugated bilirubin in the presence of a large excess of bilirubin sugar conjugates (Section VI.B.2).

VI. ANALYTICAL METHODS

This section outlines recommended analytical procedures and their limitations and significance.

A. Diazo Assays

1. Total and Direct-Reacting Rubins by Diazo Cleavage

The mechanism of reaction of *p*-diazobenzene sulfonic acid with bilirubin and a preparation enriched in glucuronide[54] has been investigated in some detail (Chapter 1). To exploit the diazo reaction for quantification of rubins, using an end-point technique, the procedure adopted should fulfil the following requirements. Diazo cleavage should be stoichiometric, quantitative, selective, and amenable to calibration. For the present, in-depth evaluation of these requirements is possible only for unconjugated bilirubin-IXα but not for other rubins, because they are not available in pure form.

a. Model Systems

Studies with solutions containing bilirubin, its mono- and diglucuronide (either alone or as suitable mixtures) are of great value in optimization of diazo assays for application to biological samples. In such model systems one can investigate the effects of various matrix components, including whole serum or purified serum albumin, and also hemoglobin, bile salt, urea, nonrubin diazo positive compounds, and other potentially interfering substances. In addition, pH and temperature should be controlled adequately, because they may critically influence the results.

How analysis in model systems can be exploited will be illustrated by discussion of a few examples. In Lucassen's diazo method (Section V.B) both bilirubin and a conjugated bilirubin preparation reacted completely and stoichiometrically with *p*-diazobenzene sulfonic acid in the presence of a caffeine/benzoate/acetate mixture. This was evident from the linear increase of A_{530} with increasing concentration of diazo reagent, until a limiting, constant value was reached. Because it was possible to determine accurately the concentrations of the diazo reagent, ε_{530} values in the reaction medium could be calculated for the unconjugated azo derivatives from bilirubin and for the conjugated azo pigments (largely azopyrromethene glucuronides) derived from conjugated pigment. The values were not different, indicating that the conjugating sugar, which is separated from the chromophore by several single bonds, has no influence on the absorbance at 530 nm. In pentan-2-one, ethyl anthranilate azo pigments showed small differences in the shape of the absorption bands around 530 nm depending primarily on the number of vinyl groups (zero, one or two) conjugated with the pyrrolic ring system.[35] It is not known whether interaction with matrix components such as albumin, bile salts, or detergents could affect differently the spectra of conjugated and unconjugated azo derivatives.

An effort should be made to prepare pure dipyrrolic azo pigments for direct determination of absorption spectra and molar absorption coefficients in any medium used for optical reading. Whether the indirect approach for determination of molar absorption coefficients, used by Lucassen,[54] can also be applied to other reaction media and diazo reagents will depend on (1) demonstration of stoichiometric and complete diazo cleavage and (2) accurate determination of the concentration of the diazo reagent. By using suitable symmetrical model compounds (Chapters 1 and 4, Volume II) the molar absorption coefficients could be determined for individual azopigment isomers, e.g.,

Indirect support for stoichiometric and complete diazo cleavage has also been given for two other procedures. Diazotized ethyl anthranilate[73] in aqueous medium at pH 2.7 and 25°C appears to react to completion with purified mono- and diglucuronides of bilirubin, since the azo color levels are independent of prolonging the reaction time after reaching a steady, maximal value. Identical, equally stable final values were obtained in parallel assays at 0°C and 25°C.[47,73] Prolongation of the reaction time beyond the period needed for maximal azo color formation did not affect the composition of the azo derivatives from bilirubin diglucuronide and monoglucuronides.[47] These observations indicate that neither hydrolysis of conjugated azo pigment, nor conversion of either azopigment to altered products, did occur. The same conclusions were reached in similar studies with diazotized *p*-iodoaniline[62,74] (reaction in the presence of normal human serum at 0°C). At 37°C, color formation from bilirubin[62] and bilirubin glucuronides[74] passed through an optimal value that was lower than the maximal, stable value found at 0°C, and then decreased, indicating destruction of azo pigment. It thus would appear that proper selection of the reaction temperature is of key importance in developing diazo assays. Obviously, destruction of rubin (e.g., by autoxidation) cannot be excluded in any of these diazo procedures since complete reaction of remaining rubin in presence of destruction of azo pigment would also give rise to stable final color levels.

The solutions should be buffered adequately as pH differently affects the course of diazo cleavage of unconjugated and conjugated bilirubins (Figure 1). The pH also influences the absorption spectrum thereby altering the colorimetric response.

For extrapolation of information about reaction conditions obtained with model systems to assays on biological samples only a few guidelines will be given. It is advisable to verify whether the reaction conditions established with model systems equally apply to the type of biological sample of interest. In particular, completeness of reaction and stability of final azo color should be verified by study of the time-course of

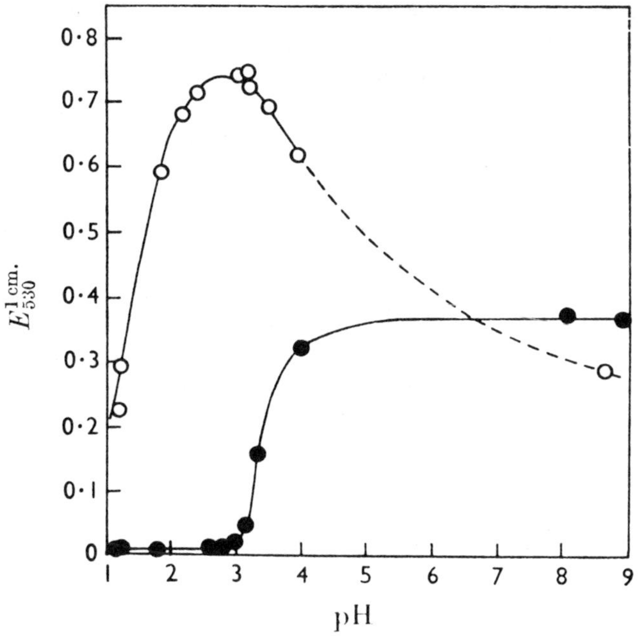

FIGURE 1. Effect of pH on diazo-cleavage of conjugated (○) and unconjugated bilirubin (●) with diazotized ethyl anthranilate. (From Van Roy, F. P. and Heirwegh, K. P. M., *Biochem. J.*, 107, 507, 1968. With permission)

azo color formation. In addition, for assays of direct-reacting bilirubins one should ascertain the extent of reaction of unconjugated bilirubin.[62,75] Studies of recovery of added rubins are straightforward. However, for the present it must be assumed that reactivity and color response of added rubins are the same as for the corresponding endogenous compounds. In general, it is recommended to test the finally adopted system with biological samples of widely different composition such as bile, serum from healthy adults, serum from jaundiced neonates and adults with hemolytic disease, and serum from patients with hepatobiliary disease.

b. Side-Reactions and Selectivity

Several types of *side-reactions* occurring on diazo treatment of model mixtures and biological samples have been noted. They can be related to (1) excessive consumption of diazo reagent, (2) isomerization and disproportionation of rubins, (3) destruction of rubins, intermediate hydroxypyrromethene carbinols and azo pigment end products, and (4) modification of the colorimetric response of azo pigment by interaction with matrix components. Finally, (5) chemical reaction of ester-linked conjugating groups may also occur. A number of papers that reflect on this topic have been discussed previously,[2,4] and only more recent developments will be discussed below.

- Sodium azide, which effectively destroys the diazonium salt reagent[70] should not be used as a preservative for reagents or biological specimens involved in diazo assays.[76] Ascorbic acid interferes similarly.[75]
- Disproportionation of monoconjugated bilirubins with formation of mixtures containing also unconjugated and diconjugated bilirubins should lead to decreased formation of azo color under conditions where reaction with unconjugated bilirubin (e.g., of direct-reacting bilirubins) is negligible. The ethyl anthranilate diazo procedure[73] is well-suited to monitor this disproportionation, because

azo color formed in the presence of a reaction accelerator should remain constant while azo color developed in the ethyl anthranilate procedure, which solely measures conjugated bilirubin, would diminish, due to conversion of bilirubin conjugates to unconjugated bilirubin. Disproportionation of rubins is probably insignificant in serum and model solutions containing an excess of albumin. Illumation of bilirubin-containing solutions may cause an increase in the fraction of direct-reacting bilirubins,[77] possibly by inducing geometric isomerization.

- Development of diazo methods coping effectively with hemolysis interference in diazo cleavage of rubins presents a major challenge.[4] Spectral error is negligible[70,78-81] in total bilirubin assays based on the procedures of Malloy and Evelyn[82] and Jendrassik and Grof.[70] Rather, destruction of rubins and possibly also of intermediate hydroxypyrromethene carbinols seems to be involved. In addition, azo color fades when alkalinization precedes optical reading, unless ascorbic acid has been added previously.[70,81] Oxyhemoglobin appears to be the primary agent causing low recovery of azo color.[80,81] Removal of molecular oxygen by gassing with carbon monoxide,[83,84] and also addition of KI or ascorbic acid[80,81] were found to decrease hemoglobin interference in several diazo assays. The protective effect of ascorbic acid, if operative at concentrations that are sufficiently low to permit complete diazo reaction of rubins, deserves further investigation. The rather small effect of hemolysis on diazo assays in the presence of caffeine or diphylline may be related to complexation with rubins, intermediate hydroxypyrromethene carbinols,[54] and heme compounds.[85] Hemolysis may lead to gross underestimation of direct-reacting bilirubin.[86] No studies with purified bilirubin conjugates have been reported.

  Destruction of azo pigment in an acidic, hemoglobin-free reaction system containing an acetone/ethanol mixture as reaction accelerator and diazotized *p*-iodoaniline as diazo reagent becomes negligible when the reaction temperature is decreased from 37 to 0°C.[62]
- Dipyrrolic azo pigments form highly colored complexes with a variety of bivalent heavy metal ions at neutral to alkaline pH.[71,72] Therefore, metal impurities in reagents may alter the colorimetric response in diazo assays in which azo color is read at neutral or alkaline pH. This interference can be eliminated by addition of 1 m*M* disodium EDTA.
- Hydrolysis of ester-conjugates (Section III) and reaction at C-1 of C-2, C-3, and C-4-*O*-acyl conjugates with aromatic amine have already been discussed (Chapter 2). It is likely that their influence on the light absorption spectra of azo derivatives will be negligible.

The *selectivity* of the diazo reaction when applied to biological samples is of major concern. Although diazo positive compounds other than rubins must be present it seems to be tacitly assumed, in general, that for serum and bile their contribution to azo color formation is negligible. Endogenous substances such as indoxyl sulfate (present in uremic serum) and a variety of drugs are diazo positive,[87-90] their response depending on the nature of the reaction accelerator and reactivity of the diazonium salt.[88,90]

Removal of interfering diazo positive material in assays on urine has been attempted by filtration on talcum[1] and by formation of azopigment/metal complexes.[70,91] In general, improvement of selectivity could be approached by establishing for the diazo system at hand, the mildest possible conditions that still allow complete color formation. Lowering of the reaction temperature and of the concentration of diazonium salt and reaction accelerator can be investigated. Further measures could consist in changing the reaction pH and the type of accelerator or diazonium salt. Reaction of unconjugated bilirubin with diazo reagent in the absence of added accelerator presents a specific problem in interpretation of values for direct-reacting bilirubins and will be discussed below.

c. Conventional Diazo Methods

Manual assays of *total bilirubin* with *p*-diazobenzene sulfonic acid have been discussed in several recent reviews.[2-5] For automation of the assays, stable diazonium salts,[88,90,92-94] accelerator agents such as detergents,[85,86,89,94-96] ethylene glycol,[88] DMSO[90,97] and single, nonaqueous reagents[88,90] have been employed. Lolehka and Limpavithayakul introduced accelerator reagents that are less viscous than the caffeine/benzoate/acetate mixture.[32]

Assay of *direct-reacting bilirubins* (Table 3) presents problems of its own.[75] A variety of reaction periods (1 to 30 min) and compositions of the aqueous acid reaction medium have been applied.[1,2,4,75] It is likely that for any well-defined type of sample and reaction conditions, an arbitrary fraction of unconjugated bilirubin, bilirubin conjugates, and possibly other diazo positive substances is determined.

In optimization of a diazo procedure for the direct-reacting fraction the following points must be considered: (1) At the time of optical reading a maximal stable azo color should have been reached, since the conversion rate may strongly depend on the rubin composition (e.g., mono- vs. diconjugates) and on matrix components such as albumin and reaction-promoting substances (e.g., bile salts or urea). Blumenfeld et al.[97] compared the 10 min-reaction procedure of Walters and Gerarde[98] and a 2 min-procedure. Both methods assayed bilirubin diglucuronide correctly but in the latter method, the response of monoglucuronide was only 50% of the expected value. Unfortunately, the extent of direct reaction of unconjugated bilirubin was not reported for the 10-min procedure. Selective underestimation of bilirubin monoglucuronide in a 1-min procedure has been invoked previously to explain discordant results obtained in assays of bilirubin UDP-glucuronyltransferase activity.[99] (2) To a certain extent unconjugated bilirubin reacts with diazo reagents in absence of a reaction accelerator. The reaction rate is expected to increase with the concentration of endogeneous accelerator substances, and possibly with reaction temperature, and concentration and reactivity of the diazo reagent. It critically depends on pH, with low reaction rates over a range of acidic pH values (Figure 1).[73,75] Therefore, construction of a curve delineating reaction of unconjugated pigment and conjugated bilirubins at various pigment concentrations is required to assess the significance of the direct-reacting fraction, particularly for samples that contain predominantly unconjugated bilirubin.[75]

d. Formation and Extraction of Organic Soluble Azo Pigments

This topic has been discussed previously, in particular with regard to the *p*-iodoaniline method for total rubins and the ethyl anthranilate method for assaying conjugated bilirubin.[4] Extraction of the azo derivatives renders the methods somewhat more complicated than single-phase procedures but offers several advantages including increased sensitivity, low blank values for hemoglobin-free reaction systems, and the possibility of separating the various azo derivatives by TLC or HPLC, thus permitting additional information about the composition of the parent rubin mixtures to be obtained (Section VI.A.3). Recovery of ethyl anthranilate azo pigment from conjugated bilirubins in liver homogenates was found to be incomplete, but could be improved by increasing the concentration of diazo reagent.[100] With the *p*-iodoaniline procedure, recovery of unconjugated bilirubin from liver homogenates is improved by adding the antioxidant, 2,6-di-tert-butyl-*p*-cresol.[101]

The power of the ethyl anthranilate diazo method to specifically measure conjugates in the presence of unconjugated bilirubin has recently been questioned on the basis of experiments involving addition of unconjugated bilirubin to undiluted bile.[102] In the standard method the reaction proceeds at 25°C in aqueous solution buffered at pH 2.7.[73] In model systems containing an aqueous bilirubinate solution, in the presence or absence of albumin, reaction of unconjugated bilirubin proved negligible at pH values below 2.7 (Figure 1), while reaction of both mono- and diglucuronides is complete.[47,73] The slow diazo cleavage of unconjugated bilirubin has been ascribed to a steric effect of the bulky carboxyethyl group in the ortho position with regard to the diazo group.[73] The reaction rate of unconjugated bilirubin is increased by the presence of liver homogenate.[103] To avoid significant reaction of unconjugated bilirubin in bile,[102] it is necessary to dilute the samples at least 20-fold with saline or distilled water.[4,104] Otherwise, the bile salts are likely to promote reaction of unconjugated pigment. Further, it is strictly necessary to buffer the samples to pH 2.7 or lower before addition of diazo reagent, as the rate of diazo reaction of bilirubin increases abruptly at slightly higher pH values (Figure 1).

An intriguing problem was disclosed by Bratlid and Winsnes,[105] who noted that purified bilirubin glucuronides added to serum reacted more completely with diazotized ethyl anthranilate than with *p*-diazobenzene sulfonic acid. Serum samples from patients with hepatobiliary disease were also examined, the value of total bilirubin with the procedure of Jendrassik and Grof[70] being put at 100%. The direct-reacting fraction obtained with *p*-diazobenzene sulfonic acid was about 76%, suggesting partial conversion of monoconjugates. However, the ethyl anthranilate method yielded only 26% of the total bilirubin value. Whether the low value found with the latter method reflects greater selectivity or loss of azo color is unresolved.

2. Total Amount of Glucuronic Acid Bound in Ester Linkage

In 1966, Brodersen[2,106] published a procedure which permits assay of the total amount of ester-linked glucuronic acid residues (sensivity 0.02 μM). The method is based on diazo treatment with diazotized [^{35}S]sulfanilic acid and scintillation counting of azopyrromethene obtained by alkaline hydrolysis from azopyrromethene glucuronide. The same principle should be applicable to other types of ester-linked conjugating groups provided adequate purification of the conjugates is developed.

3. Chromatographic Separation of Dipyrrolic Azo Derivatives

The ratios of various quantities can often be determined with acceptable accuracy whereas the absolute amounts can not. The latter have little significance when unassessed dilution may occur (e.g., bile). Pertinent recommendations for TLC have been given by McDonagh.[5] For several TLC separations, benzene-containing solvents are used to remove or separate hydrophobic compounds.[4] Keeping the volume fractions unchanged, benzene can often be replaced by the less toxic solvent toluene with minimal change in R_F values.

For separation purposes organic soluble azo derivatives are most convenient.[4] Unless stated otherwise, all work discussed in this section refers to studies done with the diazo procedure of Van Roy and Heirwegh,[73] in which the sample is treated with diazotized ethyl anthranilate for 30 min in aqueous solution at 20 to 25°C and pH 2.7. Reaction products are extracted with pentan-2-one before optical reading. The concentration of the dipyrrolic azo derivatives in the extract is calculated using ε_{530} 22.2 × 10^3 M^{-1} cm^{-1}. In calculating the corresponding rubin concentration it is important to realize that two moles of dipyrrolic azo pigment are formed for each mole of rubin. Therefore, the tetrapyrrole concentration equals half the azo pigment concentration.

The ethyl anthranilate azo pigment fractions separated by TLC have usually been denoted by Greek letters and by Roman capitals, both with subscripts (Table 5). These symbols only denote chromatographic fractions, and should not be used to refer to

Table 5
STRUCTURES AND SOURCES OF REFERENCE DIPYRROLIC AZO DERIVATIVES, AND NOTATION OF CORRESPONDING CHROMATOGRAPHIC FRACTIONS

Chromatographic fraction[a]	Reference compounds	
	Systematic name[b]	Source
α_F	Bilirubin-IXβ[35]	13,18- Vn_2-Azpm
α'_F	Bilirubin-IXδ[35]	12,17- Vn_2-Azpm
α_O	Bilirubin-IXα[35] and -XIIIα[33]	Azpm-8 (endo-vinyl isomer)
α_O	Bilirubin-IXα[35] and -IIIα[33]	Azpm-12 (exo-vinyl isomer)
G_4	Bilirubin-IXγ[35]	Azpm-2 and Azpm-18
α_2	Dog bile; enzymic synthesis	Azpm-8(Xyl) and Azpm-12(Xyl)
α_3	Dog bile; enzymic synthesis	Azpm-8(Glc) and Azpm-12(Glc)
β_x	Bilirubin-IXβ and -IXδ[35]	Azpm-3,7
δ	Mammalian bile; enzymic synthesis	Azpm-8(GlcU) and Azpm-12(GlcU)

[a] TLC separation is possible of (a) fractions ($\alpha_F + \alpha'_F$), α_O, α_2, α_3, β_x and δ,[4] (b) the isomeric pairs (13.18- Vn_2-Azpm and 12,17- Vn_2-Azpm)[23] and (Azpm-8 and Azpm-12),[4,34] and (c) derivatives of the isomeric pairs of unconjugated azo pigments, Azpm-8 and Azpm-12,[4,23,34,35] and sugar conjugates

[b] See Chapter 1.

known azo pigments. It should be realized that a similar chromatographic behaviour of an unknown azo derivative and a known reference azo pigment does not imply structural identity. Thus, a δ-fraction does not necessarily correspond with azopyrromethene glucuronide but could possibly include azopyrromethene sulfate.[107] Also, before for example an α_2 fraction is identified as azopyrromethene xyloside, conformation of the xyloside structure of the unknown α_2 pigment is required by chemical derivatization or other techniques (Chapter 2).

a. Proportion of Conjugating Groups. Ratio of Monoester to Diester Conjugates of Bilirubin. Detection of Non-α Isomers of Bilirubin-IX

When fresh bile from normal humans or rats is treated with diazotized ethyl anthranilate two major dipyrrolic azo derivatives are separated by TLC: fractions α_0 and δ which correspond with unconjugated azopyrromethene and azopyrromethene glucuronide, respectively. Similar analysis of fresh dog bile yields additional fractions, α_2 and α_3 which correspond with azopyrromethene xyloside and glucoside, respectively. In general, one also observes the fractions β_x and α_F, and occasionally small amounts of α_F, α_l and γ_l. The occurrence of β_x, α_F, and α'_F usually indicates the presence of bilirubin-IXβ and IXδ (Figure 4, Chapter 1) in the sample, since azopyrromethene-3,7 corresponds with β_x, 13,13- Vn_2-azopyrromethene with α_F, and 12,17-Vn_2- azopyrromethene with α'_F. Also, it should be noted that fractions α_0, α_1, α_2, α_3 and δ from bile each contain a mixture of exo- and endo-vinyl isomers.

Quantification of separated azo pigment bands is done either densitometrically, or by elution with methanol or pentan-2-one/formamide (9:1, v/v) followed by optical reading of the eluates.

Reference unconjugated azo pigments (Table 5) can be obtained from commercial bilirubin-IXα and synthetically prepared non-α isomers of bilirubin-IX.[35] For preparation of reference conjugated azo derivatives, enzymic synthesis of bilirubin glycoside in an incubation system with rat liver tissue preparations and UDP-sugar (xylose, glucose or glucuronic acid) followed by diazo treatment of the mixture can be exploited. Alternatively, human and rat bile (glucuronides) and dog bile (xylosides, glucosides, glucuronides) are convenient sources of reference material.

Chromatographic analysis of ethyl anthranilate azo derivatives to detect fractions α_F, α'_F, G_4 and β_x offers a convenient test for the presence of bilirubin-IXβ, IXγ, and IXδ. If such azo pigment fractions are detected, the analysis should be completed by demonstration of the parent tetrapyrroles by a direct separation technique (Section VI.B.3.d).

The molar proportion of xylosyl, glucosyl, and glucuronosyl conjugating residues can be calculated from the proportion of azo pigment fractions α_2, α_3, and δ, provided the identity of these pigments is verified.[4] In calculating the glucuronide fraction in cholestatic or stored bile, the so-called β- and γ-fractions which are artifactually formed derivatives of 2-, 3-, and 4-*O*-acyl glucuronides,[108] should be added to the δ-fraction.

The ratio of monoester to diester conjugates of bilirubin can, in principle, be calculated from the ratio R

$$R = \frac{\text{unconjugated azopyrromethenes Azpm-8 and Azpm-12}}{\text{sum of ester conjugates of azopyrromethenes Azpm-8 and Azpm-12}}$$

The R values were equal to one for isolated bilirubin monoglucuronide.[47] Further, solely azopyrromethene glucuronide was obtained when purified bilirubin diglucuronide was treated with diazo reagent, even for prolonged periods of time.[47] Thus, with these purified glucuronide preparations, the only source of azopyrromethenes Azpm-8 and Azpm-12 was the unconjugated dipyrrole half of bilirubin monoglucuronide. Reaction of the small fraction of unconjugated bilirubin present in bile can be rendered negligible by sufficient dilution of the bile samples (20-fold or more).[73,104] Under those conditions, the following ratios can be calculated:

Monoconjugated/diconjugated bilirubin $= 2 \times R/(1\text{-}R)$
Monoconjugated/total conjugated bilirubin $= 2 \times R/(1 + R)$
Diconjugated/total conjugated bilirubin $= (1 - R)/(1 + R)$

Recently, some difficulties have been encountered with this approach. In a comparative study of bile samples, the R values for some species exceeded the theoretical maximum ($R = 1$).[11,12] These aberrant results could be due to as yet unidentified direct-reacting compounds yielding unconjugated azopyrromethenes Azpm-8 and/or Azpm-12 and/or to unexpectedly high diazo cleavage of unconjugated bilirubin. As already noted, reference mono- and diglucuronides yield the predicted azo derivatives in the expected ratios.

Determination of minor azo pigment fractions (e.g., azo pigment β_x) can be rendered more accurate by applying to the same TLC plate a small and a larger volume (e.g., 25 and 500 $\mu\ell$) of azo pigment extract (double-track development). Major and minor components are eluted from the tracks corresponding with the small and large volume, respectively, of extract applied to the plate. For blank correction, appropriate areas from blank tracks are eluted. The accuracy of densitometric measurements can be improved in a similar manner.

Separation of the four major ethyl anthranilate azo pigments derived from mammalian tissues into doublets of endo- and exo-vinyl isomers by HPLC[109] and similar separation of *p*-iodoaniline azo pigments, obtained from dog bile, have been reported.[110] The isomer pairs of conjugated azopigments can be separated by TLC only after acetylation, preceded by methyl ester formation for azopyrromethene glucuronide.[4] The isomeric unconjugated azopyrromethenes are separated preferentially as methyl ester derivatives.[4,35]

b. Determination of Positional Isomers of Azopyrromethene Glucuronide[18]

The 1-, 2-, 3-, and 4-*O*-acyl glucuronides can be separated conveniently by TLC of their methyl ester derivatives. After formation of ethyl anthranilate azo derivatives at pH 6 in the absence of an excess of aromatic amine, the δ-fraction is isolated by TLC and scraped from the thin-layer plate. The pigment is eluted with pentanone/formamide (9:1, v/v), formamide is removed by washing the eluate with glycine/HCl buffer pH 2.7 and the pentanone extract is submitted to either one of the following procedures; (1) the extract is briefly treated with an excess of ethereal diazomethane and the methyl ester derivatives formed are separated on a silica-gel plate by development with chloroform/methanol (9:1, v/v). The 2-*O*-acyl isomer (R_F 0.59) moves most rapidly followed by the 3-*O*-acyl (R_F 0.55), 1-*O*-acyl (R_F 0.43), and 4-*O*-acyl (R_F 0.39) isomers. (2) On a pre-coated silane-treated silica gel plate, provided with a pad of filter paper at the upper edge, underivatized azo pigment δ is chromatographed by development with chloroform/methanol (9:1, v/v) for 12 to 15 hr. The 1-*O*-acyl isomer moves most rapidly followed by the 2-*O*-acyl isomer and a band of C-3 and C-4 isomers, in that order. The technique can be used to prepare small quantities of the free acids.

B. Tetrapyrrole Analysis

1. Direct Spectrophotometry[5]

Spectrophotometry is excellent for determination of pure rubins with known molar absorption coefficients (Table 4) and may yield satisfactory estimates of bilirubin in neonatal sera because they generally contain only small concentrations of conjugated bilirubins and interfering substances. High values may be obtained for sera of neonates after administration of lipid preparations.[111] In view of the complexity of rubin mixtures in body fluids, direct spectrophotometry is likely to remain of limited application, even when pure bilirubin conjugates become available.

2. Specific Determination of Unconjugated Bilirubin

Specific measurement of unconjugated bilirubin in serum can be achieved by chloroform extraction.[112] At 0 to 22°C recovery is optimal at pH 8.15 in the presence of ascorbate and salicylate. The latter substance improves extraction above pH 8 and a similar effect has been noted for added aniline in studies with amniotic fluid.[113] The proposed, optimal pH should be strictly adhered to.

Normal human bile contains a small fraction of unconjugated bilirubin (less than 1.2% of total bilirubins).[10,65,114] Chloroform co-extracts small amounts of conjugated bilirubin, causing relatively large errors, though correction for co-extracted bilirubins can be done by analysis of the azo derivatives prepared from the extracted pigments.[10] Similarly, 4 to 9% of conjugated bilirubin partitioned with the unconjugated bilirubin when the two-phase extraction system developed by Weber and Schalm[115] for serum samples was applied to human or rat bile.[102] Also, it is not advisable to use the alkaline methanolysis procedure (Section VI.B.3.b) for determination of a small fraction (<5%) of unconjugated bilirubin in the presence of a large excess of conjugates, since approximately 0.5% of the total conjugates in the sample are hydrolyzed, not methylated in the procedure. Accurate determination seems possible with the method of Boonyapisit et al.[65] In this procedure, bands of bilirubin and conjugates separated by TLC on a silica gel plate are eluted and quantified after conversion to azo derivatives.

3. Chromatography of Derivatized and Underivatized Rubins

For separation of labile tetrapyrroles both TLC and HPLC have specific merits and drawbacks. TLC techniques are convenient and versatile, the equipment needed is inexpensive, no special skills are required, and comparison of references and unknowns is straightforward (for pertinent recommendations, see McDonagh[5] and Chapter 4,

Volume 2). To prevent autoxidation and disproportionation of rubins it is advisable to apply the samples to thin-layer plates in a stream of nitrogen, with gentle heating of the back-side of the plate to expedite evaporation of the solvent, and to start development of the chromatogram without delay. The separated rubins should immediately be eluted or converted to azo derivatives, and determined colorimetrically. Improved stability of the chromatogram can be obtained by lightly spraying the plates with a methanolic solution of 50 mM ascorbic acid thus allowing more convenient preparation of densitometric scans. It is advisable to place the light filter between the incident light beam and the thin-layer plate.

Equipment for HPLC is expensive and efficient operation requires well-trained personnel. Otherwise, HPLC offers distinct advantages. It is not only amenable to a certain degree of automation (injection of the sample and calculation of results) but also permits exclusion of light and molecular oxygen. Also, the relatively high resolving power of HPLC may permit better separation of complex bilirubin mixtures.

a. Separation of Intact Tetrapyrroles

Only recent advances related to TLC and HPLC of rubins will be discussed. Owing to unavailability of pure reference compounds, no single direct separation technique has been validated with regard to recovery of individual rubins and calibration. Incomplete recovery could result from partial extraction of rubins from the sample and from destruction and alteration during sample application and chromatographic development. Additional problems are related to insufficient resolution and unexplained multiplicity of chromatographic bands.

Rubins extracted from dog bile can be separated on silica-gel plates into about 20 chromatographic bands by development with neutral solvent systems.[34] The following bands were detected: bilirubin-IXα, bilirubin-IXβ, the mono- and diconjugates of xylose, glucose and glucuronic acid, and diconjugates of any pair of the three sugars mentioned.[19,34,116] Each monoconjugate band contained mixtures of the two positional isomers, e.g., for the monoglucoside, bilirubin-*8*,12(Glc) and bilirubin-8, *12*(Glc). Similarly, each of the diconjugates that contain two different sugars were composed of two positional isomers, e.g., bilirubin-*8,12*(Glc; GlcU) and bilirubin-*8,12*(GlcU; Glc) in the case of the monoglucoside-monoglucuronide band. Minor bands[34] such as the monomethyl ester, bilirubin-8,12(Me), and the monomethyl-monoglucuronide diester, bilirubin-8,12(me; GlcU), were probably artifacts, formed by transesterification.[50] Additional minor mono- and diesters contained unidentified conjugating residues.[34] Occasionally, closely moving bands yielding the same pair of azo derivatives, in particular azo pigment δ, were observed.[19,34] Isomeric forms of azopyrromethene glucuronide with glucuronic acid bound to the carboxyl group of azopyrromethene at C-1, C-2, C-3, or C-4 move as azo pigment fraction δ in the TLC systems used for analysis. It is possible, therefore, that the closely moving conjugated bilirubins contained acyl-shifted glucuronyl residues.

The possibility has been considered[34] that redistribution of dipyrrole moieties by disproportionation (Section III) in the course of extraction, work up, or separation could give rise to conjugates absent from native bile; for example, diconjugates containing different sugars could be formed from different monoconjugates or diconjugates. However, semiquantitative analysis of the unconjugated bilirubin isomers obtained by saponification of isolated conjugates showed compositions similar to that in native bile.[34] Also, preincubation of dog bile with radiolabeled unconjugated bilirubin did not produce labeled monoconjugates. It may also be noted that separation of rubins from dog bile by HPLC yielded the same major rubins as observed by TLC, including the diconjugates containing two different sugar residues.[117] Therefore, gross artifactual redistribution of dipyrrole moieties is unlikely.

TLC separations, in general, are preceded by extraction of rubins into a suitable solvent. Only 50 to 70% of rubins are extracted from dog bile with chloroform by the procedure of Heirwegh et al.[34] Extraction yields have been improved by buffering the samples at pH 1.8 and adding a salting-out reagent with ascorbic acid (extraction yield: 90 to 100% for urine, liver homogenate, bile, stools and serum).[118] Gordon et al.[116] extracted bile with chloroform containing the ion-pair reagent tetraheptylammonium chloride. Extraction yields of 90% were reported.

It seems likely that in the procedure of Heirwegh et al.[34] (extraction yield for dog bile, 50 to 70%) selective losses of the more polar conjugates occur. In contrast, extraction of dog bile with chloroform containing tetraheptylammonium chloride[116] probably leads to preferential loss of less polar conjugates owing to specific interaction of the detergent with the carboxylate groups of the glucuronides. Only minor amounts of glucose and virtually no xylose conjugates were detected in dog bile with this procedure. This result conflicts with the reported distribution of conjugating residues determined with separations based on HPLC[117] and with the ethyl anthranilate diazo method, which showed the presence of approximately 30% of glucose and 10% of xylose residues.[12] Extraction at pH 1.8 in the presence of a salting-out reagent, yields a better representation of rubin composition, since the observed patterns agreed fairly well with those obtained with the alkaline methanolysis procedure (Section VI.A.3.b) and the ethyl anthranilate technique (Section VI.A.3.b).

Separations by HPLC of rubins present in bile[117,119] or model mixtures,[120] or synthetized in vitro with liver homogenate as the source of enzyme,[120] have been reported recently. In these techniques extraction is not performed and bile is applied directly to the separation column[117,119] or a fraction of the supernatant solution obtained from mixing 500 $\mu\ell$ of sample (bile or an enzymic incubation mixture) and 300 $\mu\ell$ of acetonitrile is used.[120] In studies with synthetic mixtures of mono- and diconjugates of xylose, glucose, and glucuronic acid Onishi et al.[120] achieved separation of C-8 and C-12 positional isomers of the monoconjugates.

b. Determination of Bilirubin and its Mono- and Diester Conjugates by the Alkaline Methanolysis Procedure[24,121]

Mono- and diester conjugates of bilirubin are transformed quantitatively into the corresponding mono- and dimethyl esters at room temperature by brief (60-90 s) base-catalyzed methanolysis.[121] Ascorbate and disodium EDTA are added as protective agents. Unconjugated bilirubin is not esterified and disproportionation by dipyrrole exchange does not occur under the applied reaction conditions. Dried reaction products are stable under argon at −15°C for up to 1 week.

TLC on silica gel plates with chloroform/methanol/acetic acid (97:2:1, by vol.) separates a bilirubin band (IIIα, IXα, XIIIα), four monomethyl ester bands corresponding with the IIIα, IXα-C-8, IXα-C-12 and XIIIα isomers, and a dimethyl ester band (IIIα, IXα, XIIIα), in the sequence indicated (bilirubin moves most rapidly).[121] Heme and non-α isomers of unconjugated bilirubin-IX are immobile in the TLC system used. For quantification, pigment bands are scraped from the plates, eluted with chloroform/methanol (1:1, v/v) and the eluates are read at 450 nm. Relative amounts are obtained. Pure well-characterized reference compounds are available for calibration purposes.

The reaction products can also be analyzed by HPLC using gradient elution on a silica gel column. Separation time is 14 min and 10 min is required for re-equilibration of the column with initial solvent. The limit of detection in serum (0.6 mℓ sample size) is 0.2 μM bilirubin. Hemoglobin in concentrations up to 4 mg/mℓ and non-α isomers of bilirubin-IX do not interfere. Addition to the reaction medium of xanthobilirubinic acid methyl ester as an internal standard allows direct determination of the absolute concentrations.

The method has been applied satisfactorily to a variety of aqueous samples (normal and pathological serum, normal and rubin-enriched bile, and enzymic incubation mixtures containing homogenates or microsomal fraction from liver) with and without added references (bilirubin, and its mono- and diglucuronide). For biological samples from adult humans and other mammals such as the rat the mono- and dimethyl esters are predominantly derived from bilirubin mono- and diglucuronide, respectively.

Although the procedure has been tested only with conjugates composed nearly exclusively of bilirubin glucuronides, it is likely that methanolysis of other sugar conjugates will be equally satisfactory. If so, simple or quite complex mixtures of ester conjugates could be analyzed validly. Obviously, information is lost as any mixture of bilirubin and any number of mono- and diester conjugates is reduced to the same mixture of derivatives. This, however, probably reflects a basically important biological parameter. Further, the method is likely to be applicable to any type of biological specimen.

c. Bilirubin IIIα, IXα, and XIIIα

Determination of the proportion of isomers is important for assessing the degree of purity of reference bilirubin-IXα. A chloroform solution of the free acids can be separated by TLC on silica gel with chloroform/acetic acid (99:1, v/v) and quantified by optical reading as detailed by McDonagh.[5] The IIIα isomer is particularly labile and is easily underestimated. The free acids,[21,122] and dimethyl esters[24,122] can also be separated by HPLC. The isomeric status of the bilirubin aglycone (IIIα, IXα, or XIIIα) of ester conjugates can be determined after alkaline methanolysis of bilirubin ester conjugates (Section VI.B.3.b). Alternatively, bilirubin isomers can be prepared by saponification[24] and separated and quantified as indicated above.

The IIIα and XIIIα isomers of bilirubin can be prepared by brief treatment of bilirubin-IXα in DMSO with strong acid.[123] Partial characterization of mono- and dimethyl ester derivatives of bilirubin IIIα, IXα and XIIIα has been reported.[5,121]

d. Bilirubin IXβ, IXγ, and IXδ

Assay methods have not been put on a quantitative basis. It is advisable to first submit part of the sample to diazo cleavage with diazotized ethyl anthranilate and to separate and quantify the azo derivatives (Section VI.A.3). Detection of azo pigment fraction β_x or G_4 suggests the presence of bilirubin IXβ and/or IXδ, or bilirubin-IXγ, respectively (Table 5). When β_x and G_4 are identified as Azpm-3,7 and Azpm-2 (or Azpm-18) the presence of non-α isomers of bilirubin-IX should be confirmed by analysis of tetrapyrroles. In contrast to the easy extraction of bilirubin-IXα from aqueous medium at pH 8.15 with chloroform, the more hydrophilic non-α isomers require acidification (e.g., pH 2.7) and addition of a salting-out reagent such as ammonium sulfate.[35] The isomers can be separated by TLC on silica gel plates with chloroform/methanol/water (48:9:1, by vol.). Synthesis, isolation, and partial characterization of the non-α isomers have been reported.[35]

VII. CONCLUSIONS AND PERSPECTIVE

Analytical methodology in the rubin field is passing through an important phase. Several types of unconjugated and conjugated bilirubins have been recognized and the major rubins present in bile of humans and several experimental animals have been fairly well characterized. However, unknown diazo positive pigments seem to be present in serum of patients with cholestasis and need to be identified. Consistent use of pure unconjugated bilirubin-IXα and purified preparations of mono- and diglucuronides of bilirubin-IXα in future development and evaluation of analytical procedures undoubtedly will lead to results with more clear-cut chemical significance. Such studies should be complemented with a description of the purity of the rubin preparations used. Primary standards of pure conjugated bilirubins are not available as yet and adequate conditions for storage permitting, for example, shipment to other laboratories still need to be defined. Taking account of the present knowledge of artificial changes and breakdown that can occur in rubins it is likely that appropriate conditions for storage of conjugated bilirubins can be established. While awaiting the availability of pure well-characterized bilirubin conjugates, it seems worthwhile to further characterize the more easily accessible mono- and ditaurine conjugates of bilirubin-IXα[66] and to explore the feasibility of use of these pigments as secondary standards.

Absolute reference methods that are applicable to a wide range of aqueous samples such as are obtained from mammals are not available. The notion "direct-reacting bilirubin" and, for most procedures also the notion "total bilirubin", only have operational significance. However, diazo methods such as the ethyl anthranilate technique are valuable for structure elucidation of isolated rubins. Rational application of techniques for direct separation of intact or derivatized rubins would avoid many of the shortcomings of diazo methods and is expected to lead to rapid and fundamental progress.

REFERENCES

1. **With, T. K.,** *Bile Pigments,* Academic Press, New York, 1968, 1.
2. **Brodersen, R. and Jacobsen, J.,** Separation and determination of bile pigments, *Methods Biochem. Anal.,* 17, 31, 1969.
3. **Billing, B., Haslam, R., and Wald, N.,** Bilirubin standards and the determination of bilirubin by manual and technicon autoanalyzer methods, *Ann. Clin. Biochem.,* 8, 21, 1971.
4. **Heirwegh, K. P. M., Fevery, J., Meuwissen, J. A. T. P., De Groote, J., Compernolle, F., Desmet, V., and Van Roy, F. P.,** Recent advances in the separation and analysis of diazo-positive bile pigments, *Methods Biochem. Anal.,* 22, 205, 1974.
5. **McDonagh, A. F.,** Bile pigments: bilatrienes and 5,15 biladienes, in *The Porphyrins,* Vol. 6, Biochemistry, Part A, Dolphin, D., Ed., Academic Press, New York, 1979, 293.
6. **Heirwegh, K. P. M.,** Formation, metabolism and significance of bilirubin-IXα glycosides, in *Conjugation Reactions in Drug Biotransformation,* Aitio, A., Ed., Elsevier/North Holland Biomedical Press, Amsterdam, 1978, 67.
7. **Brodersen, R., Hermann, L. S., and Vind, I.,** Normal bilirubin concentration and the occurrence of other bile pigments in human blood sera, *Scand. J. Clin. Lab. Invest.,* 15, 523, 1963.
8. **Blumenthal, S. G., Stucker, T., Rasmussen, R. D., Ikeda, R. M., Ruebner, B. H., Bergstrom, D. E., and Hanson, F. W.,** Changes in bilirubins in human prenatal development, *Biochem. J.,* 186, 693, 1980.
9. **Goresky, C. A., Gordon, E. R., Shaffer, E. A., Paré, P., Carassavas, D., and Aronoff, A.,** Definition of a conjugation dysfunction in Gilbert's syndrome: studies of the handling of bilirubin loads and of the pattern of bilirubin conjugates secreted in bile, *Clin. Sci. Mol. Med.,* 55, 63, 1978.
10. **Fevery, J., Van Damme, B., Michiels, R., De Groote, J., and Heirwegh, K. P. M.,** Bilirubin conjugates in bile of man and rat in the normal state and in liver disease, *J. Clin. Invest.,* 51, 2482, 1972.
11. **Fevery, J., Blanckaert, N., Heirwegh, K. P. M., Préaux, A.-M. and Berthelot, P.,** Unconjugated bilirubin and an increased proportion of bilirubin monoconjugates in bile of patients with Gilbert's syndrome and Crigler-Najjar disease, *J. Clin. Invest.,* 60, 970, 1977.
12. **Fevery, J., Van de Vijver, M., Michiels, R., and Heirwegh, K. P. M.,** Comparison in different species of biliary bilirubin-IXα conjugates with the activities of hepatic and renal bilirubin-IXαuridine diphosphate glycosyltransferases, *Biochem. J.,* 164, 737, 1977.
13. **Blanckaert, N.,** unpublished work, 1980.
14. **Blanckaert, N., Fevery, J., Heirwegh, K. P. M., Compernolle, F., and Dodion, J.,** Characterization of the bilirubin pigments in bile of neonates and of children with Crigler-Najjar disease, *Digestion,* 14, 468, 1976.

15. **Gollan, J. L., Huang, S. N., Billing, B. H., and Sherlock, S.,** Prolonged survival in three brothers with severe type 2 Crigler-Najjar syndrome. Ultrastructural and metabolic studies, *Gastroenterology,* 68, 1543, 1975.
16. **Gordon, E. R., Shaffer, E. A., and Sas-Kortsak, A.,** Bilirubin secretion and conjugation in the Crigler-Najjar syndrome Type II, *Gastroenterology,* 70, 761, 1976.
17. **Compernolle, F., Van Hees, G. P., Blanckaert, N., and Heirwegh, K. P. M.,** Glucuronic acid conjugates of bilirubin-IXα in normal bile compared with post-obstructive bile. Transformation of the 1-*O*-acylglucuronide into 2-, 3- and 4-*O*-acylglucuronides, *Biochem. J.,* 171, 185, 1978.
18. **Blanckaert, N., Compernolle, F., Leroy, P., Van Houtte, R., Fevery, J., and Heirwegh, K. P. M.,** The fate of bilirubin-IXα glucuronide in cholestasis and during storage *in vitro*. Intramolecular rearrangement to positional isomers of glucuronic acid, *Biochem. J.,* 171, 203, 1978.
19. **Blumenthal, S. G., Taggart, D. B., Rasmussen, R. D., Ikeda, R. M., Ruebner, B. H. Bergstrom, D. E., and Hanson, F. W.,** Conjugated and unconjugated bilirubins in humans and Rhesus monkeys — structural identity of bilirubins from biles and meconiums of newborn humans and Rhesus monkeys, *Biochem. J.,* 179, 537, 1979.
20. **McDonagh, A. F., Palma, L. A., and Lightner, D. A.,** Blue light and bilirubin excretion, *Science,* 208, 145, 1980.
21. **Onishi, S., Isobe, K., Itoh, S., Kawade, N., and Sugiyama, S.,** Demonstration of a geometric isomer of bilirubin-IXα in the serum of a hyperbilirubinaemic newborn infant and the mechanism of jaundice phototherapy, *Biochem. J.,* 190, 533, 1980.
22. **Berry, C. S., Zarembo, J. E., and Ostrow, J. D.,** Evidence for conversion of bilirubin to dihydroxyl derivatives in the Gunn rat, *Biochem. Biophys. Res. Commun.,* 49, 1366, 1972.
23. **Blanckaert, N., Fevery, J., Heirwegh, K. P. M., and Compernolle, F.,** Characterization of the major diazo-positive pigments in bile of homozygous Gunn rats, *Biochem. J.,* 164, 237, 1977.
24. **Blanckaert, N., Kabra, P. M., Farina, F. A., Stafford, B. E., Marton, L. J., and Schmid, R.,** Measurement of bilirubin and its monoconjugates and diconjugates in human serum by alkaline methanolysis and high-performance liquid chromatography, *J. Lab. Clin. Med.,* 96, 198, 1980.
25. **Berglöf, J., Grahnén, A., and Sjöholm, I.,** Determination of unconjugated bilirubin in human serum by optical rotation measurements, *Clin. Chim. Acta,* 62, 169, 1975.
26. **Lamola, A. A., Eisinger, J., Blumberg, W. E., Patel, S. C., and Flores, J.,** Fluorimetric study of the partition of bilirubin among blood components: basis for rapid microsassays of bilirubin and bilirubin binding capacity in whole blood, *Anal. Biochem.,* 100, 25, 1979.
27. **Landis, J. B. and Pardue, H. L.,** Evaluation of a kinetic method for simultaneous determination of conjugated and unconjugated bilirubin, *Clin. Chem.,* 24, 1700, 1978.
28. **Valdes, R., Brody, J. P., and Savory, J.,** New kinetic procedure for the measurement of conjugated bilirubin with a centrifugal analyzer, *Ann. Clin. Lab. Sci.,* 9, 251, 1979.
29. **Uete, T.,** Ultra-micromethods for the biochemical analysis of cutaneous capillary blood. I. Critical evaluation and application of the Roth fluorimetric determination of plasma or serum bilirubin, *Clin. Chim. Acta,* 59, 259, 1975.
30. **Ehrlich, P.,** Sulfodiazobenzol, ein Reagens auf Bilirubin, *Centralbl. Klin. Med.,* 4, 721, 1883.
31. **Hymans van den Bergh, A. A. and Muller, P.,** Über eine direkte und undirekte Diazoreaktion auf Bilirubin, *Biochem. Z.,* 77, 90, 1916.
32. **Lohehka, P. H. and Limpavithayakul, K.,** The promoting ability of five accelerating agents for diazotization of several types of bilirubin samples, *Clin. Chem.,* 23, 778, 1977.
33. **McDonagh, A. F., and Assisi, F.,** Commercial bilirubin: a trinity of isomers, *FEBS Lett.,* 18, 315, 1971.
34. **Heirwegh, K. P. M., Fevery, J., Michiels, R., Van Hees, G. P., and Compernolle, F.,** Separation by thin-layer chromatography and structure elucidation of bilirubin conjugates isolated from dog bile, *Biochem. J.,* 145, 185, 1975.
35. **Blanckaert, N., Heirwegh, K. P. M., and Compernolle, F.,** Sythesis and separation by thin-layer chromatography of bilirubin-IX isomers. Their identification as tetrapyrroles and dipyrrolic ethyl anthranilate azo derivatives, *Biochem. J.,* 155, 405, 1976.
36. **Jansen, F. H. and Billing, B. H.,** The identification of monoconjugates of bilirubin in bile as amide derivatives, *Biochem. J.,* 125, 917, 1971.
37. **Jansen, P. L. M.,** The isomerization of bilirubin monoglucuronide, *Clin. Chim. Acta.,* 49, 233, 1973.
38. **Brodersen, R.,** Bilirubin. Solubility and interaction with albumin and phospholipid, *J. Biol. Chem.,* 254, 2364, 1979.
39. **Lightner, D. A., Cu, A., McDonagh, A. F., and Palma, L. A.,** On the autoxidation of bilirubin, *Biochem. Biophys. Res. Commun.,* 69, 648, 1976.
40. **Brodersen, R. and Theilgaard, J.,** Bilirubin colloid formation in neutral aqueous solutions, *Scand. J. Clin. Lab. Invest.,* 24, 395, 1969.

41. **Lee, K.-S. and Gartner, L. M.**, Spectrophotometric characteristics of bilirubin, *Pediat. Res.*, 10, 782, 1976.
42. **Brodersen, R.**, Supersaturation with bilirubin by colloid formation and disposition, with a hypothesis on the etiology of kernicterus, *Scand. J. Clin. Lab. Invest.*, 29, 447, 1972.
43. **Jirsa, M. and Sponar, J.**, Das Absorptionsspecktrum, der physikalische Zustand und die Geschwindigkeit der Diazoreaktion des Bilirubins, *Z. Ges. Inn. Med.*, 11, 519, 1956.
44. **McDonagh, A. F.**, Thermal and photochemical reactions of bilirubin-IXα, *Ann. N. Y. Acad. Sci.*, 244, 553, 1975.
45. **Lightner, D. A.**, The photoreactivity of bilirubin and related tetrapyrroles, *Photochem. Photobiol.*, 26, 427, 1977.
46. **Blanckaert, N., Gollan, J., and Schmid, R.**, Mechanism of bilirubin diglucuronide formation in intact rats. Bilirubin diglucuronide formation in vivo, *J. Clin. Invest.*, 65, 1332, 1980.
47. **Heirwegh, K. P. M., Sieg, A., and Van Hees, G. P.**, unpublished data, 1980.
48. **Au, Y. N. and Hutchinson, D. W.**, The photoinduced isomerisation of bilirubin in cationic detergent solutions, *Biochem. J.*, 191, 657, 1980.
49. **Heirwegh, K. P. M. and Compernolle, F.**, Micro-analytic detection and structure elucidation of ester-glycosides, *Biochem. Pharmacol.*, 28, 2109, 1979.
50. **Salmon, M., Fenselau, C., Cukier, J. O., and Odell, G. B.**, Rapid transesterification of bilirubin glucuronides in methanol, *Life Sci.*, 15, 2069, 1974.
51. **Etter-Kjelsaas, H. and Kuenzle, C. C.**, A polypeptide conjugate of bilirubin from human bile, *Biochim. Biophys. Acta.*, 400, 83, 1975.
52. **Levvy, G. A. and Conchie, J.**, β-Glucuronidase and the hydrolysis of glucuronic acid, in *Glucuronic Acid. Free and Combined,* Dutton, G. J., Ed., Academic Press, New York, 1966, 301.
53. **Conchie, J., Gelman, A. L., and Levvy, G. A.**, Inhibition of glycosidases by aldonolactones of corresponding configuration. The C-4- and C-6-specificity of β-glucosidase and β-galactosidase, *Biochem. J.*, 103, 609, 1967.
54. **Lucassen, J.**, The Diazo Reaction of Bilirubin and Bilirubin Diglucuronide, Ph.D. thesis, University of Utrecht, Kemink and zoon, Utrecht, 1961, 1.
55. **Ostrow, J. D. and Murphy N.**, Isolation and properties of conjugated bilirubin from bile, *Biochem. J.*, 120, 311, 1970.
56. **Wolkoff, A. W., Scharschmidt, B. F., Plotz, P. H., and Berk, P. D.**, Purification of conjugated bilirubin: a new approach utilizing albumin-agarose gel affinity chromatography, *Proc. Soc. Exptl. Biol. Med.*, 152, 20, 1976.
57. **Fog, J.**, Bilirubin - purification - purity, *Scand. J. Clin. Lab. Invest.*, 1, 49, 1964.
58. **Ostrow, J. D., Hammaker, L., and Schmid, R.**, The prepartion of crystalline bilirubin-C^{14}, *J. Clin. Invest.*, 40, 1442, 1961.
59. **Dybkaer, R. and Hertz, H.**, A reference for determination of bilirubin concentration in serum using bilirubin in cyanide-formamide for enrichment of serum, *Scand. J. Clin. Lab. Invest.*, 25, 151, 1970.
60. **Thompson, R. P. H.**, Modification of Michaëlsson's method for the measurement of plasma total bilirubin, *J. Clin. Pathol.*, 22, 439, 1969.
61. **Doumas, B. T., Perry, B. W., Sasse, E. A., and Straumfjord, J. V.**, Standardization in bilirubin assays: evaluation of selected methods and stability of bilirubin solutions, *Clin. Chem.*, 19, 984, 1973.
62. **Van Roy, F. P., Meuwissen, J. A. T. P., De Meuter, F., and Heirwegh, K. P. M.**, Determination of bilirubin in liver homogenates and serum with diazotized *p*-iodoaniline, *Clin. Chim. Acta.*, 31, 109, 1971.
63. **Mykoniatis, M. G.**, Influence of two preparations of bovine albumin on the total bilirubin as determined by Thompson's method in its reference solution, *Clin. Biochem.*, 12, 107, 1979.
64. **Zebelman, A. M., Kenny, M. A., and Sunday, C. G.**, Bilirubin standard solutions, *Clin. Chem.*, 22, 934, 1976.
65. **Boonyapisit, S. T., Trotman, B. W., Ostrow, J. D., Olivieri, P. J., and Gallo, D.**, Measurement of conjugated and unconjugated bilirubin in bile. II. A new thin-layer chromatographic method, *J. Lab. Clin. Med.*, 88, 857, 1976.
66. **Jirsa, M. and Vecerek, B.**, Neue Bilirubinderivate. I. Ihr Vergleich mit Gallen- und Serum-Bilirubin, *Hoppe-Seyler's Z. Physiol. Chem.*, 311, 87, 1958.
67. **Talafant, E. and Appelt, J.**, Preparation of bilirubin-diglucuronide concentrates from dog bladder bile, *Clin. Chem.*, 14, 208, 1968.
68. **Jacobsen, J.**, A chromatographic separation of bilirubin glucuronides from human bile, *Acta Chem. Scand.*, 23, 3023, 1969.
69. **Blanckaert, N., Gollan, J., and Schmid, R.**, Bilirubin diglucuronide synthesis by a UDP-glucuronic acid-dependent enzyme system in rat liver microsomes, *Proc. Natl. Acad. Sci. USA,* 76, 2037, 1979.
70. **Jendrassik, L. and Grof, P.**, Vereinfachte photometrische Methoden zur Bestimmung des Blutbilirubins, *Biochem. Z.*, 297, 81, 1938.

71. **Michaëlsson, M.,** Bilirubin determination in serum and urine, *Scand. J. Clin. Lab. Invest.*, 13, (Suppl. 56), 44, 1961.
72. **Heirwegh, K. and Van Roy, F.,** Some metal-azobilirubin complexes, *Clin. Chim. Acta,* 12, 684, 1965.
73. **Van Roy, F. P. and Heirwegh, K. P. M.,** Determination of bilirubin glucuronide and assay of glucuronyltransferase with bilirubin as acceptor, *Biochem. J.*, 107, 507, 1968.
74. **Heirwegh, K. P. M. and Snowbal, S.,** unpublished work, 1980.
75. **Nosslin, B.,** The direct diazo reaction of bile pigments in serum. Experimental and clinical studies, *Scand. J. Clin. Lab. Invest.*, 12, 49, 1960.
76. **Khayam-bashi, H. and Sims, Ch.,** Effects of sodium azide on the quantitation of the chemical constituents of serum, *Am. J. Clin. Pathol.*, 69, 405, 1978.
77. **Blondheim, S. H. and Kaufmann, N. A.,** The effect of light on the direct diazo-reaction of unconjugated bilirubin, *J. Lab. Clin. Med.*, 65, 659, 1965.
78. **Brody, J. P., Valdes, R., and Savory, J.,** Centrifugal analyzer method for total bilirubin in serum by use of diazotized 2-chloroaniline-5-sulfonic acid, *Clin. Chem.*, 25, 205, 1979.
79. **Homsher, R., Wesenberg, J. C., Baginski, E. S., and Zak, B.,** Interaction of hemoglobin in elevated serum total bilirubin determinations, *Microchem. J.*, 24, 526, 1979.
80. **Shull, B. C., Lees, H., and Li, P. K.,** Mechanism of interference by hemoglobin in the determination of total bilirubin. I. Method of Malloy-Evelyn, *Clin. Chem.*, 26, 22, 1980.
81. **Shull, B. C., Lees, H., and Li, P. K.,** Mechanism of interference by hemoglobin in the determination of total bilirubin. II. Method of Jendrassik-Grof, *Clin. Chem.*, 26, 26, 1980.
82. **Malloy, H. T. and Evelyn, K. A.,** The determination of bilirubin with the photoelectric colorimeter, *J. Biol. Chem.*, 119, 481, 1937.
83. **Engel, M.,** Eine Methode zur quantitativen Bestimmung des Bilirubins im Vollblut und im hämoglobinhaltigen Plasma und Serum, *Z. Physiol. Chem.*, 259, 75, 1939.
84. **Ichida, T. and Nobuoka, M.,** Ultramicro-method for determination of total and direct bilirubin in serum by modified alkaline azobilirubin blue reaction, *Clin. Chim. Acta,* 19, 249, 1968.
85. **Novros, J. S., Koch, T. R., and Knoblock, E. C.,** Improved method for accurate quantitation of total and conjugated bilirubin in serum, *Clin. Chem.*, 25, 1891, 1979.
86. **Watanabe, F., Tsubota, N., Mukai, H., Shioyama, E., and Kawishima, H.,** Determination of total and direct bilirubin in serum with sodium dodecyl sulfate as an accelerator, *Clin. Chim. Acta,* 88, 149, 1978.
87. **Stott, A. W.,** Neonatal serum bilirubin estimation, *Br. J. Med.*, 2, 823, 1969.
88. **Ertinghausen, G., Fabiny Byrd, D. L., Tiffany, T. O., and Casey, S. J.,** Single-reagent method for rapid determination of total bilirubin with the Centrifichem analyzer, *Clin. Chem.* 19, 1366, 1973.
89. **Küffer, H., Richterich, R., Peheim, E., and Colombo, J. P.,** Die Bestimmung des Bilirubins in Plasma und Serum als Azobilirubin mit dem Greiner Electronic Selective Analyzer GSAII, *Z. Klin. Chem. Klin. Biochem.*, 12, 294, 1974.
90. **Morin, L. G.,** A single non-aqueous diazo reagent for the rapid determination of bilirubin in serum without lipemic interference, *Clin. Chim. Acta,* 71, 9, 1976.
91. **Heirwegh, K., Jansen, H., and Van Roy, F.,** Determination of total bilirubin in urine. A modification of the method of Michaëlsson, *Clin. Chim. Acta,* 14, 124, 1966.
92. **Kulhanek, V. and Appelt, J.,** A simple and rapid method for the determination of total serum bilirubin, *Clin. Chim. Acta,* 20, 29, 1968.
93. **Morin, L. G.,** Improved stable diazonium salt procedure for determination of total serum bilirubin, *Clin. Chim. Acta,* 47, 111, 1973.
94. **Pearlman, F. C. and Lee, R. T. Y.,** Detection and measurement of total bilirubin in serum, with use of surfactants as solubilizing agents, *Clin. Chem.*, 20, 447, 1974.
95. **Biggs, H. G., Ledyard, P., and Kasper, S.,** Stable diazo-*p*-benzenesulfonic acid solutions for bilirubin assays, *Clin. Chem.*, 21, 449, 1975.
96. **Colombo, J. P., Peheim, E., Kyburz, S., and Hoffmann, J. P.,** A new accelerator for the determination of total bilirubin in plasma, *Clin. Chim. Acta,* 51, 217, 1974.
97. **Blumenfeld, T. A., Steinbrink, Ch. F., Cheskin, H. S., George, J. D., and Vogl, T. P.,** Manual micromethods for bilirubin determination in sera of adults and children and investigation of reasons for observed differences, *Am. J. Clin. Pathol.*, 69, 388, 1978.
98. **Walters, M. I. and Gerarde, H. W.,** An ultramicromethod for the determination of conjugated and total bilirubin in serum and plasma, *Microchem. J.*, 15, 231, 1970.
99. **Heirwegh, K. P. M., Meuwissen, J. A. T. P., and Fevery, J.,** Critique of the assay and significance of bilirubin conjugation, *Adv. Clin. Chem.*, 16, 239, 1973.
100. **Piper, R. F. and Hargreaves, T.,** The measurement of bilirubin in liver, *Clin. Chim. Acta,* 60, 215, 1975.
101. **Mertens, B. B. E., Van de Vijver, M., and Heirwegh, K. P. M.,** Determination of bilirubin in liver homogenate with diazotized *p*-iodoaniline, *Anal. Biochem.*, 50, 652, 1972.

102. **Ostrow, J. D. and Boonyapisit, S. T.,** Inaccuracies in measurement of conjugated and unconjugated bilirubin in bile with ethyl anthranilate diazo and solvent partition methods, *Biochem. J.,* 173, 263, 1978.
103. **Heirwegh, K. P. M., Van de Vijver, M., and Fevery, J.,** Assay and properties of digitonin-activated bilirubin uridine diphosphate glucuronyltransferase from rat liver, *Biochem. J.,* 129, 605, 1972.
104. **Heirwegh, K. P. M., Van Hees, G. P., Leroy, P., Van Roy, F. P., and Jansen, F. H.,** Heterogeneity of bile pigments as revealed by chromatography of their ethyl anthranilate azo pigments, *Biochem. J.,* 120, 877, 1970.
105. **Bratlid, D. and Winsnes, A.,** Comparison between different methods for determination of bile pigments in icteric serum samples, *Scand. J. Clin. Lab. Invest.,* 31, 231, 1973.
106. **Brodersen, R.,** Bilirubin diglucuronide in normal human blood serum, *Scand. J. Clin. Lab. Invest.,* 18, 361, 1966.
107. **Noir, B. A. and Nanet, H.,** A study of ethyl anthranilate azo derivatives of bilirubin sulphate. Confirmation of the existence of bilirubin sulphate conjugates in bile, *Biochim. Biophys. Acta,* 372, 230, 1974.
108. **Compernolle, F., Van Hees, G. P., and Heirwegh, K. P. M.,** Rearranged glucuronic acid conjuates of bilirubin-IXα in post-obstructive bile. Structure elucidation of azopigments β and γ as ethyl anthranilate *N*-glycosides derived from 2-, 3-, and 4-*O*-acyl glucuronides, *Biomed. Mass. Spectrom,* 5, 453, 1978.
109. **Onishi, S., Itoh, S., and Kawade, N., Isobe, K., and Sugiyama, S.,** Accurate and sensitive analysis of ethyl anthranilate azopigments from bile by reversed-phase high-performance liquid chromatography, *J. Chromatogr.,* 182, 105, 1980.
110. **Little, G. H.,** Separation of bilirubin azopigments from bile by high-performance liquid chromatography, *J. Chromatogr.,* 163, 81, 1979.
111. **Shennan, A. T., Cherian, A. G., Angel, A., and Bryan, M. H.,** The effect of Intralipid on the estimation of serum bilirubin in the newborn infant, *J. Pediatr.,* 88, 285, 1976.
112. **Brodersen, R. and Vind, I.,** A specific method for quantitative determination of unconjugated bilirubin and mesobilirubin, *Scand. J. Clin. Lab. Invest.,* 15, 225, 1963.
113. **Mallikarjuneswara, V. R., Clemetson, C. A. B., and Carr, J. J.,** Determination of bilirubin in amniotic fluid. A new, simple and efficient method, *Clin. Chem.,* 16, 180, 1970.
114. **Nakayama, F.,** Quantitative microanalysis of bile, *J. Lab. Clin. Med.,* 69, 594, 1967.
115. **Weber, A. and Schalm, L.,** Quantitative separation and determination of bilirubin and conjugated bilirubin in human serum, *Clin. Chim. Acta,* 7, 805, 1962.
116. **Gordon, E. R., Chan, T. H., Samodai, K., and Goresky, C. A.,** The isolation and further characterization of the bilirubin tetrapyrroles in bile-containing human duodenal juice and dog gall-bladder bile, *Biochem. J.,* 167, 1, 1977.
117. **Jansen, P. L. M. and Tangerman, A.,** Separation and characterization of bilirubin conjugates by high-performance liquid chromatography, *J. Chromatogr.,* 182, 100, 1980.
118. **Fevery, J.,** unpublished work, 1980.
119. **Lim, C. K.,** The separation of conjugated and unconjugated bilirubin in bile by high-performance liquid chromatography, *J. Liquid Chromatogr.,* 2, 37, 1979.
120. **Onishi, S., Itoh, S., Kawade, N., Isobe, K., and Sugiyama, S.,** An accurate and sensitive analysis by high-pressure liquid chromatography of conjugated and unconjugated bilirubin-IXα in various biological fluids, *Biochem. J.,* 185, 281, 1980.
121. **Blanckaert, N.,** Analysis of bilirubin and bilirubin mono- and di-conjugates. Determination of their relative amounts in biological samples, *Biochem. J.,* 185, 115, 1980.
122. **Wooldridge, T. A. and Lightner, D. A.,** Separation of III-α, IX-α, and XII-α isomers of bilirubin and bilirubin dimethyl ester by high-performance liquid chromatography, *J. Liquid Chromatogr.,* 1, 653, 1978.
123. **McDonagh, A. F. and Assisi, F.,** Direct evidence for the acid-catalyzed isomeric scrambling of bilirubin-IXα, *J. Chem. Soc. Chem. Commun.,* 117, 1972.

INDEX

A

B

C

D

J

K

L

M

N

O

P

Q

R

S

T

U

V

W

X

Y

Z